Evaluation of Inflammatory Bowel Disease

Guest Editors

SAMIR A. SHAH, MD
ADAM HARRIS, MD
EDWARD FELLER, MD

GASTROENTEROLOGY CLINICS OF NORTH AMERICA

www.gastro.theclinics.com

June 2012 • Volume 41 • Number 2

SAUNDERS an imprint of ELSEVIER, Inc.

W.B. SAUNDERS COMPANY
A Division of Elsevier Inc.

Elsevier Inc. • 1600 John F. Kennedy Blvd., Suite 1800 • Philadelphia, Pennsylvania 19103-2899

http://www.theclinics.com

GASTROENTEROLOGY CLINICS OF NORTH AMERICA Volume 41, Number 2
June 2012 ISSN 0889-8553, ISBN-13: 978-1-4557-4627-9

Editor: Kerry Holland
Developmental Editor: Donald Mumford

Gastroenterology Clinics of North America (ISSN 0889-8553) is published quarterly by Elsevier Inc., 360 Park Avenue South, New York, NY 10010-1710. Months of issue are March, June, September, and December. Business and Editorial Offices: 1600 John F. Kennedy Blvd., Suite 1800, Philadelphia, PA 19103-2899. Customer Service Office: 6277 Sea Harbor Drive, Orlando, FL 32887-4800. Periodicals postage paid at New York, NY and additional mailing offices. Subscription prices are $305.00 per year (US individuals), $153.00 per year (US students), $488.00 per year (US institutions), $335.00 per year (Canadian individuals), $594.00 per year (Canadian institutions), $423.00 per year (international individuals), $211.00 per year (international students), and $594.00 per year (international institutions). Foreign air speed delivery is included in all *Clinics* subscription prices. All prices are subject to change without notice. **POSTMASTER:** Send address changes to *Gastroenterology Clinics of North America,* Elsevier Health Sciences Division, Subscription Customer Service, 3251 Riverport Lane, Maryland Heights, MO 63043. Telephone: 1-800-654-2452 (U.S. and Canada); 314-447-8871 (outside U.S. and Canada). Fax: 314-447-8029. E-mail: journalscustomerservice-usa@elsevier.com (for print support); journalsonlinesupport-usa@elsevier.com (for online support).

Reprints. For copies of 100 or more, of articles in this publication, please contact the Commercial Reprints Department, Elsevier Inc., 360 Part Avenue South, New York, New York 10010-1710. Tel. (212) 633-3813, Fax: (212) 462-1935, E-mail: reprints@elsevier.com.

Gastroenterology Clinics of North America is also published in Italian by Il Pensiero Scientifico Editore, Rome, Italy; and in Portuguese by Interlivros Edicoes Ltda., Rua Commandante Coelho 1085, 21250 Cordovil, Rio de Janeiro, Brazil.

Gastroenterology Clinics of North America is covered in *MEDLINE/PubMed (Index Medicus), Excerpta Medica, Current Contents/Clinical Medicine, Science Citation Index, ISI/BIOMED,* and *BIOSIS.*

Printed and bound by CPI Group (UK) Ltd, Croydon, CR0 4YY
Transferred to Digital Print 2012

Contributors

GUEST EDITORS

SAMIR A. SHAH, MD, FACG, FASGE, AGAF
Clinical Associate Professor of Medicine, The Warren Alpert Medical School of Brown University; Gastroenterology Associates, Inc, Providence, Rhode Island

ADAM HARRIS, MD
Clinical Assistant Professor of Medicine, Department of Gastroenterology, The Warren Alpert Medical School of Brown University, Providence, Rhode Island

EDWARD FELLER, MD, FACP, FACG
Clinical Professor of Medicine, Adjunct Professor of Community Health, Co-director, Community Health Clerkship, Brown University, Providence, Rhode Island

AUTHORS

BINCY P. ABRAHAM, MD, MS
Assistant Professor of Medicine, Section of Gastroenterology and Hepatology, Baylor College of Medicine, Houston, Texas

MARIA T. ABREU, MD
Professor of Medicine and Chief, Division of Gastroenterology, Department of Medicine, University of Miami Miller School of Medicine, Miami, Florida

ASHWIN N. ANANTHAKRISHNAN, MD, MPH
Assistant in Medicine, Massachusetts General Hospital; Instructor, Harvard Medical School, Boston, Massachusetts

WOJCIECH BLONSKI, MD, PhD
Division of Gastroenterology, University of Pennsylvania, Philadelphia, Pennsylvania; Department of Gastroenterology, Medical University, Wroclaw, Poland

ANNA M. BUCHNER, MD, PhD
Division of Gastroenterology, University of Pennsylvania, Philadelphia, Pennsylvania

GRACE CHAN, MRCPI, MRCP(UK)
Gastroenterology Department, Connolly Hospital Blanchardstown, Dublin, Republic of Ireland

ADAM S. CHEIFETZ, MD
Director, Center for Inflammatory Bowel Disease, Beth Israel Deaconess Medical Center; Assistant Professor of Medicine, Harvard Medical School, Boston, Massachusetts

THEMISTOCLES DASSOPOULOS, MD
Associate Professor and Director of Inflammatory Bowel Diseases, Gastroenterology Division, Washington University School of Medicine, St Louis, Missouri

SILVIO W. DE MELO JR, MD
Assistant Professor of Medicine, Division of Gastroenterology, University of South Alabama College of Medicine, Mobile, Alabama

SHANE M. DEVLIN, MD, FRCPC
Program Director, Adult Gastroenterology Training Program; Clinical Assistant Professor, Division of Gastroenterology and Hepatology, The University of Calgary, Calgary, Alberta, Canada

JACK A. DI PALMA, MD
Professor of Medicine and Director, Division of Gastroenterology, University of South Alabama College of Medicine, Mobile, Alabama

FRANCIS A. FARRAYE, MD, MSc
Clinical Director, Section of Gastroenterology, Boston Medical Center; Professor of Medicine, Boston University School of Medicine, Boston, Massachusetts

RICHARD J. FARRELL, MD, FRCPI
Gastroenterology Department, Connolly Hospital Blanchardstown and Royal College of Surgeons Ireland, Dublin, Republic of Ireland

DAVID S. FEFFERMAN, MD
Clinics Instructor in Medicine, Harvard Medical School, Boston; Private Practice, Digestive Health Associates, Stoneham, Massachusetts

DAVID J. GRAND, MD
Assistant Professor, Diagnostic Imaging, The Warren Alpert Medical School of Brown University, Providence, Rhode Island

ADAM HARRIS, MD
Clinical Assistant Professor of Medicine, Department of Gastroenterology, The Warren Alpert Medical School of Brown University, Providence, Rhode Island

SUNANDA KANE, MD, MSPH
Section of Gastroenterology and Hepatology, Mayo Clinic College of Medicine, Rochester, Minnesota

RALF KIESSLICH, MD, PhD
Professor of Medicine, I. Med. Klinik und Poliklinik, Johannes Gutenberg Universität Mainz, Mainz, Germany

GARY R. LICHTENSTEIN, MD
Professor of Medicine, Division of Gastroenterology, University of Pennsylvania, Philadelphia, Pennsylvania

EDWARD V. LOFTUS JR, MD
Professor of Medicine, Division of Gastroenterology and Hepatology, Mayo Clinic, Rochester, Minnesota

YUE LI, MD
Department of Gastroenterology, Peking Union Medical College Hospital, Beijing, China; Digestive Disease Institute, The Cleveland Clinic Foundation, Cleveland, Ohio

JACOB L. MCCAULEY, PhD
Assistant Professor of Human Genetics, John P. Hussman Institute for Human Genomics, Dr John T. Macdonald Foundation Department of Human Genetics, University of Miami Miller School of Medicine, Miami, Florida

MARKUS F. NEURATH, MD, PhD
Professor of Medicine, Department of Medicine I, University of Erlangen-Nuremberg, Erlangen, Germany

MIGUEL REGUEIRO, MD
Professor of Medicine, Division of Gastroenterology, Hepatology, and Nutrition, University of Pittsburgh Medical Center, Pittsburgh, Pennsylvania

DAVID A. SCHWARTZ, MD
Associate Professor of Medicine, Division of Gastroenterology, Hepatology and Nutrition, Department of Medicine, Vanderbilt University Medical Center, Nashville, Tennessee

JOSEPH H. SELLIN, MD
Professor of Medicine and Chief of Gastroenterology, Division of Gastroenterology, Ben Taub General Hospital, Baylor College of Medicine, Houston, Texas

RASHESH R. SHAH
Resident, Internal Medicine, Department of Medicine, Baylor College of Medicine, Houston, Texas

BO SHEN, MD
Digestive Disease Institute, The Cleveland Clinic Foundation, Cleveland, Ohio

COREY A. SIEGEL, MD, MS
Assistant Professor of Medicine, Dartmouth Medical School and The Dartmouth Institute for Health Policy and Clinical Practice; Director, Dartmouth-Hitchcock IBD Center, Dartmouth-Hitchcock Medical Center, Lebanon, New Hampshire

JENNIFER A. SINCLAIR, MD
Gastroenterology Fellow, Section of Gastroenterology, Boston Medical Center, Boston, Massachusetts

CHARLES A. SNINSKY, MD
Practicing Gastroenterologist, Digestive Disease Associates, Gainesville, Florida

JASON M. SWOGER, MD, MPH
Assistant Professor of Medicine, Division of Gastroenterology, Hepatology, and Nutrition, University of Pittsburgh Medical Center, Pittsburgh, Pennsylvania

SHARMEEL K. WASAN, MD
Staff Gastroenterologist, Section of Gastroenterology, Boston Medical Center; Assistant Professor of Medicine, Boston University School of Medicine, Boston, Massachusetts

PAUL E. WISE, MD
Associate Professor of Surgery, Department of Surgery, Section of Surgical Sciences, Vanderbilt University Medical Center, Nashville, Tennessee

Contents

Endoscopy plays an essential role in diagnosis, management, and surveillance of inflammatory bowel disease (IBD). Direct visual and histologic evaluation allows the distribution, severity, and disease activity to be defined. In patients with established IBD, the response to both medical and surgical therapy can be assessed. Furthermore, endoscopy has a therapeutic role in IBD in management of strictures and hemorrhage. In patients with longstanding disease, endoscopy plays an important role in dysplasia surveillance. This review aims to update the role of endoscopy in IBD, with particular reference to the initial diagnosis, disease evaluation and monitoring, dysplasia surveillance, and therapeutic functions.

Surveillance colonoscopy in patients with established ulcerative colitis is recommended because of the increased cancer risk. Chromoendoscopy has significant advantages over white light endoscopy. Chromoendoscopy using methylene blue or indigo carmine can unmask flat and circumscribed lesions, which can guide biopsies and increase the diagnostic yield for intraepithelial neoplasia. This review summarizes the recent knowledge and technique of chromoendoscopy. Clear guidance is given about the routine use of chromoendoscopy. Furthermore, additive techniques like magnifying endoscopy and confocal laser endomicroscopy are discussed.

The majority of patients with Crohn disease will undergo at least one surgical resection during their disease course. Currently, the most effective prognostic indicator of postoperative disease course is the Rutgeerts score, determined during ileocolonoscopy 6 to 12 months following surgery. Patients with endoscopic evidence of recurrence have a significant risk of symptomatic recurrence, and complications. Prophylactic therapy should be considered in patients who have risk factors for postoperative recurrence, and treatment should be escalated if there is evidence of recurrence at postoperative ileocolonoscopy. An algorithm for the evaluation and treatment of postoperative Crohn disease is presented.

Inflammatory bowel disease and, in particular, Crohn disease, can affect the small-bowel in approximately one third of patients. Capsule endoscopy plays a pivotal role in the diagnosis and monitoring of small-bowel involvement relatively noninvasively. This article discusses when capsule endoscopy may assist physicians in managing patients with inflammatory bowel disease.

Special Situations

Recent data suggest that inflammatory bowel disease (IBD) patients do not receive preventive services with the same rigor as other patients, partly because visits to the primary care physician may be infrequent. Gastroenterologists are in a unique position to provide care in both specialty and health maintenance capacities, and must consider the distinctive needs of IBD patients who are commonly immunosuppressed. This article focuses in detail on current vaccine recommendations for IBD patients, and touches on issues faced in screening for preventable diseases, including screening for cervical, skin, and colorectal cancers; depression; tobacco abuse; and maintaining appropriate bone health.

A cohort that appears to be at a higher risk for *Clostridium difficile* infection (CDI) and particularly vulnerable to the morbidity and mortality associated with it are patients with underlying inflammatory bowel diseases (IBD). Diagnosis requires demonstration of the toxin from a diarrhea stool sample. Mild CDI can be treated with oral metronidazole, whereas severe disease should be treated with oral vancomycin. Management of recurrent CDI remains challenging. Newer drugs are now available that appear to be effective with lower risk of disease recurrence. Specific treatment trials and prospective studies of CDI in patients with IBD are warranted.

Restorative proctocolectomy with ileal pouch-anal anastomosis has become the surgical treatment of choice for the majority of patients with ulcerative colitis who require colectomy. However, adverse sequelae of mechanical, inflammatory, functional, neoplastic, or metabolic conditions often occur after restorative proctocolectomy. Recognition of the disease conditions of the ileal pouch can be challenging for practicing gastroenterologists. Accurate diagnosis and classification of the disease conditions are imperative for proper management and prognosis.

Nonspecific gastrointestinal symptoms are present in both inflammatory and noninflammatory conditions. Noninvasive diagnostic tools
include the fecal markers, calprotectin and lactoferrin. These are stable
proteins that are present in the stool of patients with active and chronic
inflammation. Studies have shown their ability to discriminate in a
reproducible fashion the presence of inflammation with excellent correlation to endoscopic findings. These markers can also be used for
predicting a disease flare as well as monitoring the success of treatment. Noninvasive stool markers are a convenient and reliable clinical
tool that can be used in clinical practice.

Noninvasive imaging of inflammatory bowel disease, especially Crohn
disease, has progressed dramatically. Fluoroscopic studies including
small-bowel follow-through, the previous gold standard, have largely
been supplanted by cross-sectional techniques such as computed
tomography (CT) enterography and magnetic resonance (MR) enterography. Improved CT and MR hardware, as well as widespread use of
oral agents to distend the small bowel, now provide rapid, detailed
assessment of the small-bowel lumen in addition to extraenteric
complications such as fistula and abscess. Even greater achievements
are anticipated as imaging moves beyond simply identifying diseased
bowel segments to accurately classifying disease state and activity.

Inflammatory bowel disease (IBD) is a complex multifactorial genetic
disorder characterized by chronic inflammation of the gastrointestinal
tract. The highly variable clinical course of IBD has made the search for
genetic factors extremely challenging. However, the advent of the
genomic era and the utilization of rapidly evolving genomic technologies and analytic strategies have greatly enabled the search for genetic
factors that influence IBD pathogenesis. As the search continues to
explain the heritability of IBD, the latest in whole-genome sequencing
and so-called "gene-chip" technology will help pave the way to
practicing genomic medicine in the treatment of IBD patients.

THE CLINICS ARE NOW AVAILABLE ONLINE!

Access your subscription at:
www.theclinics.com

Preface

Evaluation of Inflammatory Bowel Disease

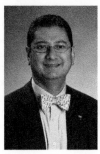 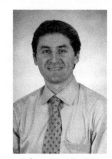 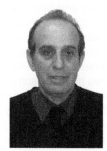

Samir A. Shah, MD	Adam Harris, MD	Edward Feller, MD
	Guest Editors	

The diagnosis and management of inflammatory bowel disease (IBD) is often complex. Better techniques for assessing IBD are needed. In this issue of *Gastroenterology Clinics of North America*, we focus on methods of diagnosing and evaluating IBD to help guide optimal treatment to maximize clinical outcomes and minimize risks. We, the guest editors, are particularly thrilled and energized to have worked with such a distinguished set of authors---highly experienced clinicians, investigators, and nationally/internationally recognized thought leaders in IBD. We asked the authors to provide a state-of-the-art update with practical information/guidelines/algorithms and cutting edge data for incorporation into practice to benefit the IBD patients we all serve.

The first set of articles deals with endoscopy: its role in diagnosis and monitoring IBD; the growing importance of chromoendoscopy in IBD surveillance exams; assessment of post-operative recurrence; and finally the emerging role of capsule endoscopy.

The second section focuses on specific scenarios that IBD physicians encounter frequently: health maintenance in IBD focusing on proper vaccinations; the growing problem of *Clostridium difficile* in IBD; assessment of pouch problems; optimal evaluation of perianal disease; the state of the art in using thiopurines including use of allopurinol to optimize metabolites and optimizing the use of infliximab by measuring levels and antibodies to infliximab; factors to consider in choosing monotherapy versus combination therapy and communication of risk/benefit to patients; and finally disability assessment in IBD.

Elsevier's style guide conforms to that of the AMA and *Dorland's Dictionary* for possessive eponyms; this means that the term *Crohn disease* appears throughout the issue instead of *Crohn's disease*.

Gastroenterol Clin N Am 41 (2012) xiii–xiv
doi:10.1016/j.gtc.2012.01.010
0889-8553/12/$ – see front matter © 2012 Elsevier Inc. All rights reserved.

The third and final section highlights noninvasive methods to evaluate IBD: clinical predictors of aggressive or disabling disease; the evolving role of specific antibodies in diagnosing, subtyping and most recently prognosticating in IBD; stool markers (calproctectin and lactoferrin) for evaluating and monitoring IBD; the growing role of imaging modalities with emphasis on MR enterography and CT enterography; and finally, the genetics of IBD and the potential role of genetic testing in the diagnosis/prognosis and tailoring of therapy.

We hope that these articles will provide clinicians with useful, state-of-the-art information in evaluating and managing IBD. Because of space restrictions, many important topics have been left out, including pregnancy in IBD and bone disease in IBD. These have been recently addressed in review articles or society guidelines. Also, we have chosen not to focus on treatment of IBD as this is recently updated in the practice guidelines published in the *American Journal of Gastroenterology* (and also a systematic review on medical therapies for IBD published as a supplement to the same journal). Finally, we thank our distinguished panel of authors for their time and contributions to this issue.

Samir A. Shah, MD
The Warren Alpert Medical School of Brown University
Gastroenterology Associates, Inc
44 West River Street
Providence, RI 02904, USA

Adam Harris, MD
The Warren Alpert Medical School of Brown University
Department of Gastroenterology
593 Eddy Street
Providence, RI 02903, USA

Edward Feller, MD
Brown University, Box G-S121
Providence, RI 02912, USA

E-mail addresses:
samir@brown.edu (S.A. Shah)
adam_harris@brown.edu (A. Harris)
Edward_Feller@brown.edu (E. Feller)

Endoscopic Assessment of Inflammatory Bowel Disease: Colonoscopy/ Esophagogastroduodenoscopy

Grace Chan, MRCPI, MRCP(UK)[a], David S. Fefferman, MD[b,c,]*,
Richard J. Farrell, MD, FRCPI[d]

KEYWORDS
- Endoscopy • Inflammatory bowel disease • Assessment
- Colonoscopy • Esophagogastroduodenoscopy

Endoscopy plays an essential role in the diagnosis, management, and surveillance of inflammatory bowel disease (IBD). Endoscopy in combination with clinical findings, blood tests, and stool analysis can help establish the diagnosis of IBD and distinguish between Crohn disease (CD) and ulcerative colitis (UC), as well as exclude other causes. Direct visual and histologic evaluation can define the distribution, severity, and disease activity. In patients with established IBD, endoscopy will help evaluate the response to treatment, thereby determining the course of medical and surgical therapy. Furthermore, endoscopy has a therapeutic role in IBD in the dilatation of strictures and management of bleeding. In patients with longstanding disease, endoscopy plays an integral role in dysplasia and colorectal cancer surveillance. This review updates the role of endoscopy in IBD, with particular reference to the initial diagnosis, disease monitoring and assessment, dysplasia surveillance, and therapeutic functions.

DIAGNOSIS OF IBD BY ENDOSCOPY

Endoscopy allows for direct visualization of the colonic mucosa and obtaining of tissue for histologic evaluation. An ileocolonoscopy is safe to perform as an initial investigation in most patients with suspected IBD. Relative contraindications for an

[a] Gastroenterology Department, Connolly Hospital Blanchardstown, Dublin, Republic of Ireland
[b] Harvard Medical School, Boston, MA, USA
[c] Private Practice, Digestive Health Associates, 3 Woodland Road #306, Stoneham, MA 02180, USA
[d] Gastroenterology Department, Connolly Hospital Blanchardstown and Royal College of Surgeons Ireland, Dublin, Republic of Ireland
* Corresponding author. Private Practice, Digestive Health Associates, 3 Woodland Road #306, Stoneham, MA 02180.
E-mail address: dfefferman@gmail.com

Gastroenterol Clin N Am 41 (2012) 271–290
doi:10.1016/j.gtc.2012.01.014
0889-8553/12/$ – see front matter © 2012 Elsevier Inc. All rights reserved.

gastro.theclinics.com

ileocolonoscopy as opposed to a sigmoidoscopy include toxic megacolon and severe colitis.[1] In severe colitis, ileocolonoscopy can be safely performed if air insufflation is minimized and difficulty in advancing the scope in a tortuous colon is avoided.[2] In patients with toxic megacolon, a sigmoidoscopy is often sufficient to provide a diagnosis. In a large retrospective study by Navaneethan and colleagues[3] in hospitalized IBD patients with severe colitis, colonoscopy was associated with a perforation rate of 1% compared with 0.6% in non-IBD patients. In IBD patients, risk factors identified for perforation include female gender, older age, and endoscopic dilatation during the procedure.[3] Adequate bowel preparation may be impossible in the unstable patient. In this setting, the benefits and risks of a sigmoidoscopy versus an unprepared colonoscopy need to be weighed. An unprepared colonoscopy may also be suitable in patients with profuse diarrhea, in whom the colon may be reasonably clear. A prospective study of 28 patients with IBD showed that an unprepared colonoscopy was often adequate to diagnose and assess the severity of IBD. It also allowed for rapid initiation or alteration in treatment and can be performed safely.[4]

Colonoscopy can provide key information to differentiate between CD and UC. This information is critical because subsequent treatment is likely to obscure initial findings such as distribution and rectal sparing.[5] During initial diagnostic evaluation, multiple biopsies from a full colonoscopy will provide further information to allow a more accurate diagnosis compared with sigmoidoscopy.[6] Optimal sampling should include at least two biopsies from the terminal ileum, cecum, ascending colon, transverse colon, descending colon, sigmoid colon, and rectum even if the mucosa appears endoscopically normal.[7] Biopsies need to be taken from the areas of erosions and ulcerations as well as from the normal adjacent areas to confirm the presence of skip lesions. In patients with CD, biopsies from the ulcer edge and aphthous erosions are more likely to demonstrate granuloma than normal-looking or cobblestoned mucosa.[8] This tendency has prognostic implications because the detection of granulomas has been associated with a more extensive and complicated disease.[9]

Modalities such as narrow band imaging (NBI) can be used to improve the yield from mucosal biopsies. In an analysis by Matsumoto and colleagues,[10] atrophic or distorted crypts and goblet cell depletion were found more frequently in the biopsy specimens taken from villous-type mucosa as oppose to crypt opening-type mucosa. Even in inactive UC, NBI seems to be able to locate areas that showed most histologic evidence of inflammatory cell infiltrate, goblet cell depletion, distorted crypts, and basal plasmacytosis. These areas are more likely to demonstrate an appearance termed "obscure mucosal vascular pattern," as opposed to "distorted mucosal vascular pattern."[11]

Ulcerative Colitis

Distribution

In UC, inflammatory changes typically begin above the anorectal junction and extend proximally in a confluent and continuous manner.[12] Inflammation may be confined to the rectum (proctitis), from the rectum up to the splenic flexure (left-sided colitis), beyond the splenic flexure (extensive colitis), or may involve the entire colon (pancolitis). There is generally a clear demarcation between inflamed and normal areas. Biopsies should be obtained from areas of inflammation as well as healthy-looking mucosa, particularly just above the proximal extent of inflammation. This strategy will allow the extent of disease to be determined accurately and can be used for monitoring disease progression.

A subgroup of UC patients develop inflammatory changes around the appendiceal orifice in conjunction with distal UC but with sparing of the right colon. These patients have a similar rate of remission, relapse, and proximal extension compared with those with no cecal patch.[13] Another subgroup of patients develop patchy right-sided colonic inflammation with left-sided disease. Again, the clinical features and outcome for these patients seem to be similar to those with classic UC.[14] However, nonspecific, isolated right-sided inflammation has been associated with normal, healthy colon and should not be misdiagnosed as IBD.[15]

Appearance

The earliest endoscopically visualized changes in UC are erythema and vascular congestion of the mucosa.[16] As edema becomes more prominent, small mounds may form resulting in a fine granular appearance.[16] The mucosa may be friable and bleed with minor contact. As inflammation becomes more severe, ulcerations form, and bleeding may occur spontaneously.[16] Coalescence of small ulcers may result in large or linear ulcerations.[12] In UC, ulcers always occur surrounded by inflamed and abnormal-appearing mucosa.

Chronic inflammation can result in mucosal atrophy with loss of the haustral folds and luminal narrowing. Mucosal atrophy may lead to pseudopolyps, which can assume diverse shapes as well as form mucosal bridges. Typically, they appear as long, glistening, fingerlike projections that are friable and bleed easily when biopsied.[17] Pseudopolyps can also be seen in CD but are typically seen in UC. Although pseudopolyps are believed not to possess malignant potential, biopsy or polypectomy should be considered if they are atypical in appearance or color or demonstrate nontraumatic bleeding. Giant pseudopolyps may not be amenable to endoscopic intervention and may cause intussusception and obstruction.[18]

Crohn Disease

Distribution

In CD, involvement is typically patchy and can affect any segment from the mouth to the anus. In the setting of colonic CD, the rectum is spared in up to 50% of patients and is often most severe in the cecum and right colon.[19] Esophageal CD can either be focal or extensive, with single or multiple erosions, often surrounded by healthy mucosa.[20] In upper gastrointestinal CD, the most frequently involved areas are the duodenum and gastric antrum.[21,22] Gastroduodenal CD occurs in 0.5% to 4% of patients with ileocolonic disease, although it occurs very rarely as an isolated entity.[23]

Double balloon enteroscopy (DBE) is superior to fluoroscopic enteroclysis (diagnostic yield of 95% vs 71%) in detecting small bowel obstruction in both Crohn-related and unrelated disease.[24] However, strictures in the small bowel are not always accessible at DBE and may require fluoroscopic imaging. The latter also has the advantage of being able to depict the site, level, and grading of obstruction more accurately than DBE.[24] If a stricture is located by DBE, tattooing of the site will assist any future surgical procedures. The risk of complications with DBE in a patient with CD is as high as 2%.[25] Care should always be taken during insertion of the endoscope. If fragile lesions such as deep ulcerations are observed, further insertion should be avoided. Diagnostic yields were similar in a study comparing DBE with capsule endoscopy in detecting small bowel lesions.[26]

Appearance

Endoscopic features of CD include aphthous ulcers, discrete ulcers, serpiginous ulcers, longitudinal ulcers, cobblestoning of mucosa, strictures, and fistulas.[27,28] In early CD, tiny aphthous ulcerations are commonly seen.[29] These ulcerations are a result of submucosal lymphoid follicle expansion. As the disease progresses, these ulcers can coalesce into larger stellate ulcers.[29] Isolated ulcerations on the ileocecal valve or in the terminal ileum are commonly seen in CD but can also represent acute colitis secondary to nonsteroidal antiinflammatory drug (NSAID) use or infection. Cobblestoning of the mucosa, which occurs more commonly in CD than UC, results from chronic submucosal edema and injury.[22] Endoscopically, gastroduodenal CD appears as mucosal edema, focal or diffuse redness, nodular lesions, erosions, ulcerations, friability, and strictures.[21,28] Biopsies demonstrating granulomas are infrequent and variable, occurring in 9% to 49% of patients with gastroduodenal CD.[21,30,31]

Endoscopic Differentiation of UC and CD

Because of the challenges in differentiating UC and CD, IBD-unclassified (IBDU) accounts for around 4% to 6% of IBD diagnosed and seems to be more common in children compared with adults.[32–34] The term *indeterminate colitis* is reserved for colectomy specimens where a diagnosis of CD or UC cannot be made based on the histology of the resected specimen. There seems to be significant interobserver variation in the classification of IBD. In a study comparing the histologic diagnosis of colonic IBD made by general pathologist versus that made by specialist gastrointestinal pathologists, 43% of cases initially diagnosed as UC were changed to CD or IC, whereas 17% initially diagnosed as CD were changed to UC or IC.[35] Odze[36] listed several reasons that lead to the diagnosis of IBDU, including failure to recognize unusual variants of UC or CD, insufficient clinical or radiologic information, fulminant colitis, presence of secondary disease such as pseudomembranous colitis, and failure to use hard criteria for CD.[36]

Endoscopic differentiation of CD from UC can be difficult, particularly in the setting of pancolitis. The combination of clinical history, serologic markers, and radiologic imaging may aid the diagnosis. Nevertheless, as many as 12% of patients who underwent surgery following initial diagnosis of either UC or IBDU were subsequently diagnosed as having CD.[37] Initial esophagogastroduodenoscopy (EGD) may be helpful in locating upper gastrointestinal (GI) disease, thereby making CD the more likely diagnosis. Lemberg and colleagues[38] described 25 children with IBDU pancolitis who were eventually diagnosed with CD following EGD. In severe colitis, the most useful discriminatory features for CD were the presence of discontinuous inflammation, anal lesions, and cobblestoning. Erosions and microulcerations within a granular mucosa were believed to be specific for UC.[39]

The terminal ileum is characteristically not involved in UC. However, up to 10% of patients with active pancolitis may develop "backwash ileitis," which can extend several centimeters into the terminal ileum.[12] The phenomenon has also been described in patients with subtotal or left-sided colitis with only mild disease activity.[40] Features that favor CD rather than UC with associated-backwash ileitis are extensive length of small bowel disease, jejunitis, proximal ileitis separated by skip regions of uninvolved cecum, transmural ileal inflammation with granulomas and neural hyperplasia, greater inflammatory activity in the terminal ileal biopsies, and mucous gland metaplasia of the ileal mucosa.[41] Recognition that CD tends to be transmural and that UC is a superficial mucosal inflammatory process has led to the use of endoscopic ultrasound (EUS) in the differentiation of IBD. However, results seem to be disappointing. EUS has only been effective in the evaluation of perirectal and perianal complications of CD.[42] For more information please refer to discussion elsewhere in this issue on examination under anesthesia, EUS, and MRI evaluation of perianal disease. In UC, EUS can also be used to evaluate the biliary tree. In one trial, a thickened common bile duct greater than 1.5 mm found by transduodenal EUS was found in patients with primary sclerosing cholangitis (PSC) but not those with uncomplicated IBD or choledocholithiasis.[43]

DISTINGUISHING IBD FROM OTHER DISORDERS

Endoscopy and histology can help distinguish IBD from infection, ischemia, diverticulitis, neoplasia, radiation, drug-induced colitis, and other causes.

Infection

In a prospective study of patients presenting with acute bloody diarrhea with suspected IBD, up to one-third were found to have an infectious cause.[44] Positive stool cultures are often indicative of infectious colitis. However, positive microbiologic results have been detected in about 20% of patients who present with IBD for the first time, an indication that infection can precipitate a flare-up in latent IBD.[45] Infections known to mimic the endoscopic and histologic appearance of IBD include salmonellosis, shigellosis, campylobacteriosis, tuberculosis (TB), *Escherichia coli* 0157:H7 infection, yersiniosis, *Clostridium difficile* infection, gonorrhea, *Klebsiella* infection, chlamydiosis, syphilis, schistosomiasis, amebiasis, herpes simplex, cytomegalovirus (CMV) and certain fungi.[46] Endoscopically, infectious colitis often has patchy inflammation unlike the continuous inflammation of UC. The discrete ulcers of CD are less common in infection but can occur with TB, CMV, and yersiniosis. Also, rectal ulcers and proctitis can be seen with gonorrhea and syphilis. Isolated ileitis, one of the many presentations of CD, can occur with *Yersinia* and *Salmonella* infection and TB.[47] Histologic features that favor IBD rather than acute self-limited colitis (ASLC) are distorted crypt architecture, increased cellularity of the lamina propria, a villous surface, epithelioid granuloma, crypt atrophy, basal lymphoid aggregates, and one or more basally located giant cells.[48] Granulomas can appear in ASLC, but these tend to be poorly formed and are associated with crypt abscesses.[47] The use of EUS in differentiating ASLC from IBD is limited. A small study demonstrated that pathologic perirectal lymph nodes on EUS have also been linked with the development of ulcerative colitis in patients initially thought to have ASLC.[49] In selected cases, EUS of the sigmoid colon helps differentiate between infectious colitis and CD. Patients with active CD have increased submucosal thickening, decreased mucosal thickening, and hypoechoic paracolonic lymph nodes compared with patients with unspecific infectious colitis.[50] However, this pattern was not observed in patients with acute UC compared with those with unspecific infectious colitis.[51]

Clinically, ASLC secondary to infection usually presents with an acute transient diarrheal illness; the short, self-limited course differentiates the condition from IBD. However, some infections such as TB run a more protracted and insidious course. Differentiation of CD from intestinal TB often poses a diagnostic challenge. Endoscopically, two factors, area of distribution and endoscopic appearance, can help distinguish between CD and intestinal TB. In terms of distribution, whereas CD and intestinal TB both seem to affect the ileocecal valve in about 60% to 70% of patients, terminal ileal involvement predominates over cecal involvement in CD, and cecal involvement predominates over terminal ileal involvement in intestinal TB.[52] Also, a fixed-open ileocecal valve was believed to be suggestive of TB over CD.[53] Makharia and colleagues[54] found no relevant difference in the involvement of the stomach and duodenum but noted that involvement of the rectum, sigmoid colon, descending colon, ascending colon, and jejunum supported the diagnosis of CD. A small prospective study from South Korea [55] formulated a scoring system to aid the differentiation between CD and intestinal TB based on eight endoscopic features. Anorectal lesions, longitudinal ulcers, aphthous ulcers, and cobblestoning supported the diagnosis of CD, whereas transverse ulcers, patulous ileocecal valve, scars, and involvement of fewer than four segments favored TB. The classical features of caseating granulomas and AFB have been found in about 30% of cases of intestinal TB.[52,56] Histologic features that suggest TB include confluent caseating granulomas, bands of epithelioid histiocytes lining ulcers, granulomas larger than 400 μm in diameter, 5 or more granulomas in biopsies from one segment, granulomas in the submucosa or in granulation tissue, and disproportionate submucosal inflammation.[52,57] In contrast, features that favor the diagnosis of CD include infrequent, small granulomas that are poorly organized and isolated and architectural distortion distant from granulomatous inflammation.[52]

Ischemia

Ischemic colitis typically affects older patients with cardiovascular risk factors. However, in younger patients, risk factors such as hypercoagulability, vasculitis, aortic surgery, infection, cocaine use, long-distance running, bowel preparation, and certain medications (eg, estrogen in women, sumatriptan and other selective serotonin agonist in patients with migraines) can all lead to bowel ischemia.[58–63] Endoscopically, ischemic colitis often spares the rectum because dual blood supply from the mesenteric and iliac arteries makes it resistant to ischemia. Other endoscopic features include loss of vascularity, erythema, friability, granularity, longitudinal ulceration, serpiginous ulceration, confluent ulceration, and submucosal hemorrhage.[64] In chronic ischemia, ulceration with granulation tissue and pseudopolyps have also been described.[65] Unlike IBD, ischemic colitis tends to occur in segments of colon, most commonly affecting the "watershed" regions at the border of the area supplied by the superior and inferior mesenteric arteries. Pancolonic involvement is rare, occurring in less than 10% of cases.[66] Histologically, iron-laden macrophages and submucosal fibrosis are characteristic of ischemic injury.[65]

Drug-Induced Colitis

Diverse drugs have been associated with colitis, with NSAIDs being the most common. Endoscopically, features associated with NSAID-induced colitis include ulcerations, inflammation, erosions, stricture formation, and even neoplastic-like masses.[67,68] Flat ulcers and the characteristic diaphragmlike stricture appear more commonly in the right colon.[69] Colonic biopsies are often indistinguishable from ischemic colitis and demonstrate patchy erosion, lamina propria fibrosis, and reactive epithelial change.[67] In upper GI biopsies, CD can mimic chemical gastropathy secondary to NSAIDs, particularly if active inflammation, erosions, and granulomas are absent.[70] The paucity of neutrophils at the base of an ulcer or erosion is typical of an NSAID lesion compared with the focal collections of numerous neutrophils that are typical of CD.[31] Follow-up endoscopies can be carried out 4 to 8 weeks following cessation of the offending NSAID to check for endoscopic resolution, which can help confirm the cause.[71,72]

Radiation

Radiation effects are related to the total dose of radiation received and frequency of radiation, as well as the total volume of tissue irradiated.[73] Chronic radiation injury can occur many years after initial exposure and in its severe form can cause narrowing of the bowel lumen, leading to obstruction. Acute radiation proctitis seems to peak 2 weeks after the onset of radiotherapy and may stabilize or regress following completion of treatment.[74] Endoscopic features in the acute setting include friability, granularity, pallor erythema, and prominent submucosal telangiectasias.[75] Histologic findings at this time will demonstrate epithelial meganucleosis, fibroblastic proliferation, and absence of mitotic activity. Conversely, chronic histologic changes include telangiectasis of capillaries, platelet thrombus formation, narrowing of the arterioles, lamina propria fibrosis, and crypt distortion.[76] It has been suggested that chronic radiation proctitis is more likely in those with initial severe acute proctitis.[77]

ENDOSCOPIC ASSESSMENT OF DISEASE EXTENT AND SEVERITY
Ulcerative Colitis

Clinical impression of UC severity was found to correlate poorly with endoscopic mucosal findings and histology, with physicians underestimating inflammatory activity in about a third of patients.[78] Osada and colleagues[79] indicated that clinical symptoms were more likely to reflect the activity of distal disease, whereas CRP and erythrocyte sedimentation rate (ESR) reflected the activity of more proximal disease.[79] When determining disease activity and severity, sigmoidoscopy can be inadequate in evaluating UC. This finding was confirmed by Kato and colleagues,[80] who showed that severe inflammatory activity was observed more frequently in patients who had maximum disease activity in the proximal colon compared with the rectum or sigmoid. Also, patients who are receiving rectal therapy may have minimal distal disease. Full colonoscopy is particularly important in the initial mapping of disease extent and severity as well as to investigate any discrepancy between clinical symptoms and rectosigmoid appearance. The extent of colonic involvement in UC is not static and can change over time. Up to a third of patients initially diagnosed with proctitis will have proximal progression of their disease.[81] Although routine colonoscopy is not usually carried out in asymptomatic patients, patients with longstanding disease require reevaluation of their disease extent because this may influence their risk of developing colorectal cancer.

Multiple clinical and endoscopic scoring methods have been designed to classify the severity of UC. The simplest clinical scoring system, introduced in 1955, is based on stool frequency, presence of fever, tachycardia, anemia, and elevated ESR.[82] Scoring systems that include endoscopic features include the Baron score, Mayo score, Powell-Tuck, Rachmilewitz endoscopic index, and the UC Disease Activity Index.[83–87] Most endoscopic scoring systems are similar in their description of inactive, mild, moderate, and severe UC. Patients with inactive UC have normal mucosa with clearly visible vascular pattern.[83] Mild disease usually consists of mild erythema, decreased vascular pattern, and mild friability.[86] Moderate disease is defined as moderate friability with mild contact bleeding, no spontaneous bleeding, and granularity.[85,88] Severe colitis is seen as spontaneous bleeding from the mucosa with pronounced mucosal damage and visible ulceration.[83,85,86]

In a study by Kiesslich and colleagues,[88] newer techniques such as chromoendoscopy (CE) and magnification endoscopy (ME) have been found to be more accurate in predicting mild disease (87%) compared with conventional endoscopy (54%), $P = .0002$.[88] The same study demonstrated that ME and CE (84.5%) were superior to conventional endoscopy (37%) in predicting the extent of UC disease activity when correlated to histologic diagnosis, $P<.0001$. For more information on CE, please refer to discussion, "CE in IBD surveillance," elsewhere in this issue.

Crohn Disease

The Crohn Disease Endoscopic Index of Severity, developed in the late 1980s, is based on the extent of disease in each of the five bowel segments (rectum sigmoid and descending, transverse, ascending and ileum) and type of lesion observed (superficial or deep ulceration, ulcerated and nonulcerated stenosis).[89] However, poor correlations were found between clinical symptoms, endoscopic scoring, and treatment outcome. This scoring system was later simplified by Daperno and colleagues[90] into the Simple Endoscopic Score for Crohn Disease (SES-CD) and evaluated ulcer size rather than depth of penetration. The SES-CD scoring system achieved better interobserver consistency and correlation with clinical symptoms as well as CRP. However, neither of these scores takes into account upper GI involvement. Following curative resection, Rutgeerts' score is the most widely used scoring system for evaluating postsurgical recurrence.[91] It takes into account the presence of aphthous ulcers, inflammation, involvement of the terminal ileum, the extent of colonic involvement, and stricturing disease.

ENDOSCOPIC ASSESSMENT OF RESPONSE TO TREATMENT

Patients who are relatively asymptomatic do not require routine follow-up colonoscopies. However, endoscopy can be useful during flares, particularly in patients who may have concurrent functional bowel disorders. Also, prior to escalation or alteration of treatment, it is often useful to obtain endoscopic and histologic documentation of disease activity to help monitor treatment response. Finally, endoscopy and biopsies can diagnose or exclude an infection that may cause a flare of IBD, such as CMV or *C difficile* infection. Detection can help determine the need for antibiotic or antiviral therapy. However, the decision to discontinue immunomodulators for the duration of infection remains unclear.[92]

Ulcerative Colitis

Endoscopic and especially histologic remission typically lag behind clinical response to treatment. Endoscopic remission has been shown to predict later symptomatic outcome and clinical remission. Early studies demonstrated that 40% of patients who achieve endoscopic remission after treatment remained symptom-free during a 1-year follow-up compared with 18% if endoscopic abnormalities persisted.[93] This finding has lead to the use of endoscopic scoring, usually in combination with patient symptoms as a clinical end point in most pharmacologic trials evaluating treatment response. These trials include the ASCEND trials and a study for patients previously treated with 5-aminosalicilyc acid (5-ASAs) by Kamm and colleagues.[94,95] More recently, the Acute Ulcerative Colitis Treatment (ACT1 and ACT2) study group evaluated the induction of mucosal healing by infliximab.[96] It was demonstrated that complete mucosal healing or a Mayo score of 0 at week 8 had a 73.7% chance of achieving symptomatic remission at week 54 and predicted a lower need for colectomy. Other than the evaluation of response to medical therapy, endoscopy is an important modality to diagnose postoperative disease such as pouchitis. (See "Evaluating pouch problems" elsewhere in this issue.)

Crohn Disease

In CD, it has been shown that there can be poor correlation between clinical and endoscopic remission. The GETAID group demonstrated that high-dose steroid therapy failed to induce mucosal healing in 29% of patients who had achieved clinical remission.[89] Also, endoscopic appearance actually worsened in 9% of patients treated with steroids despite symptomatic improvement. Endoscopic evidence of mucosal healing in CD also seems to have prognostic implications. Baert and colleagues[97] demonstrated that 70.8% of patients with a SES-CD of 0 at 2 years were found to be in steroid-free remission at years 3 and 4. In a study by Bjorkesten and colleagues,[98] mucosal healing at 3 months was successful in predicting mucosal healing at 12 months. Also, mucosal healing in CD has been shown to lead to decreased incidence of abdominal surgery and hospitalizations.[99,100] Please refer to "Evaluation for Postoperative Recurrence of CD" elsewhere in this issue for the role of endoscopy in assessing postoperative CD patients.

DYSPLASIA AND COLORECTAL CANCER SURVEILLANCE

Patients with longstanding UC and CD are at increased risk of developing dysplasia and colorectal cancer (CRC). Annual surveillance should begin after 8 years of disease duration for patients with extensive colitis and after 15 years for those with isolated left-sided disease or patchy colitis. An analysis by Lutgens and colleagues[101] involving 149 patients with UC, CD, or indeterminate colitis showed that a significantly greater proportion of patients on a surveillance program had cancers detected at an early stage. Twelve of the 23 (52.2%) surveillance-detected cancers were found to be American Joint Committee on Cancer stage 0 or 1 compared with 28 of 115 (24.3%) of those not on surveillance. This difference also correlated with a statistically significant 5-year survival advantage ($P = .0042$).[101]

The risk for CRC is increased in active and extensive disease, severe disease, longer disease duration, young age of onset, backwash ileitis, family history of CRC, and with concurrent PSC.[102,103] A metaanalysis by Eaden and colleagues[104] found the prevalence of CRC in patients with UC to be 3.7% overall and 5.4% in those with pancolitis. Patients with CD also have increased risk of CRC compared with the general population, particularly those with extensive disease.[105,106] The relative risk of adenocarcinoma of the small bowel is significant in those with ileal CD. However, because of the rarity of this condition in healthy individuals, the absolute risk is very small.[107] Current guidelines do not provide clear recommendations for small bowel endoscopic surveillance; any proposed screening would likely be in the form of radiologic imaging. Furthermore, small bowel CD can be complicated by fistulas and strictures, which would increase the risk of any endoscopic surveillance.

Endoscopically, dysplasia can appear either flat or elevated. In a study by Rutter and colleagues[108] it was noted that 85 (77.3%) out of 110 neoplastic lesions were macroscopically visible, of which 16 were dysplasia or dysplasia-associated lesions or masses (DALMs), 64 were sporadic adenomas, and five were CRCs.[108] However, flat dysplasia can often be difficult to detect macroscopically. Therefore, it is essential that a sufficient number of samples are provided for histologic evaluation. The accuracy in predicting dysplasia has been found to be around 90% with 33 biopsies and increases to 95% when 64 biopsies are obtained.[109] Guidelines suggest that four quadrantic biopsies should be taken from every 10 cm of the colon. However, the adherence to biopsy recommendations is poor and highly variable between gastro-enterologists.[110,111] Some have even suggested that the current guidelines on biopsy protocol are not worthwhile, because on average, only one episode of intraepithelial neoplasia is detected for every 1266 random biopsies taken.[112]

Elevated DALM can appear as a polyp, a cluster of polyps, nodules, plaques or velvety patches.[113,114] Endoscopically, DALMs can be difficult to distinguish from sporadic adenomatous polyps unrelated to colitis. However, the latter are usually encountered in a disease-free bowel segment. Multiple biopsies should be taken from contiguous mucosa to ensure that microscopic disease is not missed. DALMs are also more commonly sessile, poorly circumscribed, possess an irregular surface, and are associated with ulceration, stricturing, and tethering.[17] Schneider and Stolte[115] found that patients with DALMs were younger in age (43 vs 66 years) and had a longer duration of disease (12.6 vs 7.2 years) compared with patients with sporadic adenomas. Those who developed DALMs were also more likely to have multiple lesions (73% vs 35%).[115] DALMs can also be differentiated from sporadic adenomas using immunophenotyping and molecular criteria. DALMs usually show nuclear positivity for p53 protein, membranous beta catenin, and lack of Bcl2 protein.[116] Nevertheless, the combination of these three immunohistochemical markers is not entirely specific for differentiating DALMs from sporadic adenomas.[36,117]

Identification of flat dysplasia and DALMs is typically an indication for colectomy because of likelihood of finding synchronous CRC.[113] In spite of this likelihood, many physicians believe that a diagnosis of DALM-associated indefinite for dysplasia (IND) or low-grade dysplasia (LGD) is insufficient to justify prophylactic colectomy. Previous studies suggest that adenomalike lesions, encompassing both sporadic adenomas and DALMs, can be managed more conservatively.[118] A retrospective analysis supported the strategy of endoscopic resection for adenomalike lesions, which can be removed fully followed by aggressive surveillance, regardless of grade of dysplasia.[108]

The decision to proceed to prophylactic colectomy depends on the rate of progression from IND or LGD to CRC. However, supporting evidence has been remarkably inconsistent. In a recent retrospective study of 124 patients, Ullman and colleagues[119] found that the 5-year rate for developing CRC for IND was 4% compared with 6.4% for LGD and 43% for high-grade dysplasia (HGD). The same study demonstrated that DALMs had similar rates of progression to CRC as flat dysplasia found by nontargeted biopsies.[119] A separate retrospective study by Lim and colleagues[120] also found that the rate of progression from LGD to HGD or CRC after 10 years was around 10%. In contrast, much higher figures have been reported elsewhere, for example Connell and colleagues[121] found that at 5 years, 54% of LGD had progressed to either HGD or CRC. The decision to proceed with a colectomy in patients with endoscopically resectable, DALM-associated LGD should not be taken lightly. The decision should only be made following a thorough discussion with the patient while taking into account the patient's age and comorbidities. In the presence of IND, the patient should be rebiopsied in 6 to 12 months or sooner if the suspicion of dysplasia is high.[104,122] All biopsies should be reviewed by at least two expert GI pathologists. If IND persists, repeat surveillance colonoscopies should be repeated at a 3–6 month interval following intensive medical therapy to control inflammation and symptoms.[123] All flat confirmed dysplasia should be considered an indication for colectomy.

Several advances in endoscopic technology may improve the detection of dysplasia including NBI, CE, virtual CE, confocal endomicroscopy, and autofluorescence imaging. The role for NBI in dysplasia surveillance is debatable. Matsumoto and colleagues[124] found that in raised lesions, an NBI-determined tortuous surface pattern was likely to indicate dysplasia, but the presence of the same surface pattern in flat mucosa was unreliable. A randomized crossover trial in 42 patients with UC did not find any significant difference between NBI and conventional colonoscopy in dysplasia surveillance.[125] See the discussion on CE elsewhere in this issue for other techniques.

THERAPEUTIC ENDOSCOPY

Endoscopy has a limited but valuable role in the treatment of IBD-related complications such as strictures and bleeding.

Strictures

Strictures in IBD can occur because of longstanding inflammation and are more commonly seen in CD compared with UC. According to the National Cooperative Crohn Disease Study, 101 of 403 patients (25%) had at least one small bowel stricture and 42 (10%) had at least one colonic stricture.[126] Because of recent advances in IBD treatment, these figures are likely to have improved significantly as more patients are maintained in remission. In small bowel CD, the terminal ileum was the most common site for stricture formation.[127] However, the prevalence of colorectal stricture has been shown to be higher in patients with colonic involvement alone (19%) compared with those with ileocolonic involvement (11%).[128]

Colonic strictures in IBD patients should be considered malignant until proven otherwise. In a study at Mount Sinai,[129] malignant change was found in 17 of 59 (29%) UC patients with colonic strictures. The same study cited duration of disease greater than 20 years, location of stricture proximal to splenic flexure, and strictures resulting in obstructive symptoms as features associated with malignancy. Even though stricturing disease is more prevalent in CD, malignant change seems to be far less common than in UC. Only 9 of 132 (6.8%) CD patients with colorectal strictures were found to have malignancy.[128] There have also been case reports of malignancy arising at previous stricturoplasty sites.[130,131]

Stricture dilatation should be avoided if fistulous tracts are present or if strictures are located in areas of actively inflamed colon.[132] Incidental findings of strictures in an asymptomatic IBD patient, with no associated prestenotic dilatation, do not typically warrant dilatation.[132] However, it has been suggested that dilatation should be considered in asymptomatic patients with longstanding IBD to allow for dysplasia surveillance.[133] Balloon dilatation of strictures typically involves balloons between 5 and 8 cm in length and up to 25 mm in diameter. Larger balloons are more likely to be associated with complications such as perforation.[134] A metaanalysis involving 574 endoscopic balloon dilatations found a technical success rate of 90% with a 3% major complication rate.[135] In a single-center analysis of the long-term outcome following dilatation, it was demonstrated that 46% of patients required further dilatation and another 24% of patients required surgery.[136] A stricture length of equal to or less than 4 cm has been associated with better dilatation outcome.[137] In a retrospective multicenter study, balloon dilatation of small bowel CD-related strictures using DBE had a long-term success rate of 70% (22 of 31 patients).[127] Gastroduodenal strictures may not benefit from dilatation because of the fibrotic nature of the tissue and resistance to dilatation.[138] It has been suggested that endoscopy in combination with EUS may allow estimation of the wall structure and depth of surrounding ulcerations, improving risk stratification prior to balloon dilatation.[139]

Several small trials have studied the use of intrastricture injections of antiinflammatory agents to achieve a more sustained response. Studies using concurrent balloon dilatation with either steroids[140,141] or triamcinolone[142] injections seem to demonstrate good response. However, larger, adequately powered trials are required before these practices can be applied routinely. A small study successfully used a sphincterotome to produce radial incisions as an adjunct to balloon dilatation with no added complications.[143] A case study of 2 patients who underwent metallic stenting of colonic and anastomotic strictures found that surgical intervention was delayed despite early stent migration.[144,145]

Bleeding

The role of endoscopy in the treatment of hemorrhage in IBD is limited because most patients with recurrent major hemorrhage require more definitive therapy with surgery. Acute major hemorrhage occurs in 0.6% to 3.8% of patients with CD[146–148] and 1.4% to 4.2% of those with UC.[149–151] In CD, hemorrhage occurs more frequently in those with colonic disease than in isolated small bowel disease.[152] Published case reports of endoscopic intervention during hemorrhage in IBD include the injection of ethanol and 1% polidocanol[153] as well as placement of clips.[154] When the bleeding site is overt and localized, such as in the setting of an actively bleeding visible vessel or solitary bleeding ulcer, standard endoscopic management is probably sufficient. More commonly, endoscopy serves only to diagnose the bleeding site prior to surgical resection.

SUMMARY

Endoscopy plays an important role in the initial diagnosis of IBD, including the evaluation of disease severity, activity, and extent. The implications of complete mucosal healing further confirm the function of endoscopy in the follow-up of IBD patients. The use of therapeutic endoscopy, for example stricture dilatation, can avoid the need for bowel resection. Modalities such as capsule endoscopy, EUS, NBI, CE, and other emerging techniques are likely to have an increasing role in the management of IBD, particularly in the area of dysplasia surveillance and treatment.

REFERENCES

1. American Society for Gastrointestinal Endoscopy guideline: endoscopy in the diagnosis and treatment of inflammatory bowel disease. Gastrointest Endosc 2006;63: 558–65.
2. Carbonnel F, Lavergne A, Lemann M, et al. Colonoscopy of acute colitis. A safe and reliable tool for assessment of severity. Dig Dis Sci 1994;39:1550–7.
3. Navaneethan U, Parasa S, Venkatesh PG, et al. Prevalence and risk factors for colonic perforation during colonoscopy in hospitalized inflammatory bowel disease patients. J Crohns Colitis 2011;5:189–95.
4. Raza SH, Sultan N, Sabir M, et al. Value of unprepared colonoscopy in the management of inflammatory bowel disease. Presented at the Irish Society Gastroenterology meeting. Galway, Ireland, June 2–3, 2011.
5. Bernstein C, Shanahan F, Anton P, et al. Patchiness of mucosal inflammation in treated ulcerative colitis: a prospective study. Gastrointest Endosc 1995;42:232–7.
6. Bentley E, Jenkins D, Campbell F, et al. How could pathologists improve the initial diagnosis of colitis? Evidence from an international workshop. J Clin Pathol 2002; 55(12):955–60.
7. Cornaggia M, Leutner M, Mescoli C, et al. Chronic idiopathic inflammatory bowel diseases: the histology report. Dig Liver Dis 2011;43:S293–303.
8. Potzi R, Walgram M, Lochs H, et al. Diagnostic significance of endoscopic biopsy in Crohn's disease. Endoscopy 1989;21:60–2.
9. Ramzan NN, Leighton JA, Heigh RI, et al. Clinical significance of granuloma in Crohn's disease. Inflamm Bowel Dis 2001;8:168–73.
10. Matsumoto T, Kudo T, Yao T, et al. Magnifying NBI colonoscopic findings in ulcerative colitis. Stomach Intestine 2007;42:877–81.

11. Kudo T, Matsumoto T, Esaki M, et al. Mucosal vascular pattern in ulcerative colitis: observations using narrow band imaging colonoscopy with special reference to histologic inflammation. Int J Colorectal Dis 2009;24:495–501.

12. Chutkan RK, Waye JD. Endoscopy in inflammatory bowel disease. In: Kirsner JB, editor. Inflammatory bowel disease. 5th edition. Baltimore (MD): Williams and Wilkins; 2000. p. 453–77.

13. Byeon J-S, Yan S-K, Myung S-J, et al. Clinical course of distal ulcerative colitis in relation to appendiceal orifice inflammation status. Inflamm Bowel Dis 2005;11: 366–71.

14. Mutinga ML, Odze RD, Wang HH, et al. The clinical significance of right-sided colonic inflammation in patients with left-sided chronic ulcerative colitis. Inflamm Bowel Dis 2004;10(3):215–9.

15. Paski SC, Wightman R, Robert ME, et al. The importance of recognizing increased cecal inflammation in health and avoiding the misdiagnosis and non-specific colitis. Am J Gastroenterol 2007;102:2294.

16. Fefferman DS, Farrell RJ. Endoscopy in inflammatory bowel disease: indications, surveillance, and use in clinical practice. Clin Gastroenterol Hepatol 2005;3:11–24.

17. Friedman S. Endoscopic evaluation of polypoid lesions in patients with inflammatory bowel disease. Tech Gastrointest Endosc 2004;6:175–81.

18. Maldonado TS, Firoozi B, Stone D, et al. Colocolonic intussusception of a giant pseudopolyp in a patient with ulcerative colitis: a case report and review of the literature. Inflamm Bowel Dis 2004;10:41–4.

19. Fujimura Y, Kamoi R, Lida M. Pathogenesis of aphthoid ulcers in Crohn's disease: correlative findings by magnifying colonoscopy, microscopy, and immunohisto-chemistry. Gut 1996;38:724–32.

20. Geboes K, Janssens J, Rutgeerts P, et al. Crohn's disease of the esophagus. J Clin Gastroenterol 1986;8:31–7.

21. Nugent FW, Roy MA. Duodenal Crohn's disease: an analysis of 89 cases. Am J Gastroenterol 1989;84:249–54.

22. Reynolds HL Jr, Stellate TA. Crohn's disease of the foregut. Surg Clin North Am 2001;81:117–35.

23. Rao KV, Sterling MJ, Klein KM. Isolated gastroduodenal Crohn's disease presenting with acute pancreatitis. Gastroenterol Hepatol 2008;4(7):494–9.

24. Ohmiya N, Arakawa D, Nakamura M, et al. Small-bowel obstruction: diagnostic comparison between double-balloon endoscopy and fluoroscopic enteroclysis, and the outcome of enteroscopic treatment. Gastrointest Endosc 2009;69:84–93.

25. Oshitani N, Yukawa T, Yamagami H, et al. Evaluation of deep small bowel involvement by double-balloon enteroscopy in Crohn's disease. Am J Gastroenterol 2006;101:1484–9.

26. Fukumoto A, Tanaka S, Shishido T. Comparison of detectability of small-bowel lesions between capsule endoscopy and double-balloon endoscopy for patients with suspected small-bowel disease. Gastrointest Endosc 2009;69:857–65.

27. Matsui T, Yao T, Sakurai T, et al. Clinical features and pattern of indeterminate colitis: Crohn's disease with ulcerative colitis-like clinical presentation. J Gastroenterol 2003;38:647–55.

28. Wagtmans MJ, Van Hogezand RA, Verspaget HW, et al. Crohn's disease of the upper gastrointestinal tract. Neth J Med 1997;50:S2–7.

29. Lee SD, Cohen R. Endoscopy in inflammatory bowel disease. Gastroenterol Clin N Am 2002;31:119–32.

30. Gad A. The diagnosis of gastroduodenal Crohn's disease by endoscopic biopsy. Scand J Gastroenterol Suppl 1989;167:23–8.

31. Wright CL, Riddell RH. Histology of the stomach and duodenum in Crohn's disease. Am J Surg Pathol 1998;22:383–90.

32. Prenzel F, Uhlig HH. Frequency of indeterminate colitis in children and adults with IBD - a metaanalysis. J Crohns Colitis 2009;3(4):277–81.

33. Zhou N, Chen WX, Chen SH, et al. Inflammatory bowel disease unclassified. J Zhejiang Univ Sci B 2011;12:280–6.

34. Bardhan KD, Simmonds N, Royston C, et al. A United Kingdom inflammatory bowel disease database: making the effort worthwhile. J Crohns Colitis 2010;4:405–12.

35. Farmer M, Petras RE, Hunt LE, et al. The importance of diagnostic accuracy in colonic inflammatory bowel disease. Am J Gastroenterol 2000;95:3184–8.

36. Odze R. Diagnostic problems and advances in inflammatory bowel disease. Mod Pathol 2003;16:347–58.

37. Murrell ZA, Melmed GY, Ippoliti A, et al. A prospective evaluation of the long term outcome of ileal pouch-anal anastomosis in patients with inflammatory bowel disease-unclassified and indeterminate colitis. Dis Colon Rectum 2009;52:872–8.

38. Lemberg DA, Clarkson CM, Bohane TD, et al. Role of esophagogastroduodenoscopy in the initial assessment of children with inflammatory bowel disease. J Gastroenterol Hepatol 2005;20:1696–700.

39. Pera A, Bellando P, Caldera D, et al. Colonoscopy in inflammatory bowel disease. Diagnostic accuracy and proposal of an endoscopic score. Gastroenterology 1987; 92:181–5.

40. Haskell H, Andrews CW Jr, Reddy SI, et al. Pathologic features and clinical significance of "backwash" ileitis in ulcerative colitis. Am J Surg Pathol 2005;29:1472–81.

41. Goldstein N, Dulai M. Contemporary morphologic definition of backwash ileitis in ulcerative colitis and features that distinguish it from Crohn's disease. Am J Clin Pathol 2006;126:365–76.

42. Lew RJ, Ginsberg GG. The role of endoscopic ultrasound in inflammatory bowel disease. Gastrointest Endosc Clin N Am 2002;12:561–71.

43. Mesenas S, Vu C, Doig L, et al. Duodenal EUS to identify thickening of the extrahepatic biliary tree wall in primary sclerosing cholangitis. Gastrointest Endosc 2006;63:403–8.

44. Tedesco FJ, Hardin RD, Harper RN, et al. Infectious colitis endoscopically simulating inflammatory bowel disease: a prospective evaluation. Gastrointest Endosc 1983; 29:195–7.

45. Schumacher G, Kollberg B, Sandstedt B, et al. A prospective study of first attacks of inflammatory bowel disease and non-relapsing colitis: microbiologic findings. Scand J Gastroenterol 1993;28:1077–85.

46. Farrell RJ, LaMont JT. Microbial factors in inflammatory bowel disease. Gastroenterol Clin North Am 2002;31:41–62.

47. Surawicz CM. What's the best way to differentiate infectious colitis (acute self-limited colitis) from IBD? Inflamm Bowel Dis 2008;14:S157–8.

48. Holdsworth CD. Acute self limited colitis. Br Med J (Clin Res Ed) 1984;289:270–1.

49. Gast P. Endorectal ultrasound in infectious colitis may predict development of chronic colitis. Endoscopy 1999;31:265–8.

50. Ellrichmann M, Wietzke-Braun P, Wintermeyer L, et al. Endoscopic ultrasound of the sigmoid colon for the differentiation of Crohn's disease from unspecific infectious colitis and healthy controls - a prospective, blinded, comparative study. Gastroenterology 2011;140:S-692.

51. Wietzke-Braun P, Ellrichman M, Wintermeyer L, et al. Quantification of the level of inflammation in patients with ulcerative colitis compared to unspecific infectious

colitis and healthy controls by endoscopic ultrasound of the sigmoid colon - a prospective, blinded, comparative study. Gastroenterology 2011;140:S-693.

52. Pulimood AB, Peter S, Ramakrishna BS, et al. Segmental colonoscopic biopsies in the differentiation of ileocolic tuberculosis from Crohn's disease. J Gastroenterol Hepatol 2005;20:688–96.

53. Li X, Liu X, Zou Y, et al. Predictors of clinical and endoscopic findings in differentiating Crohn's disease from intestinal tuberculosis. Dig Dis Sci 2011;56:188–96.

54. Makharia GK, Srivastava S, Das P, et al. Clinical, endoscopic, and histological differentiations between Crohn's disease and intestinal tuberculosis. Am J Gastroenterol 2010;105:642–51.

55. Lee YJ, Yang S-K, Byeon J-S, et al. Analysis of colonoscopic findings in the differential diagnosis between intestinal tuberculosis and Crohn's disease. Endoscopy 2006;38:592–7.

56. Kim KM, Lee A, Choi KY, et al. Intestinal tuberculosis: clinicopathologic analysis and diagnosis by endoscopic biopsy. Am J Gastroenterol 1998;93:606–9.

57. Pulimood AB, Ramakrishna BS, Kurian G. Endoscopic mucosal biopsies are useful in distinguishing granulomatous colitis due to Crohn's disease from tuberculosis. Gut 1999;45:537–41.

58. Baudet JS, Castro V, Redondo I. Recurrent ischemic colitis induced by colonoscopy bowel lavage. Am J Gastroenterol 2010;105:700–1.

59. Koutrobakis IE, Sfiridaki A, Theodoropoulou A, et al. Role of acquired and hereditary thrombotic risk factors in colon ischemia of ambulatory patients. Gastroenterology 2001;121:561–5.

60. Maupin GE, Rimar SD, Villalba M. Ischemic colitis following abdominal aortic reconstruction for rupture aneurysm. A 10 year experience. Ann Surg 1989;55:378–80.

61. Su C, Brandt L, Sigal SH, et al. The immunohistochemical diagnosis of E. coli 0157:H7 colitis: possible association with colon ischemia. Am J Gastroenterol 1998;93:1055–9.

62. Linder J, Monkemuller K, Raijman I, et al. Cocaine-associated ischemic colitis. South Med J 2000;93:909–13.

63. Lucas W, Schroy PC. Reversible ischemic colitis in a high endurance athlete. Am J Gastroenterol 1998;93:2231–4.

64. Lozano-Maya M, Ponferrada-Diaz A, Gonzalez-Asanza C, et al. Usefulness of colonoscopy in ischaemic colitis. Rev Esp Enferm Dig 2010;102:478–83.

65. Toursarkissian B, Thompson RW. Ischemic colitis. Surg Clin North Am 1997;77: 461–70.

66. Brandt LJ, Feuerstadt P, Blaszka MC. Anatomic patterns, patient characteristics, and clinical outcomes in ischemic colitis: a study of 313 cases supported by histology. Am J Gastroenterol 2010;105:2245–52.

67. Margolius D, Cataldo TE. Nonsteroidal anti-inflammatory drug colopathy mimicking masses of the colon: a report of three cases and review of the literature. Am Surg 2010;76:1282–6.

68. Kurahara K, Matsumoto T, Lida M. Characteristics of nonsteroidal an-inflammatory drugs-induced colopathy. Nihon Rinsho 2011;69:1098–103.

69. Puspok A, Kiener H-P, Oberhuber G. Clinical endoscopic, and histologic spectrum of nonsteroidal anti-inflammatory drug-induced lesions in the colon. Dis Colon Rectum 2000;43:685–91.

70. Riddell RH. Pathology of idiopathic inflammatory bowel disease. In: Kirsner JB, Shorter RG, editors. Inflammatory bowel disease, 4th edition. Baltimore (MD): Williams & Wilkins; 1995. p. 517–52.

71. Stolte M, Karimi D, Vieth M, et al. Strictures, diaphragms, erosions or ulcerations of ischemic type in the colon should always prompt consideration of nonsteroidal anti-inflammatory drug induced lesions. World J Gastroenterol 2005;11:5828–33.

72. Nagar AB. Isolated colonic ulcers: diagnosis and management. Curr Gastroenterol Rep 2007;9:422–8.

73. Kennedy GD, Heise CP. Radiation proctitis and colitis. Clin Colon Rect Surg 2007;20:64–72.

74. Hovdenak N, Fajardo LF, Hauer-Jensen M. Acute radiation proctitis: a sequential clinicopathologic study during pelvic radiotherapy. Int J Radiat Oncol Biol Phys 2000;48:1111–7.

75. Reichelderfer M, Morrisey JF. Colonoscopy in radiation colitis. Gastrointest Endosc 1980;26:41–3.

76. Habouchi NY, Schofield PF, Rowland PL. The light and electron microscopic features of early and late phase radiation-induced proctitis. Am J Gastroenterol 1988;83:1140–4.

77. Denham JW, O'Brien PC, Dunstan RH, et al. Is there more than one late radiation proctitis syndrome? Radiother Oncol 1999;51:43–53.

78. Regueiro M, Rodemann J, Kip KE, et al. Physician assessment of ulcerative colitis correlates poorly with endoscopic disease activity. Inflamm Bowel Dis 17;2011: 1008–14.

79. Osada T, Ohkusa T, Okayasu I, et al. Correlations among total colonoscopic findings, clinical symptoms, and laboratory markers in ulcerative colitis. J Gastroenterol Hepatol 2008;23:S262–7.

80. Kato J, Kuriyama M, Hiraoka S, et al. Is sigmoidoscopy sufficient for evaluating inflammatory status of ulcerative colitis patients? J Gastroenterol Hepatol 2011;26: 683–7.

81. Meucci G, Vecchi M, Astegiano M, et al. The natural history of ulcerative proctitis: a multicenter, retrospective study. Gruppo di Studio per le Malattie Inflammatorie Intestinali (GSMII). Am J Gastroenterol 2000;95:469–73.

82. Truelove SC, Witts LJ. Cortisone in ulcerative colitis; final report on a therapeutic trial. Br Med J 1955;ii:1041–8.

83. Baron JH, Connell AM, Lemmard-Jones JE. Variation between observers in describing mucosal appearances in proctocolitis. Br Med J 1964;1:89–92.

84. Powell-Tuck J, Day DW, Buckell NA, et al. Correlations between defined sigmoidoscopic appearances and other measures of disease activity in ulcerative colitis. Dig Dis Sci 1982;27:533–7.

85. Rachmilewitz D. Coated mesalazine (5-aminosalicylic acid) versus sulphasalazine in the treatment of active ulcerative colitis: a randomised control trial. Br Med J 1989;298:82–6.

86. Schroeder KW, Tremaine W, Ilstrup DM. Coasted oral 5-aminosalycylic acid therapy for mildly to moderately active ulcerative colitis. New Engl J Med 1987;317:1625–9.

87. Sutherland LR, Martin F, Greer S, et al. 5-aminosalicylic acid enema in the treatment of distal ulcerative colitis, proctosigmoiditis, and proctitis. Gastroenterol 1987;92: 1894–8.

88. Kiesslich R, Fritsch J, Holtmann M, et al. Methylene blue-aided chromoendoscopy for the detection of intraepithelial neoplasia and colon cancer in ulcerative colitis. Gastroenterology 2003;124:880–8.

89. Modigliani R, Mary JY, Simon JF, et al. Clinical, biological and endoscopic picture of attacks of Crohn's disease. Evolution of prednisolone. Groupe d'Etude Therapeutiques des Affections Inflammatoires Digestives. Gastroenterology 1990;98:811–8.

90. Daperno M, D'Haens G, van Assche G, et al. Development and validation of a new and simple endoscopic activity score for Crohn's disease: the SES-CD. Gastrointest Endosc 2004;60:505–12.
91. Rutgeerts P, Geboes K, Vantrappen G, et al. Predictability of the postoperative course of Crohn's disease. Gastroenterology 1990;99:956–63.
92. Yanai H, Nguyen GC, Yun L, et al. Practice of gastroenterologists in treating flaring inflammatory bowel disease patients with clostridium difficile: antibiotics alone or combined antibiotics/immunomodulators? Inflamm Bowel Dis 2011;17:1540–6.
93. Wright R, Truelove SR. Serial rectal biopsy in ulcerative colitis during the course of a controlled therapeutic trial of various diets. Am J Dig Dis 1966;11:847–57.
94. Lichtenstein GR, Ramsey D, Rubin DT. Randomised clinical trial: delayed-release oral mesalazine 4.8g/day vs. 2.4g/day in endoscopic mucosal healing – ASCEND I and II combined analysis. Aliment Pharmacol Ther 2011;33:672–8.
95. Kamm MA, Lichtenstein GR, Sandborn WJ, et al. Effect of extended MMX mesalamine therapy for acute, mild-to-moderate ulcerative colitis. Inflamm Bowel Dis 2009;15:1–8.
96. Colombel JF, Rutgeerts P, Reinisch W, et al. Mucosal healing in patients with ulcerative colitis associates with a reduced colectomy risk, high incidence of symptomatic remissions, and corticosteroid-free state. Gut 2010;59(Suppl III):A411.
97. Baert F, Moortgat L, Van Assche G, et al. Mucosal healing predicts sustained clinical remission in patients with early-stage Crohn's disease. Gastroenterology 2010;138:463–8.
98. Bjorkesten C-GA, Nieminen U, Turunen U, et al. Endoscopic monitoring of infliximab therapy in Crohn's disease. Inflamm Bowel Dis 2010;17:947–53.
99. Schnitzler F, Fidder H, Ferrante M, et al. Mucosal healing predicts long-term outcome of maintenance therapy with infliximab in Crohn's disease. Inflamm Bowel Dis 2009;15:1295–301.
100. Rutgeerts P, Feagan BG, Lichtenstein GR, et al. Comparison of scheduled and episodic treatment strategies of infliximab in Crohn's disease. Gastroenterology 2004;126:402–13.
101. Lutgens MW, Oldenburg B, Siersema PD, et al. Colonoscopic surveillance improves survival after colorectal cancer diagnosis in inflammatory bowel disease. Br J Cancer 2009;101:1671–5.
102. Rutter M, Saunders B, Wilkinson K, et al. Severity of inflammation is a risk factor for colorectal neoplasia in ulcerative colitis. Gastroenterology 2004;126:451–9.
103. Itzkowitz SH, Harpaz N. Diagnosis and management of dysplasia in patients with inflammatory bowel diseases. Gastroenterol 2004;126:1634–48.
104. Eaden J, Abrams KR, Mayberry JF. The risk of colorectal cancer in ulcerative colitis: a meta-analysis. Gut 2001;48:526–35.
105. Sachar DB. Cancer in Crohn's disease: dispelling the myths. Gut 1994;35:1507–8.
106. Gillen CD, Anfrews HA, Prior P, et al. Crohn's disease and colorectal cancer. Gut 1994;35:651–5.
107. Bernstein CN, Blanchard JF, Kliewer E, et al. Cancer risk in patients with inflammatory bowel disease: a population based study. Cancer 2001;91:854–62.
108. Rutter MD, Saunders BP, Wilkinson KH, et al. Most dysplasia in ulcerative colitis is visible at colonoscopy. Gastrointest Endosc 2004;60:334–9.
109. Rubin C, Haggitt R, Burner G. DNA aneuploidy in colonic biopsies predicts future development of dysplasia in ulcerative colitis. Gastroenterology 1992;103:1611–20.

110. Eaden JA, Ward BA, Mayberry JF. How gastroenterologists screen for colonic cancer in ulcerative colitis: an analysis of performance. Gastrointest Endosc 2000; 51:123–8.

111. Gearry RB, Wakeman CJ, Barclay ML, et al. Surveillance for dysplasia in patients with inflammatory bowel disease: a national survey of colonoscopic practice in New Zealand. Dis Colon Rectum 2004;47:314–22.

112. Rutter MD. Surveillance programmes for neoplasia in colitis. J Gastroenterol 2011; 46:S1–5.

113. Blackstone MO, Riddell RH, Rogers BH, et al. Dysplasia-associated lesion or mass (DALM) detected by colonoscopy in long-standing ulcerative colitis: an indication for colectomy. Gastroenterology 1981;80:366–74.

114. Butt JH, Konishi F, Morson BC, et al. Macroscopic lesions in dysplasia and carcinoma complicating ulcerative colitis. Dig Dis Sci 1983;28:18–26.

115. Schneider A, Stolte M. Differential diagnosis of adenomas and dysplastic lesions in patients with ulcerative colitis. Z Gastroenterol 1993;31:653–6.

116. Cross SS, Vergani P, Stephenson T, et al. Dysplasia-associated mass or lesion (DALM) and sporadic adenomas in patients with chronic idiopathic inflammatory bowel disease. Diagnostic Histopathology 2007;14:110–5.

117. Odze RD, Brown CA, Hartmann CJ, et al. Genetic alterations in ulcerative colitis-associated adenoma-like DALMs are similar to non-colitic sporadic adenomas. Am J Surg Pathol 2000;24:1209–16.

118. Rubin PH, Firedman S, Harpaz N, et al. Colonoscopic polypectomy in chronic colitis: conservative management after endoscopic resection of dysplastic polyps. Gastroenterology 1999;117:1295–300.

119. Ullman TA, Wild D, Murphy SJ, et al. The natural history of dysplasia in inflammatory bowel disease: influence of disease type and dysplasia morphology and grade on cancer risk. Gastroenterology 2008;134:A-346.

120. Lim CH, Dixon MF, Vail A, et al. Ten year follow up of ulcerative colitis patients with and without low grade dysplasia. Gut 2003;52:1127–32.

121. Connell WR, Lennard-Jones JE, Williams CB, et al. Factors affecting the outcome of endoscopic surveillance for cancer in ulcerative colitis. Gastroenterology 1994;107: 934–44.

122. Itzkowitz SH, Present DH. Consensus conference: Colorectal cancer screening and surveillance in inflammatory bowel disease. Inflamm Bowel Dis 2005;11:314–21.

123. Chan EP, Lichtenstein GR. Endoscopic evaluation for cancer and dysplasia in patients with inflammatory bowel disease. Tech Gastrointest Endosc 2004;6: 169–74.

124. Matsumoto T, Kudo T, Jo Y, et al. Magnifying colonoscopy with narrow band imaging system for the diagnosis of dysplasia in ulcerative colitis: a pilot study. Gastrointest Endosc 2007;66:957–65.

125. Dekker E, van den Broek FJ, Reitsma JB, et al. Narrow-band imaging compared with conventional colonoscopy for the detection of dysplasia in patients with longstanding ulcerative colitis. Endoscopy 2007;39:216–21.

126. Goldberg HI, Caruthers SB Jr, Nelson JA, et al. Radiographic findings of the National Cooperative Crohn's Disease study. Gastroenterology 1979;77:925–37.

127. Fukumoto A, Tanaka S, Yamamoto H, et al. Diagnosis and treatment of small-bowel stricture by double balloon endoscopy. Gastrointest Endosc 2007;66:S108–12.

128. Yamazaki Y, Ribeiro MB, Sachar DB, et al. Malignant colorectal strictures in Crohn's disease. Am J Gastroenterol 1991;86:882–5.

129. Gumaste V, Sachar DB, Greenstein AJ. Benign and malignant colorectal strictures in ulcerative colitis. Gut 1992;33:938–41.

130. Menon AM, Mirza AH, Moolla S, et al. Adenocarcinoma of the small bowel arising from a previous strictureplasty for Crohn's disease: report of a case. Dis Colon Rectum 2006;50:257–9.
131. Jaskowiak NT, Michelassi F. Adenocarcinoma at a strictureplasty site in Crohn's disease: report of a case. Dis Colon Rectum 2001;44:284–7.
132. Erkelens GW, van Deventeer SJH. Endoscopic treatment of strictures in Crohn's disease. Best Pract Res Clin Gastroenterol 2004;18:201–7.
133. Bernstein CN. The role of an endoscopy in inflammatory bowel disease. Clinical Update 2008;15:1–4.
134. Couckuyt H, Gevers AM, Coremans G, et al. Efficacy and safety of hydrostatic balloon dilatation of ileocolonic Crohn's strictures: A prospective longterm analysis. Gut 1995;36:577–80.
135. Wibmer AG, Kroesen AJ, Grone J, et al. Comparison of strictureplasty and endo-scopic balloon dilatation for structuring Crohn's disease-review of the literature. Int J Colorectal Dis 2010;25:1149–57.
136. Thienpont C, D'Hoore A, Vermeire S, et al. Long-term outcome of endoscopic dilatation in patients with Crohn's disease is not affected by disease activity or medical therapy. Gut 2010;59:320–4.
137. Hassan C, Zullo A, De Francesco V, et al. Systematic review: endoscopic dilatation in Crohn's disease. Aliment Pharmacol Ther 2007;26:1457–64.
138. Grubel P, Choi Y, Schneider D, et al. Severe isolated Crohn's-like disease of the gastroduodenal tract. Dig Dis Sci 2003;48:1360–5.
139. Oka S, Tanaka S, Fukumoto A, et al. Endoscopic ultrasonography with double balloon enteroscopy for small bowel diseases. Tech Gastrointest Endosc 2008;10: 113–8.
140. Ramboer C, Verhamme M, Dhondt E, et al. Endoscopic treatment of stenosis in recurrent Crohn's disease with balloon dilation combined with local corticosteroid injection. Gastrointest Endosc 1993;42:252–5.
141. Brooker JC, Beckett CG, Saunders BP, et al. Long-acting steroid injection after endoscopic dilation of anastomotic Crohn's strictures may improve the outcome. A retrospective case series. Endoscopy 2003;35:333–7.
142. Lavy A. Triamcinolone improves outcome in Crohn's disease strictures. Dis Colon Rectum 1997;40:184–6.
143. Bloomberg B, Rolny P, Jarnerot G. Endoscopic treatment of anastomotic strictures in Crohn's disease. Endoscopy 1991;23:195–8.
144. Matsuhashi N, Nakajima A, Suzuki A, et al. Nonsurgical strictureplasty for intestinal strictures in Crohn's disease: preliminary report of two cases. Gastrointest Endosc 1997;45:176–8.
145. Matsuhashi N, Nakajima A, Suzuki A, et al. Long-term outcome of non-surgical strictureplasty using metallic stents for intestinal strictures in Crohn's disease. Gastrointest Endosc 2000;51:343–5.
146. Greenstein AJ, Kark AE, Dreiling DA. Crohn's disease of the colon. II. Controversial aspects of hemorrhage, anaemia and rectal involvement in granulomatous disease involving the colon. Am J Gastroenterol 1975;63:40–8.
147. Cirocco WC, Reilly JC, Rusin LC. Life threatening hemorrhage and exsanguinations from Crohn's disease. Report of four cases. Dis Colon Rectum 1995;38:85–95.
148. Kostka R, Lukas M. Massive, life threatening bleeding in Crohn's disease. Acta Chir Belg 2005;105:168–74.
149. Robert JH, Sachar DB, Aufses AH, et al. Management of severe hemorrhage in ulcerative colitis. Am J Surg 1990;159:550–5.

150. Edwards FC, Truelove SC. The course and prognosis of ulcerative colitis. III. Complications. Gut 1964;5:1–26
151. Bruce D, Cole WH. Complications of ulcerative colitis. Ann Surg 1962;155:768–81.
152. Belaiche J, Louis E, D'Haens G, et al. Acute lower gastrointestinal bleeding in Crohn's disease: characteristics of a unique series of 34 patients. Belgian IBD research Group. Am J Gastroenterol 1999;94:2177–81.
153. Hirana H, Atsumi M, Sawai N, et al. A case of ulcerative colitis with local bleeding treated by endoscopic injection of absolute ethanol and 1% polidocanol. Gastroenterol Endosc 1999;4:969–73.
154. Yoshida Y, Kawaguchi A, Mataki N, et al. Endoscopic treatment of massive lower GI hemorrhage in two patients with ulcerative colitis. Gastrointest Endosc 2001;54: 779–81.

Chromoendoscopy in Inflammatory Bowel Disease

Ralf Kiesslich, MD, PhD[a],*, Markus F. Neurath, MD, PhD[b]

KEYWORDS

- Chromoendoscopy • Confocal laser endoscopy
- Crohn disease • Endomicroscopy • Inflammatory bowel disease
- Magnification • Narrow band imaging • Ulcerative colitis

Patients with longstanding, extensive ulcerative colitis are at increased risk of developing colorectal cancer.[1] The risk is lower than previously reported, but colonoscopic surveillance is recommended still to detect intraepithelial neoplasia early and to reduce colitis-associated mortality.[2] Surveillance relies on the detection of premalignant dysplastic tissue. Here, adenomatous changes should be differentiated from colitis-associated dysplasia, because the management is fundamentally different. Adenomas can be removed safely endoscopically, whereas multiple low-grade or at least 1 high-grade, colitis-associated dysplastic tissue requires proctocolectomy.[3–5]

DETECTION OF ADENOMAS AND COLITIS-ASSOCIATED DYSPLASIA IN INFLAMMATORY BOWEL DISEASE

Adenomas occur usually as clearly demarcated lesions using white light colonoscopy. Adenomas can be either polypoid, flat, or depressed. The development follows the adenoma–carcinoma sequence and adenomas are increasingly prevalent with age.

Colitis-associated neoplasia can occur in addition to adenomas in patients with longstanding ulcerative colitis. These lesions are triggered by inflammation and the macroscopic appearances are often flat and multifocal.[3] The borders of the lesions are often ill defined and biopsies of the subtle changes as well as of the surrounding mucosa are recommended.

There are no clear-cut, endoscopic, histologic, or immunohistochemical discriminators to permit absolute accurate stratification between adenomas and colitis-associated

The authors have nothing to disclose.
[a] I. Med. Klinik und Poliklinik, Johannes Gutenberg Universität Mainz, Langenbeckstrasse 1, 55131 Mainz, Germany
[b] Department of Medicine I, University of Erlangen-Nuremberg, Ulmenweg 18, 91054 Erlangen, Germany
* Corresponding author.
E-mail address: kiesslich@uni-mainz.de

Gastroenterol Clin N Am 41 (2012) 291–302
doi:10.1016/j.gtc.2012.01.016
0889-8553/12/$ – see front matter © 2012 Elsevier Inc. All rights reserved.

dysplasia. However, optimal diagnosis combines endoscopic and histologic features. The term "intraepithelial neoplasia" in accordance to the new Vienna classification was established, which summarizes adenomas and colitis-associated neoplasia.[4]

Multiple, untargeted, random biopsies are recommended to diagnose intraepithelial neoplasia. Four random biopsies per site over 9 sites throughout the colon should be undertaken, with increased sampling from the rectosigmoid and with additional biopsies from raised or suspicious lesions.[2] However, this approach is time consuming and dysplastic lesions might still be overlooked.

Chromoendoscopy can help greatly to identify premalignant and malignant lesions. A multitude of randomized, controlled trials, as well as a recently published meta-analysis, have underscored the value of chromoendoscopy.[5] Chromoendoscopy-guided biopsies have a significantly higher diagnostic yield compared with random biopsies.[5] Furthermore, magnifying endoscopy enables analysis of surface structure, whereas confocal laser endomicroscopy (CLE) enables in vivo histology, which further decreases the number of biopsies needed per patient.[6]

CHROMOENDOSCOPY

Intravital staining is the oldest and simplest method used to improve the diagnosis of epithelial changes. Chromoendoscopy, vital staining, and contrast endoscopy are synonyms for the same technique: Dye solutions are applied to the mucosa of the gastrointestinal tract, enhancing the recognition of details to uncover mucosal changes not perceivable by purely optical methods before targeted biopsy and histology[7] (**Fig. 1**). Three classes of dyes used for chromoendoscopy are mainly differentiated.[7,8]

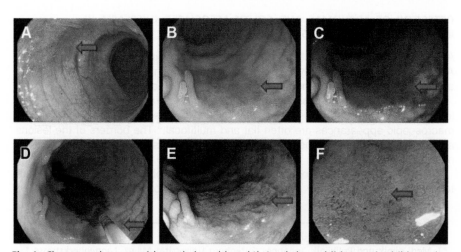

Fig. 1. Chromoendoscopy with methylene blue. (*A*) A subtle, reddish area is visible underneath remnants of stool (*arrow*). (*B*) A reddish lesion becomes visible after thorough cleaning (*arrow*). (*C*) Virtual chromoendoscopy using i-scan highlights the overall appearance of the lesion (*arrow*). (*D*) A spraying catheter is advanced and intravital staining with methylene blue is applied using a spraying catheter (*arrow*). (*E*) Methylene blue clearly highlights the border of the lesion. The absorption of dye is less intense throughout the lesions, which indicated neoplastic changes (*arrow*). (*F*) Magnifying inspection and crypt analysis shows irregular pattern architecture which also indicated neoplasia. Endoscopic resection was performed and high-grade intraepithelial neoplasia could be was confirmed (*arrow*).

Contrast Dyes

Contrast dyes coat the colonic mucosal surface and highlight tissue architecture because of the higher contrast of pooled dye within the small grooves between the colonic crypts and within the colonic pits. An example is indigo carmine, which is commonly used throughout the gastrointestinal tract. When indigo carmine (concentration, 0.2%–0.4%) is sprayed on the surface, the pit pattern of the colonic surface becomes evident, and disruption, indicating inflammation or changes of the normal pattern indicating hyperplasia or intraepithelial neoplasia, can be readily identified. Contrast staining lasts for few minutes and disappears owing to dilution throughout the colon.

Absorptive Dyes

Absorptive dyes are absorbed by different cells to different degrees, highlighting distinct cell types. An example is methylene blue (concentration, 0.1%), which avidly stains noninflamed mucosa, but is poorly taken up by areas of active inflammation and intraepithelial neoplasia. Methylene blue reacts initially as a contrast stain and is subsequently absorbed. The absorption requires about 60 seconds. However, stable staining patterns occur, which allows examination times of up to 20 minutes of the stained area (see **Fig. 1**).

Reactive Dyes

The binding of reactive coloring agents with certain mucosal areas is used to identify reactions. Their use is less common and their diagnostic relevance is low.

In patients with ulcerative colitis, the most commonly used dyes are indigo carmine and methylene blue. Chromoendoscopy has 2 main goals. First, it improves the detection of subtle colonic lesions, raising the sensitivity of the endoscopic examination; this is important in ulcerative colitis, because flat dysplastic lesions can be difficult or impossible to detect with white light endoscopy. Second, once a lesion is detected, chromoendoscopy can improve lesion characterization, increasing the specificity of the examination. This can be further refined with magnifying and/or high-definition colonoscopes. Surface analysis of colorectal lesions using magnifying endoscopes has led to new optical impression for endoscopists. First in 1996, Kudo and associates[9] described that some of the regular staining patterns are often seen in hyperplastic polyps or normal mucosa, whereas unstructured surface architecture was associated with malignancy. Also, the kind of adenoma (tubular or villous) can be seen by detailed inspection. This experience has led to a categorization of the different staining patterns in the colon. The so-called pit-pattern classification[9] differentiated 5 types and several subtypes. Types 1 and 2 are staining patterns predicting non-neoplastic lesions, whereas types 3 to 5 are predicting neoplastic lesions. With the help of this classification, the endoscopist can predict histology with good accuracy in patients with ulcerative colitis.[10]

Several prospective, randomized trials using methylene blue or indigo carmine for panchromoendoscopy in patients with longstanding ulcerative colitis have shown the unique benefit of chromoendoscopy for the diagnosis of intraepithelial neoplasia[5,10–14] (**Table 1**).

SURFACE GUIDELINES AND EXAMINATIONTECHNIQUE[8]

The *SURFACE* guidelines[15] were established for the use and standardization of this new technique in inflammatory bowel disease patients (**Box 1**). Patients with

Table 1
Value of chromoendoscopy in ulcerative colitis

Author	Year	Country	Dye	Staining	Endoscopy	Design	No of Patients	Patients with Dysplasia	Outcome Chromo vs Standard
Kiesslich et al	2003	Germany	MB	Pancolonic	Magnification	Randomized 1:1	165	19	32 vs 10 dysplastic lesions
Matsumoto et al	2003	Japan	IC	Pancolonic	WLE	Prospective cohort	57	12	86% vs 38% sensitivity
Rutter et al	2004	UK	IC	Pancolonic	WLE	Prospective cohort	100	7	9 vs 2 dysplastic lesions
Hurlstone et al	2005	UK	IC	Targeted	Magnification	Prospective cohort	700	81	69 vs 24 dysplastic lesions
Kiesslich et al	2007	Germany	MB	Pancolonic	CLE	Randomized 1:1	153	15	19 vs 4 dysplastic lesions
Marion et al	2008	US	MB	Pancolonic	WLE	Tandem colonoscopy	102	19	17 vs 3 patients with dysplastic lesions
Günther et al	2011	Germany	IC	Pancolonic	CE	Randomized 1:1:1	150	6	0 vs 6 patients with dysplastic lesions
Hlavaty et al	2011	Slovakia	IC	Pancolonic	CE	Tandem colonoscopy	30	7	0 vs 7 dysplastic lesions

Abbreviations: CE, chromoendoscopy; IC, indigo carmine; MB, methylene blue; WLE, white light endoscopy.

Box 1
SURFACE guidelines for chromoendoscopy in patients with ulcerative colitis

Strict patient selection.

- Patients with histologically proven ulcerative colitis and at least eight years' duration in clinical remission.
- Avoid patients with active disease.

Unmask the mucosal surface.

- Excellent bowel preparation is needed. Remove mucus and remaining fluid in the colon when necessary.

Reduce peristaltic waves.

- When drawing back the endoscope, a spasmolytic agent should be used (if necessary).

Full length staining of the colon.

- Perform full length staining of the colon (panchromoendoscopy) in ulcerative colitis rather than local staining

Augmented detection with dyes.

- Intravital staining with 0.4% indigo carmine or 0.1% methylene blue should be used to unmask flat lesions more frequently than with conventional colonoscopy.

Crypt architecture analysis.

- All lesions should be analyzed according to the pit pattern classification.
- Whereas pit pattern types I–II suggest the presence of nonmalignant lesions, staining patterns III–V suggest the presence of intraepithelial neoplasia and carcinomas.

Endoscopic targeted biopsies.

- Perform targeted biopsies of all mucosal alterations, particularly of circumscript lesions with staining patterns indicative of intraepithelial neoplasia and carcinomas (pit patterns III–V).

---

longstanding colitis in clinical remission and with mucosal healing are ideal candidates for chromoendoscopy (see **Box 1**).

Before the procedure, 100 mL of 0.1% indigo carmine or 0.1% methylene blue is drawn into 50- or 200-mL syringes. Thorough bowel preparation is crucial and prerequisite for chromoendoscopy and any other enhanced imaging technique. On insertion, all fecal fluid should be aspirated to ensure optimal mucosal views (see **Box 1**). After the cecum has been reached, meticulous inspection of the colonic mucosa is performed on withdrawal. To reduce spasm and haustral fold prominence (thus reducing blind spots), intravenous butyl-scopolamine 20 mg (or intravenous glucagon 1 mg) can be given when the cecum al pole is reached. Further increments can be given as required (**Box 1**). Adequate air insufflation is necessary, and if the lumen remains collapsed, the patient should be turned. A dye-spray catheter is inserted down the instrumentation channel, and the tip protruded 2 to 3 cm. Under the direction of the endoscopist, an assistant firmly squeezes the syringe, generating a fine mist of dye, which is then painted onto the mucosa by withdrawing the colonoscope in a spiral fashion. Subsequently, the stained area is reinspected. Chromoendoscopy greatly reduces the risk of overlooking subtle abnormalities (see **Box 1**), and adds about 11 minutes to the duration of the procedure in experienced hands.[5]

Spraying should be done in a segmental fashion (every 20–30 cm). Once a segment has been sprayed, excess dye is suctioned, and the colonoscope reinserted to the proximal extent of the segment. It is occasionally necessary to wait a few seconds for indigo carmine to settle into the mucosal contours; methylene blue takes about 60 seconds to be absorbed. Once that segment has been examined, the next segment is sprayed, and so on until the anal margin is reached. On average, 60 to 100 mL of solution are required to spray the entire colorectal mucosa. Dye-spraying greatly aids the detection of intraepithelial neoplasia (see **Box 1**).

Chromoendoscopy can unmask flat and depressed lesions, completely delineating the borders. Thus, targeted biopsies can easily be performed or complete endoscopic resection is facilitated. Furthermore, the combination of chromoendoscopy and new-generation, high-definition colonoscopes with magnification enables detailed mucosal surface analysis (see **Box 1**). Neoplastic changes are characterized by an irregular, tubular, or villous crypt arc hitecture staining pattern. Non-neoplastic changes are characterized by stellar or regular round pits. The different staining patterns are categorized using the "pit pattern" classification.[9]

By targeting biopsies toward mucosal abnormalities (see **Box 1**), the specificity of each biopsy for dysplasia is increased and the total number of biopsies taken per colonoscopic examination can be reduced in comparison with random biopsies with standard colonoscopy.[5]

Efficiency

The first randomized, controlled trial was published 2003 to test whether chromo- and magnifying endoscopy might facilitate early detection of intraepithelial neoplasia in patients with ulcerative colitis by using magnifying chromoendoscopy.[10] One hundred sixty-five patients with long-standing ulcerative colitis were randomized in a 1:1 ratio to undergo conventional colonoscopy or colonoscopy with chromoendoscopy using 0.1% methylene blue. Circumscript lesions in the colon were evaluated according to a modified pit pattern classification. In the chromoendoscopy group, there was a significantly better correlation between the endoscopic assessment of degree and extent of colonic inflammation and the histopathologic findings compared with the conventional colonoscopy group. More targeted biopsies were possible, and significantly more intraepithelial neoplasia were detected in the chromoendoscopy group (32 vs 10). Using the modified pit pattern classification, both the sensitivity and specificity for differentiation between non-neoplastic and neoplastic lesions were 93%. The overall sensitivity of magnifying chromoendoscopy to predict neoplasia was 97% with a specificity of 93%, respectively. Subsequently, 4 studies followed, which all confirmed the advantages of chromoendoscopy.[11–14]

The ability of the dye technique to distinguish neoplastic from non-neoplastic lesions to enhance detection of more dysplastic lesions in flat mucosa is a potential major advance in dysplasia surveillance. The difference in yield of dysplasia between chromoendoscopy and white light endoscopy was 7% (95% confidence interval [CI], 3.2–11.3) on a per-patient analysis with a number needed to treat of 14.3. The difference in proportion of lesions detected by targeted biopsies was 44% (95% CI, 28.6–59.1) and flat lesions was 27% (95% CI, 11.2–41.9) in favor of chromoendoscopy, as a recent meta-analysis including 1277 patients clearly pointed out.[5] **Table 1** summarizes the relevant studies and specifies the design and the used dye.

The diagnosis of flat dysplastic lesions is particularly increased using intravital staining. The pooled increase based on the meta-analysis[5] in flat dysplastic (low- or high grad-) lesion detection of chromoendoscopy over white light endoscopy was 27% (95% CI, 11.2–41.9). Chromoendoscopy prolongs the length of the procedure time by an additional 11 minutes.[5] However, this length depends on the biopsy protocol. The probability of finding dysplasia is increased and it might be justified to perform targeted biopsies only. However, random biopsies diagnose additional dysplastic lesion and recommendations about the right biopsy protocol varies between chromoendoscopic guided biopsies only or the combination of chromoendoscopic-guided and random biopsies.[16] Magnifying endoscopy and CLE are possible conjuncts of chromoendoscopy, which can further reduce the amount of biopsies based on surface tissue analysis or in vivo histology.

Chromoendoscopy also guides endoscopic treatment toward suspicious unmasked lesions. The diagnosis of dysplasia (adenoma versus colitis-associated dysplasia versus cancer) is facilitated and proper pathology can better define whether endoscopic therapy was sufficient (adenomas) and complete or whether proctocolectomy (colitis associated dysplasia) might be mandatory.

Limitations

Until now, there were no severe side effects reported from local use of indigo carmine. However, Olliver and colleagues[17] raised some concerns about the intravital dye methylene blue, despite a harmless transient discoloration of stool and urine. In patients with Barrett's esophagus, they found oxidative DNA damage after chromoendoscopy (as measured by single cell gel electrophoresis) and argued that methylene blue together with white light during endoscopy could also be a risk for patients to drive carcinogenesis. Subsequently, the same group showed in 10 patients with ulcerative colitis that only methylene blue but not indigo carmine causes DNA damage to colonocytes *in* vitro and in vivo at concentrations used in clinical chromoendoscopy.[18]

However, a follow-up report (median follow-up, 23 months) about the safety of methylene blue staining patients with previous chromoendoscopies showed fewer intraepithelial neoplasia compared with patients who were screened by colonoscopy. These data suggest that chromoendoscopy with methylene blue is a safe and highly effective approach for the detection of flat colonic lesions in ulcerative colitis. The reported increase of DNA lesions upon methylene blue-light treatment is unlikely to have biologic significance in vivo, and unwanted side effects seem to be negligible.[19]

The visual evaluation of minute detail allowed by magnification endoscopy in conjunction with chromoendoscopy is promising, but some limitations exist. Inflammation can cause significant disturbance of the image when magnifying endoscopy is used to look for the minute changes indicative of neoplasia, and there is a danger of false-positive results. Inflamed epithelium should be treated before final endoscopic evaluation whenever possible. Moreover, patients with multiple pseudopolyps are still very difficult to survey because not all visible lesions can be inspected in a reasonable time frame. All studies dealing with the value of chromoendoscopy were using standard resolution colonoscopies with or without magnification. The introduction of high-definition endoscopes has further improved the resolution and the ability to identify surface details has dramatically increased even without additional zoom. It is unclear whether these newly available endoscopes still require chromoendoscopy or magnification to increase the diagnostic yield of intraepithelial neoplasia. Here, further studies are warranted.

NARROW BAND IMAGING

Narrow band imaging (NBI) is an innovative optical technology that can clearly enhance and visualize the microvascular structure of the mucosal layer.[19] NBI illuminates the tissue surface using special filters that narrow the respective red–green–blue bands, while simultaneously increasing the relative intensity of the blue band. This enhances the tissue microvasculature, mainly as a result of the differential optical absorption of light by hemoglobin in the mucosa associated with initiation and progression of dysplasia, particularly in the blue range. The resulting images look like "chromoendoscopy without dye" focusing on capillaries.

NBI is particularly useful to characterize colorectal lesions and adenomas can be differentiated from nonadenomatous tissue with high accuracy.[20,21] However, 2 randomized, controlled trials from The Netherlands have clearly pointed out that NBI is not useful for increasing the detection rate of intraepithelial neoplasia over conventional colonoscopy.[22,23]

The first study included 42 patients with a prospective, randomized, crossover design. With NBI, 52 suspicious lesions were detected in 17 patients, compared with 28 suspicious lesions in 13 patients detected during conventional colonoscopy. Histopathologic evaluation of targeted biopsies revealed 11 patients with neoplasia: In 4 patients, the neoplasia was detected by both techniques, in 4 patients neoplasia was detected only by NBI, and in 3 patients neoplasia was detected only by conventional colonoscopy. More recently, with an identical study design, the same group compared the diagnostic value of high-definition endoscopy with and without NBI. Twenty-five patients were randomized to undergo high-definition endoscopy first and 23 to undergo NBI first. Of 16 neoplastic lesions, 11 (69 %) were detected by high-definition endoscopy and 13 (81 %) by NBI, a difference that was not significant. Only the use of trimodal imaging, which combines white light endoscopy with autofluorescence and NBI, showed a significant increase of intraepithelial neoplasia in a single study.[24]

Therefore, there is no proven value for the use of NBI in in patients with ulcerative colitis. It can be speculated that focusing on capillary structures might be difficult owing to background inflammation in patients with chronic inflammation.

CLE

Another newly available technology is endomicroscopy, which provides in vivo histology during ongoing endoscopy. The difference with chromoendoscopy is fundamental. Histology is not predicted; it can be seen.

CLE offers in vivo imaging of the mucosal layer at cellular and even subcellular resolution (**Figs. 2** and **3**). This new imaging modality provides more than conventional histology; because cellular interaction can be observed over time (physiology) and distinct changes like cell regeneration or mucosal barrier dysfunction can be identified in inflammatory bowel disease in vivo (pathophysiology).[25]

CLE can be currently achieved with 2 different endoscopic models. First, a miniaturized confocal scanner has been integrated into the distal tip of a flexible endoscope.[26] Second is the use of confocal microscopy miniprobes.[27] These probes can be fitted through the working channel of standard endoscopes. Endomicroscopy with both techniques provides in vivo histology during endoscopy at subcellular resolution (see **Fig. 2**).

CLE mandates the use of fluorescent agents. Most studies in humans have been performed with intravenous fluorescein sodium. Fluorescein quickly distributes within all compartments of the tissue, and CLE is possible within seconds after injection. It contrasts cellular and subcellular details, connective tissue, and vessel architecture at high resolution, but does not stain nuclei.[28] Acriflavine as an alternative or additional contrast medium is applied topically to the colonic mucosa and predominantly stains nuclei and, to a lesser extent, cytoplasm.[29]

A multitude of trials have proven the high accuracy with which CLE can differentiate non-neoplastic from neoplastic tissue by using fluorescein aided endomicroscopy, and simplified endomicroscopic criteria have been established[26,30–33] (see **Fig. 3**).

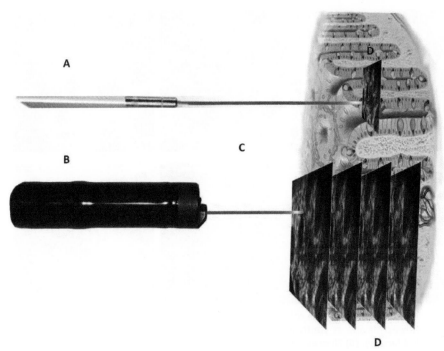

Fig. 2. Scheme of endomicroscopy. Two different confocal endomicroscopic systems are currently available. The mini-probe (*A*) can be passed over the working channel of standard endoscopes. (*Courtesy of* MaunaKea, France; with permission.) Or the endomicroscope (*B*) is embedded in an otherwise standard endoscope. (*Courtesy of* PENTAX Europe GmbH, Hamburg; with permission.) The blue laser light is applied onto and into the mucosa (*C*). The fluorescence and reflected light is measures and grey-scale images of mucosal micro-architecture are displayed on an additional monitor. The mini-probe has a fixed imaging plane depth (*D*), whereas the confocal endoscope can vary the imaging plane depth during imaging from the surface up to the deepest parts of the mucosal layer (imaging plane depth ranges from 0 to 250 μm).

The combination of topical acriflavine and systemic fluorescein administration also allowed reliable differentiation of low-grade from high-grade intraepithelial neoplasia with high accuracy.[34] Endomicroscopy is well-suited for patients with longstanding ulcerative colitis. Chromoendoscopy in combination with endomicroscopy enabled a significant increase in the diagnostic yield of intraepithelial neoplasia.[12]

CLE was able to predict the presence of intraepithelial neoplasia in vivo with an accuracy of 98% when used in such a targeted fashion. If endomicroscopy suggested normal mucosa, histopathology confirmed normal mucosa in 99% of optical biopsy sites. These results further support the notion of taking fewer targeted ("smart") biopsies rather than untargeted random biopsies: The combined use of CLE with chromoendoscopy reduced the number of biopsies in comparison to white light endoscopy surveillance to 3.9 biopsies per patient instead of 40 to 50, but still demonstrated a more than 4-fold increased diagnostic yield for intraepithelial neoplasia on a per-lesion basis.

Two further studies have confirmed the additional value of endomicroscopy in conjunction with chromoendoscopy. Chromoendoscopy was able to define areas of interest, and endomicroscopy allowed accurate histologic diagnosis.[32,35]

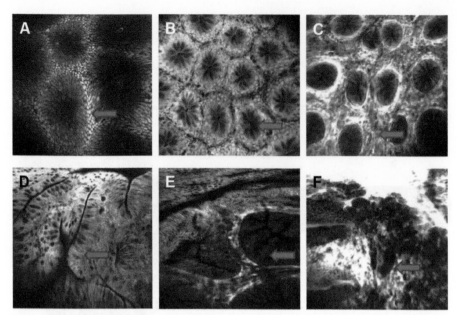

Fig. 3. Endomicroscopy of the colon. (*A*) Normal colonic crypts are visible using endomicroscopy with acriflavine as contrast medium. Single epithelial cells including nuclei can be identified (*arrow*). (*B*) Fluorescein aided endomicroscopy reveals normal crypt architecture. Here, mucin containing cells can be identified based on the black color, which represent goblet cells (*arrow*). (*C*) Increased vasculature with leakage of fluorescein in the lamina propria as well as infiltration of inflammatory cells characterizes inflammation in ulcerative colitis (*arrow*). (*D*) Hyperplastic changes can be identifies based on the stellar architecture of crypts with normal amount of goblet cells (*arrow*). (*E*) Adenomatous glands can be identifies based on their distinct shape and colorization. The number of goblet cells is decreased (*arrow*). (*F*) Colitis associated cancer can be identified based on the dark irregular cells which are invading in deeper parts of the tissue (*see arrow*).

SUMMARY

Chromoendoscopy with methylene blue or indigo carmine significantly increases the diagnostic yield of finding intraepithelial neoplasia in patients with longstanding colitis. The number needed to treat is 14 for panchromoendoscopy to identify 1 additional patient with dysplasia. Chromoendoscopy can greatly facilitate the identification of flat lesions harboring intraepithelial neoplasia. Chromoendoscopy can guide biopsies and clearly reduces the amount of biopsies that are needed per patient. Magnifying endoscopy or CLE are additional techniques, which can be used in conjunction with chromoendoscopy to further reduce the amount of biopsies and to further increase the diagnostic yield.

Chromoendoscopy is an established clinical procedure and recommended by many gastroenterological societies for surveillance of patients with longstanding ulcerative colitis. Thus, intravital staining should be an essential part of the diagnostic armamentarium of every colonoscopist.

REFERENCES

1. Ullman TA, Itzkowitz SH. Intestinal inflammation and cancer. Gastroenterology 2011; 140:1807–16.

2. Triantafillidis JK, Nasioulas G, Kosmidis PA. Colorectal cancer and inflammatory bowel disease: epidemiology, risk factors, mechanisms of carcinogenesis and prevention strategies. Anticancer Res 2009;29:2727–37.
3. Odze RD, Farraye FA, Hecht JL, et al. Long-term follow-up after polypectomy treatment for adenoma-like dysplastic lesions in ulcerative colitis. Clin Gastroenterol Hepatol 2004;2:534–41.
4. Stolte M. The new Vienna classification of epithelial neoplasia of the gastrointestinal tract: advantages and disadvantages. Virchows Arch 2003;442:99–106.
5. Subramanian V, Mannath J, Ragunath K, et al. Meta-analysis: the diagnostic yield of chromoendoscopy for detecting dysplasia in patients with colonic inflammatory bowel disease. Aliment Pharmacol Ther 2011;33:304–12.
6. Goetz M, Watson A, Kiesslich R. Confocal laser endomicroscopy in gastrointestinal diseases. J Biophotonics 2011;4:498–508.
7. Kiesslich R, Neurath MF. Chromoendoscopy and other novel imaging techniques. Gastroenterol Clin North Am 2006;35:605–19.
8. Rutter M, Bernstein C, Matsumoto T, et al. Endoscopic appearance of dysplasia in ulcerative colitis and the role of staining. Endoscopy 2004;36:1109–14.
9. Kudo S, Tamura S, Nakajima T, et al. Diagnosis of colorectal tumorous lesions by magnifying endoscopy. Gastrointest Endosc 1996;44:8–14.
10. Kiesslich R, Fritsch J, Holtmann M, et al. Methylene blue-aided chromoendoscopy for the detection of intraepithelial neoplasia and colon cancer in ulcerative colitis. Gastroenterology 2003;124:880–8.
11. Hurlstone DP, Sanders DS, Lobo AJ, et al. Indigo carmine-assisted high-magnification Chromoscopic colonoscopy for the detection and characterisation of intraepithelial neoplasia in ulcerative colitis: a prospective evaluation. Endoscopy 2005;37: 1186–92.
12. Kiesslich R, Goetz M, Lammersdorf K, et al. Chromoscopy-guided endomicroscopy increases the diagnostic yield of intraepithelial neoplasia in ulcerative colitis. Gastroenterology 2007;132:874–82.
13. Marion JF, Waye JD, Present DH, et al. Chromoendoscopy-targeted biopsies are superior to standard colonoscopic surveillance for detecting dysplasia in inflammatory bowel disease patients: a prospective endoscopic trial. Am J Gastroenterol 2008; 103:2342–9.
14. Matsumoto T, Nakamura S, Jo Y, et al. Chromoscopy might improve diagnostic accuracy in cancer surveillance for ulcerative colitis. Am J Gastroenterol 2003;98: 1827–33.
15. Kiesslich R, Neurath MF. Chromoendoscopy: an evolving standard in surveillance for ulcerative colitis. Inflamm Bowel Dis 2004;10:695–6.
16. Neumann H, Vieth M, Langner C, et al. Cancer risk in IBD: how to diagnose and how to manage DALM and ALM. World J Gastroenterol 2011;17:3184–91.
17. Olliver JR, Wild CP, Sahay P, et al. Chromoendoscopy with methylene blue and associated DNA damage in Barrett's oesophagus. Lancet 2003;362:373–4.
18. Davies J, Burke D, Olliver JR, et al. Methylene blue but not indigo carmine causes DNA damage to colonocytes in vitro and in vivo at concentrations used in clinical chromoendoscopy. Gut 2007;56:155–6.
19. Kiesslich R, Burg J, Kaina B, et al. Safety and efficacy of methylene blue aided chromoendoscopy in ulcerative colitis: a prospective pilot study upon previous chromoendoscopies. Gastrointest Endosc 2004;59:AB97.
20. Gono K, Obi T, Yamaguchi M, et al. Appearance of enhanced tissue features in narrow-band endoscopic imaging. J Biomed Opt 2004;77:568–77.

21. Sauk J, Hoffman A, Anandasabapathy S, et al. High-definition and filter-aided colonoscopy. Gastroenterol Clin North Am 2010;39:859–81.
22. Dekker E, van den Broek FJ, Reitsma JB, et al. Narrow-band imaging compared with conventional colonoscopy for the detection of dysplasia in patients with longstanding ulcerative colitis. Endoscopy 2007;39:216–21.
23. van den Broek FJ, Fockens P, van Eeden S, et al. Narrow-band imaging versus high-definition endoscopy for the diagnosis of neoplasia in ulcerative colitis. Endoscopy 2011;43:108–15.
24. van den Broek FJ, Fockens P, van Eeden S, et al. Endoscopic tri-modal imaging for surveillance in ulcerative colitis: randomised comparison of high-resolution endoscopy and autofluorescence imaging for neoplasia detection; and evaluation of narrow-band imaging for classification of lesions. Gut 2008;57:1083–9.
25. Kiesslich R, Duckworth CA, Moussata D, et al. Local barrier dysfunction identified by confocal laser endomicroscopy predicts relapse in inflammatory bowel disease. Gut 2011. [Epub ahead of print].
26. Kiesslich R, Burg J, Vieth M, et al. Confocal laser endoscopy for diagnosing intraepithelial neoplasias and colorectal cancer in vivo. Gastroenterology 2004;127:706–13.
27. Wallace MB, Fockens P. Probe-based confocal laser endomicroscopy. Gastroenterology 2009;136:1509–13.
28. Wallace MB, Meining A, Canto MI, et al. The safety of intravenous fluorescein for confocal laser endomicroscopy in the gastrointestinal tract. Aliment Pharmacol Ther 2010;31:548–52.
29. Kiesslich R, Goetz M, Vieth M, et al. Confocal laser endomicroscopy. Gastrointest Endosc Clin North Am 2005;5:715–31.
30. Shahid MW, Buchner AM, Heckman MG, et al. Diagnostic accuracy of probe-based confocal laser endomicroscopy and narrow band imaging for small colorectal polyps: a feasibility study. Am J Gastroenterol 2011. [Epub ahead of print].
31. Kuiper T, van den Broek FJ, van Eeden S, et al. New classification for probe-based confocal laser endomicroscopy in the colon. Endoscopy 2011;43:1076–81.
32. Günther U, Kusch D, Heller F, et al. Surveillance colonoscopy in patients with inflammatory bowel disease: comparison of random biopsy vs. targeted biopsy protocols. Int J Colorectal Dis 2011;26:667–72.
33. Xie XJ, Li CQ, Zuo XL, et al. Differentiation of colonic polyps by confocal laser endomicroscopy. Endoscopy 2011;43:87–93.
34. Sanduleanu S, Driessen A, Gomez-Garcia E, et al. In vivo diagnosis and classification of colorectal neoplasia by chromoendoscopy-guided confocal laser endomicroscopy. Clin Gastroenterol Hepatol 2010;8:371–8.
35. Hlavaty T, Huorka M, Koller T, et al. Colorectal cancer screening in patients with ulcerative and Crohn's colitis with use of colonoscopy, chromoendoscopy and confocal endomicroscopy. Eur J Gastroenterol Hepatol 2011;23:680–9.

Evaluation for Postoperative Recurrence of Crohn Disease

Jason M. Swoger, MD, MPH, Miguel Regueiro, MD*

KEYWORDS
- Crohn disease • Postoperative • Surgery
- Endoscopic recurrence • Treatment • Prevention

Crohn disease is a chronic inflammatory condition, affecting the entire gastrointestinal tract, that follows a relapsing and remitting course. Approximately two-thirds of patients with Crohn disease undergo a resective surgery during their lifetime, often because of complications associated with the disease, including fistula, abscess, fibrostenotic stricture.[1–4] Once patients undergo a surgical resection, they are at an increased risk for future reoperation, and 30% to 70% of patients with Crohn disease require reoperation within 10 years of their initial surgery.[3,5–7] Although some risk factors have been associated with need for reoperation, the complexities of the timing and severity of disease recurrence are not well-understood.

Currently, the gold standard for postoperative Crohn disease evaluation is performing an ileocolonoscopy within 1 year of a resective surgery. During this evaluation, the severity of endoscopic recurrence in the neoterminal ileum can be determined (Rutgeerts score), providing prognostic information regarding the risk of future symptomatic recurrence, as well as the development of complications, and the need for reoperation.[2] Recently, noninvasive strategies to assess for early disease recurrence have been described, including wireless capsule endoscopy (WCE), small intestinal contrast ultrasonography (SICUS), and magnetic resonance enterography (MRE).[8–11] However, ileocolonoscopy remains the procedure of choice because of its well-described prognostic score.

Recent reviews have focused on stratifying patients based on their risk factors for postoperative recurrence, and considering prophylactic therapy for those patients who are at higher risk for disease progression.[12] The timing of treatment initiation in the postoperative period remains controversial, although an ileocolonoscopy should be performed within12 months postoperatively regardless of a patient's treatment

Financial disclosures: Dr Swoger – none. Dr Regueiro – none.
Division of Gastroenterology, Hepatology, and Nutrition, University of Pittsburgh Medical Center, 200 Lothrop Street, C-Wing, Mezzanine, Pittsburgh, PA 15213, USA
* Corresponding author.
E-mail address: Mdr7@pitt.edu

regimen. Several classes of medications have been evaluated in the postoperative setting, with the strongest data supporting the use of nitroimidazole antibiotics, immunomodulators (azathioprine [AZA]/6-mercaptopurine [6-MP]), and antitumor necrosis factor (anti-TNF) medications.[13–20]

This article discusses the evaluation of postoperative Crohn disease, focusing on endoscopic evaluation with ileocolonoscopy and WCE. Risk factors for recurrence are reviewed, as well as recommendations for risk stratification. Finally, an algorithm for the evaluation and treatment of postoperative Crohn disease is presented.

DEFINITION AND PATTERNS OF RECURRENCE

Postoperative Crohn disease recurrence has been defined in several different manners, including endoscopic, histologic, symptomatic (clinical), radiographic, and surgical. Early studies demonstrated that reconstitution of the fecal stream is critical for the development of postoperative recurrence, and evidence of histopathologic Crohn disease has been described as soon as 7 days following resective surgery.[21] The timing of recurrence follows a well-described pattern, with endoscopic recurrence always a precursor to symptomatic recurrence.[2] Endoscopic recurrence rates are 73% to 95% at 1 year, and 83% to 100% at 3 years, with symptomatic recurrence rates being only 20% to 37% and 34% to 86% at these respective time points.[2,7,22–24] This clinically silent disease has been best described in the postoperative Crohn disease setting, but elucidates the natural history of Crohn disease; most disease is asymptomatic until intestinal inflammation is severe, often corresponding with the development of complications requiring surgery. Endoscopic recurrence follows a predictable pattern, with the initial postoperative ulcers presenting in the neoterminal ileum, proximal to the ileocolonic anastomosis.[2,22] The postoperative disease pattern tends to mimic that of the preoperative period, meaning that patients who undergo resective surgery for a stricturing or penetrating complication are likely to have those respective disease behaviors recur postoperatively.[25]

RISK FACTORS FOR RECURRENCE

Multiple studies have attempted to describe patient and disease characteristics that are associated with a higher risk for disease recurrence. Data concerning many of these risk factors are conflicting, although several risk factors have consistently been shown to be associated with early and severe disease recurrence (**Box 1**).[3,26,27–32] Cigarette smoking, a penetrating disease phenotype, and a history of prior surgical resections are the strongest risk factors for postoperative disease recurrence.[25,33,34–36] In addition, short disease duration prior to initial surgery may be a risk factor for postoperative recurrence.[7,37] Several other risk factors have been studied, with conflicting results, including gender, indication for surgery, length of resected segment, presence of granulomas in resected segment, involvement of resected margin with active disease, genetic factors (NOD2/CARD15), serologic profile anti-saccharomyces cerevisiae antibodies, corticosteroid treatment at time of surgery, and a perioperative blood transfusion requirement.[7,29,30,38–40] Although not yet described, it is the authors' opinion that patients failing to respond to immunomodulators/biologics who progress to surgery are also at high risk for postoperative recurrence.

Box 1
Risk factors for postoperative Crohn disease recurrence

High Quality Evidence:

- Smoking
- Penetrating disease
- Prior Crohn disease resection
- Short duration of disease

Conflicting Evidence:

- Perioperative complications
- Young age at disease onset
- Family history of IBD
- Anatomical site of disease (ileal vs colonic vs ileocolonic)
- Disease extent (>100 cm)
- Disease activity at time of resection
- Type of anastomosis

ENDOSCOPIC EVALUATION OF POSTOPERATIVE CROHN DISEASE
Ileocolonoscopy

Rutgeerts and colleagues[24] initially described a scoring system for the endoscopic evaluation of postoperative Crohn disease in 1984. The Rutgeerts score, grading the severity of endoscopic lesions 1 year postoperatively, is currently the best predictor of postoperative Crohn disease course (**Table 1** and **Fig. 1**).[2] Mild endoscopic recurrence includes patients with no evidence of aphthous ulcerations (i0), and patients with less than 5 aphthous ulcerations in the neoterminal ileum (i1). Patients with i2 disease had a postoperative clinical behavior between those with mild disease and those with more severe lesions, and had an endoscopic appearance of greater than 5 aphthous ulcerations, with normal intervening mucosa, or skip areas of larger lesions, or lesions confined to the ileocolonic anastomosis. Finally, patients with i3 or

---

Table 1
Rutgeerts postoperative Crohn disease endoscopic scoring system

Endoscopic Score	Endoscopic Findings
i0	No lesions
i1	≤5 aphthous lesions
i2	>5 aphthous lesions with normal mucosa between the lesions, or skip areas of larger lesions or lesions confined to the ileocolonic anastomosis (ie, <1 cm in length)
i3	Diffuse aphthous ileitis with diffusely inflamed mucosa
i4	Diffuse inflammation with already larger ulcers, nodules, and/or narrowing

Data from Rutgeerts P, Geboes K, Vantrappen G, et al. Predictability of the postoperative course of Crohn's disease. Gastroenterology 1990;99(4):956–63.

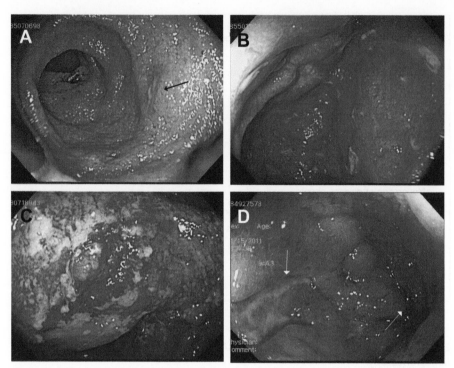

Fig. 1. Differing severities of endoscopic recurrence in postoperative Crohn disease. (*A*) i1 endoscopic recurrence, with a single aphthous ulcer (*arrow*), and otherwise normal mucosa; (*B*) i2 endoscopic recurrence, more than 5 aphthous ulcers, and normal intervening mucosa; (*C*) i3 endoscopic recurrence, with multiple aphthous ulcers and diffusely inflamed mucosa; (*D*) i4 endoscopic recurrence, with larger ulcer (*arrow*), nodularity, and evidence of stenosis (*arrow*).

i4 endoscopic scores had a more severe appearance. Patients with diffuse aphthous ileitis with diffusely inflamed mucosa were categorized as i3, whereas the presence of diffuse inflammation with larger ulcers, nodules, and/or narrowing were categorized as i4.

In 1990, the same group reported on a cohort of 122 patients who had been prospectively followed after undergoing bowel resection for Crohn disease.[2] The aims of this study were to describe the evolution of endoscopic lesions found during postoperative ileocolonoscopy and to determine if these lesions were left behind at surgery, or represented de novo lesions. At 1 year postoperatively, 73% of patients had evidence of endoscopic recurrence, whereas only 20% had symptoms suggestive of recurrence. Multivariate analysis, stratified for the preoperative disease activity score, found that the only factor significantly associated with symptomatic recurrence was the endoscopic index.

Clinical outcome was then analyzed based on endoscopy score, with i0 and i1 patients grouped together. The 39% of the cohort who were included in the mild endoscopic activity (i0/i1) group did very well, with 80% of these patients having no endoscopic lesions after 3 years of follow-up. There were also few cases of clinical recurrence in this group during follow-up. Conversely, patients with evidence of more significant endoscopic recurrence (i3–i4) tended to have a more severe disease course, developing early symptoms and progressing to complications. At 12 months postoperatively, 70% of patients with i4 disease had already experienced symptomatic recurrence, and all but one patient had experienced symptomatic recurrence by 3 years. Whereas 80% of patients with mild endoscopic lesions had unchanged lesions at 3 years, 92% of those with severe lesions at initial ileocolonoscopy had progression or very severe evolution at 3 years.

These investigators and others have been able to describe a biphasic pattern to postoperative recurrence, which can be explained by the findings of this study.[2,41] Patients with severe disease (i3/i4) tend to have early symptomatic recurrence and experience complications, including penetrating disease, which require early reoperation. Another group of patients experiences slower disease progression, ultimately leading to fibrostenotic stricturing, and often requires reoperation 5 to 7 years later.

The Crohn disease activity index (CDAI) is often used in clinical trials in order to assess for disease activity and to monitor for disease recurrence.[42] However, in the postoperative setting, the usefulness of the CDAI has been questioned, and the Rutgeerts score has proved to be a better predictor of disease evolution.[2]

Regueiro and colleagues[43] studied the correlation between CDAI and endoscopic recurrence as part of their postoperative infliximab study. Endoscopic recurrence was defined as a score of i2 to i4, clinical recurrence was CDAI greater than 200, and clinical remission was CDAI greater than 150. At 1-year postoperatively, 50% of the 24 patients were in endoscopic remission, with 50% showing evidence of endoscopic recurrence. There was no relationship found between mean CDAI score and endoscopy score at 1 year. In fact, mean CDAI scores at 1 year were identical (134) in both groups, and the agreement between CDAI scores and endoscopy was poor (Pearson $R = 0.07$). When a CDAI greater than 200 was used as a cutoff for clinical recurrence, sensitivity and specificity with endoscopy was 33% and 91%, respectively. Therefore, most endoscopic recurrences did not meet criteria for clinical recurrence using the CDAI score, which had a 67% false-negative rate. Interestingly, neither C-reactive protein nor erythrocyte sedimentation rate was associated with endoscopic recurrence in this study, although histologic scores were found to correlate with endoscopic recurrence.

This study demonstrates that the CDAI score is not an effective measure of postoperative disease recurrence, and, although CDAI is not routinely used clinically, these results support the observations that patients do not experience symptomatic recurrence until later in their postoperative course.

Wireless Capsule Endoscopy

Although ileocolonoscopy remains the recommend modality for the assessment of postoperative disease recurrence, several studies have begun to evaluate a possible role for WCE in this setting[8,9,11] (**Fig. 2**). The advantages of noninvasive tests to evaluate for postoperative recurrence include greater patient acceptance, lack of sedation, less bowel preparation, and a decreased risk (perforation, bleeding) than with colonoscopy.[8] In addition, there may be technically difficult anatomy encountered during postoperative ileocolonoscopy, and the neoterminal ileum cannot always be accessed. Finally, WCE allows examination of a greater area of small bowel mucosa.[9]

Bourreille and colleagues[8] prospectively studied WCE compared with ileocolonoscopy for the diagnosis of postoperative Crohn disease recurrence.[8] In addition, the investigators reported on lesions in the proximal small bowel detected by WCE and assessed interobserver variability in the detection and description of lesions found during WCE. Patients underwent an imaging study prior to capsule ingestion to rule out the presence of stricturing disease if it was more than 5 months since their surgery (50%), and 1 L of polyethylene glycol was ingested to improve visualization.

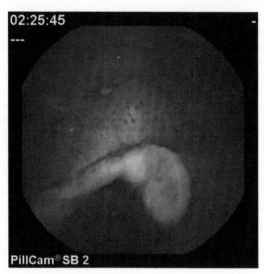
02:25:45

PillCam® SB 2

Fig. 2. Wireless capsule endoscopy image showing large ulcer consistent with active postoperative small bowel Crohn disease.

Thirty-two patients were included in the study, and the procedures were performed a median of 6 months following surgery. No strictures were identified among the patients who underwent imaging evaluation prior to capsule ingestion. Overall, 21 patients (68%) had evidence of recurrence in the neoterminal ileum, although the investigators used a definition of endoscopic recurrence of any Rutgeerts score at or greater than i1. Depending on the modality used to classify patients in this study, 19 to 21 of the 31 patients were i0/i1, with only 2 to 6 patients in the i3 group and no patients found to have an i4 endoscopic score. Ileocolonoscopy detected recurrence in 19 patients (61%). Therefore, WCE detected recurrence in 2 additional patients, not identified during ileocolonoscopy. The grading of lesions by WCE and ileocolonoscopy were well-correlated, although there was a trend for underestimation of severity by WCE. WCE detected jejunal lesions in 10 of 21 patients with recurrence in their neoterminal ileum, but did not detect any proximal lesions (0/10) in patients without distal ileal recurrence.

The sensitivity and specificity of WCE were 62% to 76% and 91% to 100%, depending on how discordant WCE findings were classified. The sensitivity and specificity of ileocolonoscopy were 90% and 100%, respectively. These operating characteristics did not dramatically change if the definition of endoscopic recurrence was changed to a score at or above i2. Interobserver concordance was high for the description of erythema, denudation, erosions, and ulcerations (kappa coefficient 0.7–1.0). However, for description of ileal ulceration, concordance was slightly lower, with a kappa coefficient of 0.6. Based on these findings, the investigators did not recommend that WCE take the place of ileocolonoscopy in the routine assessment of postoperative Crohn disease.

Pons Beltran and colleagues[11] evaluated WCE compared with ileocolonoscopy in 24 patients with Crohn disease who underwent bowel resection with a side-to-side anastomosis. The investigators compared the diagnostic yield of WCE with that of ileocolonoscopy for the detection of preanastomotic mucosal lesions. All patients were asymptomatic, and none were prescribed postoperative Crohn disease medications. All patients had a patency capsule examination prior to undergoing WCE. The investigators also reported patient preferences, therapeutic changes based on the examinations, and proximal small bowel lesions detected by WCE. A Rutgeerts score at or above i2 was considered evidence of endoscopic recurrence. Patients followed a clear liquid diet and fasted for 8 hours prior to WCE but did not use a bowel purgative.

The patency capsule was delayed in 2 patients (8.3%), and the complete small bowel was visualized during WCE in all but 1 patient. Of the 22 patients who underwent WCE, 15 (68%) had evidence of recurrence in the neoterminal ileum, with proximal small bowel lesions visualized in 13 patients (59%). Ileocolonoscopy was technically successful in 21 patients (88%), with evidence of endoscopic recurrence identified in 6 (28%). These results are significant for the high rate of recurrence in the WCE examinations (68%), compared with ileocolonoscopy. There were no false-negative WCE examinations, although ileocolonoscopy did not detect recurrence in 8 patients who had evidence of lesions on WCE. As would be expected, patients preferred WCE to ileocolonoscopy.

Biancone and colleagues[9] performed a prospective study to determine the usefulness of noninvasive tests for postoperative recurrence, specifically evaluating WCE and SICUS, and using ileocolonoscopy as the gold standard. Twenty-two patients were followed for up to 1 year postoperatively, and were prophylactically treated with mesalamine (2.4 g/d) following ileocolonic resection. Patients underwent SICUS, followed by ileocolonoscopy, followed by WCE, if no evidence of stricture or stenosis was found during the prior studies. In this study, lesions found above the ileum were not considered compatible with Crohn disease recurrence. All but 1 patient had evidence of recurrence on ileocolonoscopy (95.4%), with 18 patients having i2-i4 disease.

SICUS detected lesions in all patients, for a sensitivity of 100% and a specificity of 0%. The degree of wall thickening noted on SICUS was not highly correlated with the endoscopic recurrence score ($r = 0.42$). Of the 22 patients in the study, 5 (22.8%) did not undergo WCE because of findings of luminal narrowing or stricture. Findings suggestive of recurrence were noted in 16 of 17 patients (94.1%) who underwent WCE. Lesions proximal to the distal ileum were noted in 13 patients (76.4%), but these were not considered compatible with recurrence. In this study, WCE had a sensitivity and specificity of 100%. When anastomotic lesions were excluded, the sensitivity and specificity of SICUS was 86% and 33% (positive predictive value [PPV] 86%, negative predictive value [NPV] 33%), with respective findings for WCE of 93% and 67% (PPV 93%, NPV 67%).

There are limitations associated with WCE for the evaluation of postoperative disease that make it a less accepted modality than ileocolonoscopy. Studies have reported on the presence of lesions in the proximal small bowel, but these lesions are of unknown clinical significance.[44] In addition, it is unknown if these lesions were present preoperatively, or if they have the potential to affect the clinical course.

Currently, there is no standardized scoring system for WCE in the postoperative setting, although most investigators have adopted the Rutgeerts score for this emerging modality.[2,44] The Rutgeerts score was developed specifically for the assessment of postoperative endoscopic recurrence and has been correlated with disease and histologic activity. At this time, WCE findings in the postoperative setting have not been correlated with subsequent clinical course. In addition, the Rutgeerts score requires a careful and precise evaluation, which may not be possible with WCE because the physician cannot control the instrument. If WCE has a greater sensitivity for detecting mucosal lesions, which may or may not be clinically relevant, an

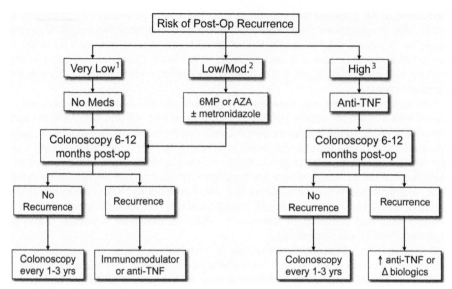

Fig. 3. Algorithm for the evaluation and treatment of postoperative Crohn disease. 1. Long-standing Crohn disease, first surgery, short stricture. 2. Less than 10 years Crohn disease, long stricture or inflammatory Crohn disease. 3. Penetrating disease, more than two surgeries, smoking, complicated peri- and postoperative course. (*From* Regueiro M. Management and prevention of postoperative Crohn's disease. Inflamm Bowel Dis 2009;15(10):1588. Reproduced with permission.)

alternate scoring system will be necessary to more accurately determine prognosis. Interobserver variability in the interpretation of WCE has also been reported, especially with ileal lesions, which adds to diagnostic uncertainty.[45]

Finally, there is a risk of capsule retention, as mentioned with each of the individual studies, and use of either a radiographic imaging technique or a patency capsule may be necessary prior to performing WCE. The rate of capsule retention in patients with known Crohn disease may be as high as 13%, although it is not clear what the risk is in the postoperative setting.[46,47]

PROPOSED ALGORITHM FOR EVALUATION AND TREATMENT OF POSTOPERATIVE CROHN DISEASE RECURRENCE

The authors have proposed an algorithm for the evaluation and treatment of postoperative Crohn disease recurrence (**Fig. 3**).[12]

At the time of surgery, patients should be stratified into groups based on their risk for early disease recurrence. Patients who smoke, have a history of penetrating complications, or have had more than two resective surgeries should be considered at high risk for disease recurrence, and postoperative anti-TNF therapy should be considered. Additionally, patients who had been on appropriate doses of 6-MP/AZA or methotrexate preoperatively, and progressed to surgery, may also represent a group to consider for postoperative anti-TNF therapy.

The authors consider moderate risk patients as those who have had a diagnosis of Crohn disease for less than 10 years, or underwent surgery for a long (>10 cm) stricture or segment of inflammatory Crohn disease. Postoperative prophylactic therapy with an immunomodulator, with or without a nitroimidazole antibiotic, should be considered in this moderate risk group.

Finally, patients with longstanding Crohn disease (>10 years), who undergo their initial resective surgery for a short, fibrostenotic stricture, are at very low risk for early disease recurrence. In this low-risk group, the authors do not recommend that prophylactic medications should be initiated postoperatively.

All patients, regardless of risk stratification, should undergo ileocolonoscopy 6 to 12 months postoperatively, and further treatment decisions should be based on the degree of endoscopic recurrence in the neoterminal ileum.[2,12] If no endoscopic recurrence is found (i0, i1), colonoscopy should be repeated on an every 1 to 3 year basis. However, should endoscopic recurrence be visualized (i2–i4), treatment should be escalated, and colonoscopy repeated in 1 year. In the low and moderate risk groups, considerations would be for adding an immunomodulator and/or anti-TNF agent. For high risk patients with evidence of endoscopic recurrence who are receiving an anti-TNF medication, considerations include adding an immunomodulator, dose escalation of the anti-TNF, or switching to an alternate anti-TNF medication or alternate biologic agent.

Finally, the question of whether a score of i1 documented at an interval prior to 1 year postoperatively represents a high risk for progression is not known. At present, the Rutgeerts scoring and postoperative endoscopy data have been established for a 1-year end point.[2] Whether a colonoscopy at 3 to 6 months, with findings of an endoscopic score of i1, should be included as a high risk for recurrence and treatment adjusted accordingly, is debatable.

SUMMARY

Disease recurrence following resective surgery for Crohn disease remains a challenging clinical problem, and more studies are needed to better define risk stratification and treatment recommendations in the postoperative setting. Endoscopy remains the gold standard for the assessment of postoperative disease recurrence, and all Crohn disease patients who undergo surgery should undergo ileocolonoscopy within 6 to 12 months of surgery.[12] The degree of endoscopic recurrence in the neoterminal ileum during this procedure provides prognostic information regarding the severity of the future disease course.[2] WCE, MRE, and SICUS are all promising noninvasive modalities to assess for postoperative Crohn disease activity.[8–11] However, further studies are needed to better define scoring systems, operating characteristics and variability, and prognostic data for each of these modalities. In patients at risk for early disease recurrence, more aggressive prophylactic therapy should be considered, in hopes of delivering true "top-down" therapy that may offer maximum impact in altering the natural history of Crohn disease.

REFERENCES

1. Cosnes J, Nion-Larmurier I, Beaugerie L, et al. Impact of the increasing use of immunosuppressants in Crohn's disease on the need for intestinal surgery. Gut 2005;54(2):237–41.
2. Rutgeerts P, Geboes K, Vantrappen G, et al. Predictability of the postoperative course of Crohn's disease. Gastroenterology 1990;99(4):956–63.
3. Bernell O, Lapidus A, Hellers G. Risk factors for surgery and postoperative recurrence in Crohn's disease. Ann Surg 2000;231(1):38–45.
4. Solberg IC, Vatn MH, Hoie O, et al. Clinical course in Crohn's disease: results of a Norwegian population-based ten-year follow-up study. Clin Gastroenterol Hepatol 2007;5(12):1430–8.
5. Landsend E, Johnson E, Johannessen HO, et al. Long-term outcome after intestinal resection for Crohn's disease. Scand J Gastroenterol 2006;41(10):1204–8.

6. Lock MR, Farmer RG, Fazio VW, et al. Recurrence and reoperation for Crohn's disease: the role of disease location in prognosis. N Engl J Med 1981;304(26): 1586–8.
7. Chardavoyne R, Flint GW, Pollack S, et al. Factors affecting recurrence following resection for Crohn's disease. Dis Colon Rectum 1986;29(8):495–502.
8. Bourreille A, Jarry M, D'Halluin PN, et al. Wireless capsule endoscopy versus ileocolonoscopy for the diagnosis of postoperative recurrence of Crohn's disease: a prospective study. Gut 2006;55(7):978–83.
9. Biancone L, Calabrese E, Petruzziello C, et al. Wireless capsule endoscopy and small intestine contrast ultrasonography in recurrence of Crohn's disease. Inflamm Bowel Dis 2007;13(10):1256–65.
10. Koilakou S, Sailer J, Peloschek P, et al. Endoscopy and MR enteroclysis: equivalent tools in predicting clinical recurrence in patients with Crohn's disease after ileocolic resection. Inflamm Bowel Dis 2010;16(2):198–203.
11. Pons Beltran V, Nos P, Bastida G, et al. Evaluation of postsurgical recurrence in Crohn's disease: a new indication for capsule endoscopy? Gastrointest Endosc 2007;66(3):533–40.
12. Regueiro M. Management and prevention of postoperative Crohn's disease. Inflamm Bowel Dis 2009;15(10):1583–90.
13. Rutgeerts P, Hiele M, Geboes K, et al. Controlled trial of metronidazole treatment for prevention of Crohn's recurrence after ileal resection. Gastroenterology 1995;108(6): 1617–21.
14. Rutgeerts P, Van Assche G, Vermeire S, et al. Ornidazole for prophylaxis of postoperative Crohn's disease recurrence: a randomized, double-blind, placebo-controlled trial. Gastroenterology 2005;128(4):856–61.
15. D'Haens GR, Vermeire S, Van Assche G, et al. Therapy of metronidazole with azathioprine to prevent postoperative recurrence of Crohn's disease: a controlled randomized trial. Gastroenterology 2008;135(4):1123–9.
16. Ardizzone S, Maconi G, Sampietro GM, et al. Azathioprine and mesalamine for prevention of relapse after conservative surgery for Crohn's disease. Gastroenterology 2004;127(3):730–40.
17. Hanauer SB, Korelitz BI, Rutgeerts P, et al. Postoperative maintenance of Crohn's disease remission with 6-mercaptopurine, mesalamine, or placebo: a 2-year trial. Gastroenterology 2004;127(3):723–9.
18. Reinisch W, Angelberger S, Petritsch W, et al. Azathioprine versus mesalazine for prevention of postoperative clinical recurrence in patients with Crohn's disease with endoscopic recurrence: efficacy and safety results of a randomised, double-blind, double-dummy, multicentre trial. Gut 2010;59(6):752–9.
19. Regueiro M, Schraut W, Baidoo L, et al. Infliximab prevents Crohn's disease recurrence after ileal resection. Gastroenterology 2009;136(2):441–50 e441 [quiz: 716].
20. Sorrentino D, Terrosu G, Avellini C, et al. Infliximab with low-dose methotrexate for prevention of postsurgical recurrence of ileocolonic Crohn disease. Arch Intern Med 2007;167(16):1804–7.
21. D'Haens GR, Geboes K, Peeters M, et al. Early lesions of recurrent Crohn's disease caused by infusion of intestinal contents in excluded ileum. Gastroenterology 1998; 114(2):262–7.
22. Olaison G, Smedh K, Sjodahl R. Natural course of Crohn's disease after ileocolic resection: endoscopically visualised ileal ulcers preceding symptoms. Gut 1992; 33(3):331–5.
23. Sachar DB. The problem of postoperative recurrence of Crohn's disease. Med Clin North Am 1990;74(1):183–8.

24. Rutgeerts P, Geboes K, Vantrappen G, et al. Natural history of recurrent Crohn's disease at the ileocolonic anastomosis after curative surgery. Gut 1984;25(6):665–72.
25. Greenstein AJ, Lachman P, Sachar DB, et al. Perforating and non-perforating indications for repeated operations in Crohn's disease: evidence for two clinical forms. Gut 1988;29(5):588–92.
26. Lautenbach E, Berlin JA, Lichtenstein GR. Risk factors for early postoperative recurrence of Crohn's disease. Gastroenterology 1998;115(2):259–67.
27. Mekhjian HS, Switz DM, Watts HD, et al. National Cooperative Crohn's Disease Study: factors determining recurrence of Crohn's disease after surgery. Gastroenterology 1979;77(4 Pt 2):907–13.
28. Scarpa M, Ruffolo C, Bertin E, et al. Surgical predictors of recurrence of Crohn's disease after ileocolonic resection. Int J Colorectal Dis 2007;22(9):1061–9.
29. Unkart JT, Anderson L, Li E, et al. Risk factors for surgical recurrence after ileocolic resection of Crohn's disease. Dis Colon Rectum 2008;51(8):1211–6.
30. Yamamoto T. Factors affecting recurrence after surgery for Crohn's disease. World J Gastroenterol 2005;11(26):3971–9.
31. McLeod RS, Wolff BG, Ross S, et al. Recurrence of Crohn's disease after ileocolic resection is not affected by anastomotic type: results of a multicenter, randomized, controlled trial. Dis Colon Rectum 2009;52(5):919–27.
32. Caprilli R, Corrao G, Taddei G, et al. Prognostic factors for postoperative recurrence of Crohn's disease. Gruppo Italiano per lo Studio del Colon e del Retto (GISC). Dis Colon Rectum 1996;39(3):335–41.
33. Reese GE, Nanidis T, Borysiewicz C, et al. The effect of smoking after surgery for Crohn's disease: a meta-analysis of observational studies. Int J Colorectal Dis 2008;23(12):1213–21.
34. Kane SV, Flicker M, Katz-Nelson F. Tobacco use is associated with accelerated clinical recurrence of Crohn's disease after surgically induced remission. J Clin Gastroenterol 2005;39(1):32–5.
35. Cosnes J, Carbonnel F, Beaugerie L, et al. Effects of cigarette smoking on the long-term course of Crohn's disease. Gastroenterology 1996;110(2):424–31.
36. Avidan B, Sakhnini E, Lahat A, et al. Risk factors regarding the need for a second operation in patients with Crohn's disease. Digestion 2005;72(4):248–53.
37. Poggioli G, Laureti S, Selleri S, et al. Factors affecting recurrence in Crohn's disease. Results of a prospective audit. Int J Colorectal Dis 1996;11(6):294–8.
38. Maconi G, Colombo E, Sampietro GM, et al. CARD15 gene variants and risk of reoperation in Crohn's disease patients. Am J Gastroenterol 2009;104(10):2483–91.
39. Hollaar GL, Gooszen HG, Post S, et al. Perioperative blood transfusion does not prevent recurrence in Crohn's disease. A pooled analysis. J Clin Gastroenterol 1995;21(2):134–8.
40. Anseline PF, Wlodarczyk J, Murugasu R. Presence of granulomas is associated with recurrence after surgery for Crohn's disease: experience of a surgical unit. Br J Surg 1997;84(1):78–82.
41. De Dombal FT, Burton I, Goligher JC. Recurrence of Crohn's disease after primary excisional surgery. Gut 1971;12(7):519–27.
42. Best WR, Becktel JM, Singleton JW, et al. Development of a Crohn's disease activity index. National Cooperative Crohn's Disease Study. Gastroenterology 1976;70(3):439–44.
43. Regueiro M, Kip KE, Schraut W, et al. Crohn's disease activity index does not correlate with endoscopic recurrence one year after ileocolonic resection. Inflamm Bowel Dis 2011;17(1):118–26.

44. Katz JA. Postoperative endoscopic surveillance in Crohn's disease: bottom up or top down? Gastrointest Endosc 2007;66(3):541–3.
45. Lai LH, Wong GL, Chow DK, et al. Inter-observer variations on interpretation of capsule endoscopies. Eur J Gastroenterol Hepatol 2006;18(3):283–6.
46. Cave D. Capsule endoscopy and Crohn's disease. Gastrointest Endosc 2005;61(2): 262–3.
47. Triester SL, Leighton JA, Leontiadis GI, et al. A meta-analysis of the yield of capsule endoscopy compared to other diagnostic modalities in patients with non-stricturing small bowel Crohn's disease. Am J Gastroenterol 2006;101(5):954–64.

The Role of Capsule Endoscopy in Evaluating Inflammatory Bowel Disease

Silvio W. de Melo Jr, MD, Jack A. Di Palma, MD*

KEYWORDS
- Capsule endoscopy • Crohn disease
- Inflammatory bowel disease • Small-bowel evaluation

Inflammatory bowel disease (IBD) is a generic term used to describe Crohn disease (CD), ulcerative colitis (UC) or IBD type unclassified (IBDU), formerly known as indeterminate colitis. By definition, only CD has the possibility to involve the whole gastrointestinal tract. However, in 10% to 15% of cases, a change in diagnosis is made from UC to CD or vice versa.

There is no absolute diagnostic test for IBD. The correct classification for CD and UC relies in the use of a combination of endoscopic, histologic, radiologic, and biochemical investigations.[1–4]

The terminal ileum is the most common area affected by CD and it is usually accessible at the time of colonoscopy. In approximately one third of patients with ileocolonic CD, the proximal small-bowel (SB) may be the only area of the gastrointestinal tract affected.[5] Therefore, it is important to maintain a high degree of suspicion in the appropriate clinical setting, even with a normal colonoscopy with terminal ileal intubation.

In the past, the endoscopic visualization of the small intestine was limited to the terminal ileum during colonoscopy and to the proximal jejunum during push enteroscopy. The majority of the SB was not seen endoscopically and was evaluated with radiologic tests such as small bowel follow-through (SBFT) or enteroclysis.

Our current armamentarium for the investigation of the gastrointestinal tract involves cross-sectional radiologic imaging tests, such as computed tomographic enterography (CTE) and magnetic resonance enterography (MRE; see the article on the radiologic

Disclosure: Jack A. Di Palma, MD, discloses that his daughter is a capsule endoscopy sales representative for Olympus Corp.
Division of Gastroenterology, University of South Alabama College of Medicine, USA Pavilion at Infirmary West, 5600 Girby Road, Mobile, AL 36693, USA
* Corresponding author.
E-mail address: jdipalma@usouthal.edu

Gastroenterol Clin N Am 41 (2012) 315–323
doi:10.1016/j.gtc.2012.01.005
0889-8553/12/$ – see front matter © 2012 Elsevier Inc. All rights reserved.

evaluation of IBD), deep enteroscopy with balloon-assisted or overtube-assisted endoscopy, collectively called device-assisted enteroscopy, and wireless video capsule (capsule endoscopy). Each technology has its own strengths and weaknesses. They should be viewed as complementary studies and not mutually exclusive.[6,7]

This article focuses on the role of capsule endoscopy in IBD in adults. We discuss the use of capsule endoscopy in suspected CD, established CD, UC (including ileal–anal pouch anastomosis), and IBDU.

PREPARATION

Capsule endoscopy, as opposed to regular endoscopy, does not have the ability to clean the mucosa or eliminate bubbles, debris, or bile during the procedure. Thus, bowel preparation should be used. There is no consensus about patient preparation for capsule endoscopy. In the setting of IBD, especially in established CD patients, SB strictures should be considered before proceeding with capsule endoscopy.[2] Some clinicians perform SBFT, CTE, or MRE before capsule endoscopy. A patency capsule (a capsule that dissolves in case of impaction) can also be used to investigate for significant stenosis. Others advise to use the patency evaluation only in those individuals where an obstruction is suspected or highly probable.

Each practice seems to use a different combination of dietary fasting, laxatives, and medications to stimulate peristalsis. Our group uses a full bowel preparation in a split dose regimen, followed by 10 mg of metoclopramide and 80 mg of simethicone orally 30 minutes before capsule ingestion. This regimen had good to excellent cleansing in 94% of patients versus 76% ($P<.001$) with fasting alone in the proximal SB and 55% versus 37% ($P = .01$) in the distal SB.[8] A meta-analysis evaluating purgative preparation versus clear liquids diet found similar results where purgative preparations had a higher diagnostic yield (odds ration [OR], 1.813; 95% confidence interval [CI], 1.251–2.628; $P = .002$), and SB visualization quality (OR, 2.113; 95% CI, 1.252–3.566; $P = .005$).[9]

There is no standardized method to report SB cleansing in capsule endoscopy. The examination is enhanced when clear of debris, air bubbles, and bile. A popular technique for formal evaluation of cleansing during clinical investigation is to observe the images every 5 minutes (2-minute duration) and report the quality of the preparation analogously to the colon cleansing score on colonoscopy. For research purposes and patient quality measures, an ideal score should be easy to use, quick, and with excellent reproducibility.

A recent score has been suggested using the proportion of the visualized mucosal and the degree of bubbles, debris, and bile obscuring the mucosa in 1 frame every 5 minutes. The investigators compared it with the standard 2 minutes of assessment every 5 minutes. The concordance with the standard method, the interobserver agreement and intrapatient agreement were excellent ($\kappa = 0.82$, $\kappa = 0.8$, and $\kappa = 0.76$, respectively).[10]

After ingestion of the capsule device, the patient should monitor its passage. If the patient does not notice the passage of the capsule after 14 days or has symptoms of partial or complete SB obstruction, radiologic examination is recommended. Unpassed capsules can be retrieved endoscopically or surgically.

CAPSULE ENDOSCOPY FINDINGS ARE NONSPECIFIC

IBD is diagnosed by clinical, pathologic, radiologic and endoscopic means. There is no single test to diagnose CD or UC. Physicians rely on all the information obtained to being able to correctly diagnose a patient. Endoscopy allows for mucosal evaluation, and also permits tissue acquisition and performance of therapeutics, such as stricture dilation. Capsule endoscopy is able to provide image acquisition, but it cannot obtain biopsies or perform therapeutics.

The SB has limited ways to demonstrate injury: Mucosal disruption (erosions and ulcers), erythema, villous blunting, and strictures. These findings are easily captured by capsule endoscopy, but are not pathognomonic of IBD. Any type of injury can produce similar findings such as nonsteroidal anti-inflammatory drugs (NSAIDs), ischemia, and celiac disease, and these findings may be present in normal individuals.[11,12] Even as little as 2 weeks of standard dose NSAID use can cause SB injury in 75% of asymptomatic individuals.[12] Moreover, 20% of normal individuals may have mild mucosal abnormalities.[11]

One can then appreciate that capsule endoscopy findings are very nonspecific and should not be used solely to diagnose IBD. It is very important to exclude the use of NSAIDs, even in usually prescribed or over-the-counter doses.

SPECIFIC SITUATIONS
Suspected and Established CD

In the majority of patients with suspected CD, the diagnosis can be confirmed by colonoscopy with ileal intubation. In approximately 30%, the proximal SB may be the only affected area.[5]

A study examining the performance characteristics of different combinations of colonoscopy (with ileal intubation), CTE, capsule endoscopy, and SBFT found that colonoscopy with either CTE or SBFT was more accurate than capsule endoscopy with CTE, SBFT, or colonoscopy, secondary to the low specificity of capsule endoscopy.[13] This suggests that capsule endoscopy may be reserved for patients with strong clinical suspicion for CD with unremarkable colonoscopy and radiologic evaluations.[6,7] Conversely, capsule endoscopy has a high negative predictive value (96%–100%). In other words, an unremarkable capsule endoscopy evaluation virtually excludes SB CD.[14–16]

The findings on capsule endoscopy in CD are nonspecific and should be interpreted with caution. Studies define the primary endpoint as the "diagnostic yield" (number of examinations with abnormal findings divided by the number of total examinations), which should not be confused with sensitivity (the number of true-positive examinations divided by the number of true-positive and false-negative examinations), or specificity (the number of true-negative examinations divided by the number of true-negative and false-positive tests). A test with high diagnostic yield does not mean that it is a sensitive or specific test. Moreover, there is no standard definition of what constitutes CD on capsule endoscopy. The most common accepted definition for SB involvement in CD is the presence of 3 or more ulcerations.[14] This definition had a 50% positive predictive value for a diagnosis of CD.[15] The significance of minor mucosal changes is uncertain and caution should be applied not to overdiagnose CD and expose the patient to unnecessary risk from escalation of therapy.

There are 2 scoring systems to quantify the extent of small intestinal disease in CD. The Lewis Index uses 3 parameters: villous edema, ulceration, and stenosis (weight based on severity and extent).[17] The other system is called Capsule Endoscopy Crohn Disease Activity Index (CECDAI). It divides the SB into proximal and distal segments and uses different weights for 3 parameters: Inflammation, extent of disease, and stricture. The final score is the sum of the proximal and distal segmental numbers. It ranges from 0 (normal study) to 36 (severe disease). The agreement for the CECDAI score was excellent at 0.867.[18] External validation of these scores is awaited but the CECDAI appears easy to use and has a high degree of interobserver agreement.

It seems that capsule endoscopy is a better study to exclude SB involvement in CD rather than confirming it.

Capsule Endoscopy and Plain Abdominal Radiology

SBFT x-ray and enteroclysis remain available, but there has been a trend toward using more accurate diagnostic tests, such as CTE and MRE. Overall, capsule endoscopy has a higher mucosal diagnostic yield for patients with suspected or established CD compared with SBFT and enteroclysis, ranging from 49% to 93% versus 12% to 67%, respectively.[19–26] These studies have excluded patients with suspected or known SB strictures.

Meta-analyses evaluating the performance of CE versus SBFT/enteroclysis showed better performance of capsule endoscopy with an incremental yield (IY) of 32% favoring capsule endoscopy ($P<.0001$; 95% CI, 16%–48%).[27–29]

Capsule Endoscopy and MRE

Earlier studies with small numbers of patients with suspected and established CD suggested that capsule endoscopy and MRE had similar performance characteristics with good correlation between the 2 techniques. Capsule endoscopy detected slightly more mucosal disease and MRE identified more extraintestinal manifestations, such as strictures, fistulae, and abscesses.[30–32] A meta-analysis did not show a difference between the 2 studies.[29]

A prospective trial of 93 patients compared the diagnostic accuracy of capsule endoscopy, MRE, and CTE for terminal ileal disease in patients with suspected or established CD using ileocolonoscopy with biopsy as the gold standard. Sensitivity for capsule endoscopy, MRE, and CTE was 100% (95% CI, 79%–100%), 81% (95% CI, 58%–95%), and 76% (95% CI, 53%–92%), respectively; specificity of 91% (95% CI, 79%–97%), 86% (95% CI, 74%–94%), 85% (95% CI, 72%–93%), respectively. There was statistical difference in sensitivity compared with CTE, but only a trend compared with MRE and no statistical difference was seen in the specificity.[16]

Capsule Endoscopy and Computed Tomography Enterography

Computed tomography enterography is the most commonly used technique to investigate SB involvement in CD given its ease to use, reliability, and lower cost compared with MRE. It has the disadvantage of ionizing radiation exposure. Studies comparing CTE and capsule endoscopy showed a higher diagnostic yield of capsule endoscopy but no significant difference was seen.[13,33,34] However, the prospective study mentioned did show a higher sensitivity of capsule endoscopy versus CTE for terminal ileal involvement with CD (100% vs. 76%; $P = .3$), but no difference was found for specificity.[16]

A meta-analysis found that capsule endoscopy had a higher diagnostic yield than CTE in both suspected and established CD patients (IY, 47%; 95% CI, 31%–63% [$P<.00001$] and IY, 32%; 95% CI, 16%–47% [$P<.0001$]).[29]

Capsule Endoscopy and Other Endoscopic Techniques

There are several other endoscopic techniques to evaluate the SB mucosa: Push enteroscopy, intraoperative enteroscopy, balloon-assisted deep enteroscopy, and device-assisted deep enteroscopy. Capsule endoscopy is less invasive compared

---

Box 1
Indications for CE in CD

Monitor the extent and activity of established CD.

After negative ileocolonoscopy and SB radiologic evaluation with high clinical suspicion for CD.

Evaluation of postoperative recurrence of CD.

Investigation of IBDU.

Evaluation of iron-deficiency anemia or thrombocytosis in patients with inflammatory bowel disease and unremarkable endoscopic and radiologic tests.

Investigation of weight loss, biochemical or fecal markers of inflammation after inconclusive colonoscopy and radiologic procedures.

---

with the other techniques, but does not allow for tissue acquisition or for therapeutics to be performed.

The results of CE seem to be comparable to both push enteroscopy and balloon-assisted enteroscopy in the assessment of SB disease.[35,36] In the cases where an intervention is planned, such as stricture dilation or retrieval of a foreign body, capsule endoscopy findings are useful to suggest which route to take: Antegrade or retrograde.[37] Specifically for patients with suspected or established CD, capsule endoscopy has a higher diagnostic yield than push enteroscopy with enteroclysis and, in this study, led to a change of management in 70% of patients.[38]

IBDU

Formerly known as "indeterminate colitis," the term IBDU represents a colonic IBD, without SB involvement, for which a definite diagnosis of either CD or UC could not be made after ileocolonoscopy, biopsies, and SB radiology.[6] Indeterminate colitis is reserved for colectomy specimens where a diagnosis of CD or UC cannot be made. It is unclear at this time the role of capsule endoscopy in patients with IBDU. Studies have shown that, in patients with IBDU, the SB may show changes suggestive of CD in 16% to 39% of patients, but it resulted in no change in management in the majority of patients.[39-41] In patients with UC and IBDU undergoing colectomy, preoperative capsule endoscopy findings do not predict ileal–anal pouch outcomes, such as pouchitis or pouch dysfunction.[42]

UC

A diagnosis of UC does not involve the SB; thus, capsule endoscopy is generally not recommended. Some experts suggest that a SB evaluation should be considered, particularly in patients with severe refractory UC before colectomy.[6] This is supported by 1 study of patients with equivocal diagnosis of UC, including a patient with ileal–anal anastomosis, which showed that 61% had changes suggestive of CD.[14]

Potential Indications

The role of capsule endoscopy in the management of IBD is still unclear. Some potential indications for capsule endoscopy are shown in **Box 1**.

Complications

Overall, capsule endoscopy is tolerated very well. Some patients report abdominal discomfort and pain, which are usually transient. The main concern of using capsule endoscopy in IBD, particularly CD, is capsule retention, suggested by the nonvisualization of the cecum during the examination. Up to 25% of patients with CD may have stricturing or penetrating disease at presentation.[43] By performing a SB radiographic study, the risk of capsule retention may be minimized to approximately 1%.[44] It is important to inform patients that they have a small risk of capsule retention, even in the setting of a normal radiologic evaluation. A dissolvable patency capsule can be used to assess for significant strictures before capsule endoscopy, but it can also cause symptoms such as abdominal discomfort and retention.[45] Retention risk is higher (4%–6.7%)[14,46] in patients with established CD and approaches the risk in the general population in patients with suspected CD (approximately 1%). Persistent capsule retention (symptomatic patient or >14 days from ingestion) can be managed medically, endoscopically, or surgically.[47–50]

Because it is a metallic device, MRI testing should not be performed until capsule passage is ensured clinically or radiologically. A warning remains for performing capsule endoscopy in patients with cardiac pacemakers or other implanted electromedical devices. Recent data show no significant interaction between capsule endoscopy and pacemakers or implantable cardioversion devices.[51]

SUMMARY

Capsule endoscopy is a relatively new technology available in the investigation of IBD. Its place in the algorithm of evaluating IBD is being refined. Capsule endoscopy has the ability to visualize the entire SB with very few complications. It is a sensitive test for the diagnosis of mucosal changes, but should be viewed as complementary to other radiologic evaluations, such as CTE and MRE.

Capsule endoscopy is nonspecific and its findings have to be interpreted with caution and in the right clinical setting, because up to one fifth of normal individuals may have subtle changes in the small intestine. Care should also be taken to exclude NSAID use because it mimics findings seen in CD.

Capsule endoscopy is an exciting technology that opened the possibility of the evaluation of the SB in the era of "deep remission." It is best applied in patients with a high clinical suspicion for IBD after unremarkable colonoscopy with terminal ileal intubation and radiologic investigation.

REFERENCES

1. Stange EF, Travis SP, Vermeire S, et al. European evidence-based Consensus on the diagnosis and management of ulcerative colitis: definitions and diagnosis. J Crohns Colitis 2008;2:1–23.
2. Van Assche G, Dignass A, Panes J, et al. The second European evidence-based Consensus on the diagnosis and management of Crohn's disease: definitions and diagnosis. J Crohns Colitis 2010;4:7–27.
3. Dignass A, Van Assche G, Lindsay JO, et al. The second European evidence-based Consensus on the diagnosis and management of Crohn's disease: current management. J Crohns Colitis 2010;4:28–62.
4. Van Assche G, Dignass A, Reinisch W, et al. The second European evidence-based Consensus on the diagnosis and management of Crohn's disease: special situations. J Crohns Colitis 2010;4:63–101.
5. Farmer RG, Hawk WA, Turnbull RB Jr. Clinical patterns in Crohn's disease: a statistical study of 615 cases. Gastroenterology 1975;68:627–35.
6. Bourreille A, Ignjatovic A, Aabakken L, et al. Role of small-bowel endoscopy in the management of patients with inflammatory bowel disease: an international OMED-ECCO consensus. Endoscopy 2009;41:618–37.

7. Doherty GA, Moss AC, Cheifetz AS. Capsule endoscopy for small-bowel evaluation in Crohn's disease. Gastrointest Endosc 2011;74:167–75.
8. Landreneau SW, Black TP, Manolakis CS, et al. Does bowel cleansing enhance capsule endoscopy? Gastroenterology 2011;140:S-757.
9. Rokkas T, Papaxoinis K, Triantafyllou K, et al. Does purgative preparation influence the diagnostic yield of small bowel video capsule endoscopy? A meta-analysis. Am J Gastroenterol 2009;104:219–27.
10. Park SC, Keum B, Hyun JJ, et al. A novel cleansing score system for capsule endoscopy. World J Gastroenterol 2010;16:875–80.
11. Goldstein JL, Eisen GM, Lewis B, et al. Video capsule endoscopy to prospectively assess small bowel injury with celecoxib, naproxen plus omeprazole, and placebo. Clin Gastroenterol Hepatol 2005;3:133–41.
12. Maiden L, Thjodleifsson B, Theodors A, et al. A quantitative analysis of NSAID-induced small bowel pathology by capsule enteroscopy. Gastroenterology 2005;128:1172–8.
13. Solem CA, Loftus EV Jr, Fletcher JG, et al. Small-bowel imaging in Crohn's disease: a prospective, blinded, 4-way comparison trial. Gastrointest Endosc 2008;68:255–66.
14. Mow WS, Lo SK, Targan SR, et al. Initial experience with wireless capsule enteroscopy in the diagnosis and management of inflammatory bowel disease. Clin Gastroenterol Hepatol 2004;2:31–40.
15. Tukey M, Pleskow D, Legnani P, et al. The utility of capsule endoscopy in patients with suspected Crohn's disease. Am J Gastroenterol 2009;104:2734–9.
16. Jensen MD, Nathan T, Rafaelsen SR, et al. Diagnostic accuracy of capsule endoscopy for small bowel Crohn's disease is superior to that of MR enterography or CT enterography. Clin Gastroenterol Hepatol 2011;9:124–9.
17. Gralnek IM, Defranchis R, Seidman E, et al. Development of a capsule endoscopy scoring index for small bowel mucosal inflammatory change. Aliment Pharmacol Ther 2008;27:146–54.
18. Gal E, Geller A, Fraser G, et al. Assessment and validation of the new capsule endoscopy Crohn's disease activity index (CECDAI). Dig Dis Sci 2008;53:1933–7.
19. Buchman AL, Miller FH, Wallin A, et al. Videocapsule endoscopy versus barium contrast studies for the diagnosis of Crohn's disease recurrence involving the small intestine. Am J Gastroenterol 2004;99:2171–7.
20. Costamagna G, Shah SK, Riccioni ME, et al. A prospective trial comparing small bowel radiographs and video capsule endoscopy for suspected small bowel disease. Gastroenterology 2002;123:999–1005.
21. Dubcenco E, Jeejeebhoy KN, Petroniene R, et al. Capsule endoscopy findings in patients with established and suspected small-bowel Crohn's disease: correlation with radiologic, endoscopic, and histologic findings. Gastrointest Endosc 2005;62:538–44.
22. Efthymiou A, Viazis N, Vlachogiannakos J, et al. Wireless capsule endoscopy versus enteroclysis in the diagnosis of small-bowel Crohn's disease. Eur J Gastroenterol Hepatol 2009;21:866–71.
23. Eliakim R, Fischer D, Suissa A, et al. Wireless capsule video endoscopy is a superior diagnostic tool in comparison to barium follow-through and computerized tomography in patients with suspected Crohn's disease. Eur J Gastroenterol Hepatol 2003;15:363–7.
24. Eliakim R, Suissa A, Yassin K, et al. Wireless capsule video endoscopy compared to barium follow-through and computerised tomography in patients with suspected Crohn's disease: final report. Dig Liver Dis 2004;36:519–22.

25. Marmo R, Rotondano G, Piscopo R, et al. Capsule endoscopy versus enteroclysis in the detection of small-bowel involvement in Crohn's disease: a prospective trial. Clin Gastroenterol Hepatol 2005;3:772–6.

26. Park CH, Kim JO, Choi MG, et al. Utility of capsule endoscopy for the classification of Crohn's disease: a multicenter study in Korea. Dig Dis Sci 2007;52:1405–9.

27. Marmo R, Rotondano G, Piscopo R, et al. Meta-analysis: capsule enteroscopy vs. conventional modalities in diagnosis of small bowel diseases. Aliment Pharmacol Ther 2005;22:595–604.

28. Triester SL, Leighton JA, Leontiadis GI, et al. A meta-analysis of the yield of capsule endoscopy compared to other diagnostic modalities in patients with non-stricturing small bowel Crohn's disease. Am J Gastroenterol 2006;101:954–64.

29. Dionisio PM, Gurudu SR, Leighton JA, et al. Capsule endoscopy has a significantly higher diagnostic yield in patients with suspected and established small-bowel Crohn's disease: a meta-analysis. Am J Gastroenterol 2010;105:1240–8.

30. Crook DW, Knuesel PR, Froehlich JM, et al. Comparison of magnetic resonance enterography and video capsule endoscopy in evaluating small bowel disease. Eur J Gastroenterol Hepatol 2009;21:54–65.

31. Tillack C, Seiderer J, Brand S, et al. Correlation of magnetic resonance enteroclysis (MRE) and wireless capsule endoscopy (CE) in the diagnosis of small bowel lesions in Crohn's disease. Inflamm Bowel Dis 2008;14:1219–28.

32. Albert JG, Martiny F, Krummenerl A, et al. Diagnosis of small bowel Crohn's disease: a prospective comparison of capsule endoscopy with magnetic resonance imaging and fluoroscopic enteroclysis. Gut 2005;54:1721–7.

33. Hara AK, Leighton JA, Heigh RI, et al. Crohn disease of the small bowel: preliminary comparison among CT enterography, capsule endoscopy, small-bowel follow-through, and ileoscopy. Radiology 2006;238:128–34.

34. Hara AK, Leighton JA, Sharma VK, et al. Small bowel: preliminary comparison of capsule endoscopy with barium study and CT. Radiology 2004;230:260–5.

35. Pasha SF, Leighton JA, Das A, et al. Double-balloon enteroscopy and capsule endoscopy have comparable diagnostic yield in small-bowel disease: a meta-analysis. Clin Gastroenterol Hepatol 2008;6:671–6.

36. Sidhu R, McAlindon ME, Kapur K, et al. Push enteroscopy in the era of capsule endoscopy. J Clin Gastroenterol 2008;42:54–8.

37. Gay G, Delvaux M, Fassler I. Outcome of capsule endoscopy in determining indication and route for push-and-pull enteroscopy. Endoscopy 2006;38:49–58.

38. Chong AK, Taylor A, Miller A, et al. Capsule endoscopy vs. push enteroscopy and enteroclysis in suspected small-bowel Crohn's disease. Gastrointest Endosc 2005;61:255–61.

39. Lopes S, Figueiredo P, Portela F, et al. Capsule endoscopy in inflammatory bowel disease type unclassified and indeterminate colitis serologically negative. Inflamm Bowel Dis 2010;16:1663–8.

40. Maunoury V, Savoye G, Bourreille A, et al. Value of wireless capsule endoscopy in patients with indeterminate colitis (inflammatory bowel disease type unclassified). Inflamm Bowel Dis 2007;13:152–5.

41. Mehdizadeh S, Chen G, Enayati PJ, et al. Diagnostic yield of capsule endoscopy in ulcerative colitis and inflammatory bowel disease of unclassified type (IBDU). Endoscopy 2008;40:30–5.

42. Murrell Z, Vasiliauskas E, Melmed G, et al. Preoperative wireless capsule endoscopy does not predict outcome after ileal pouch-anal anastomosis. Dis Colon Rectum 2010;53:293–300.

43. Louis E, Collard A, Oger AF, et al. Behaviour of Crohn's disease according to the Vienna classification: changing pattern over the course of the disease. Gut 2001;49: 777–82.
44. Cave D, Legnani P, de Franchis R, et al. ICCE consensus for capsule retention. Endoscopy 2005;37:1065–7.
45. Signorelli C, Rondonotti E, Villa F, et al. Use of the Given Patency System for the screening of patients at high risk for capsule retention. Dig Liver Dis 2006;38:326–30.
46. Voderholzer WA, Beinhoelzl J, Rogalla P, et al. Small bowel involvement in Crohn's disease: a prospective comparison of wireless capsule endoscopy and computed tomography enteroclysis. Gut 2005;54:369–73.
47. Irkorucu O, Tascilar O, Emre AU, et al. Small-bowel obstruction secondary to wireless capsule enteroscopy: extraction of the capsule without enterotomy. Endoscopy 2007;39(Suppl 1):E286–7.
48. Tanaka S, Mitsui K, Shirakawa K, et al. Successful retrieval of video capsule endoscopy retained at ileal stenosis of Crohn's disease using double-balloon endoscopy. J Gastroenterol Hepatol 2006;21:922–3.
49. Bai Y, Gao J, Song B, et al. Surgical intervention for capsule endoscope retained at ileal stricture. Endoscopy 2007;39(Suppl 1):E268–9.
50. Van Weyenberg SJ, Van Turenhout ST, Bouma G, et al. Double-balloon endoscopy as the primary method for small-bowel video capsule endoscope retrieval. Gastrointest Endosc 2010;71:535–41.
51. Leighton JA, Srivathsan K, Carey EJ, et al. Safety of wireless capsule endoscopy in patients with implantable cardiac defibrillators. Am J Gastroenterol 2005;100: 1728–31.

Health Maintenance in the Inflammatory Bowel Disease Patient

Jennifer A. Sinclair, MD[a], Sharmeel K. Wasan, MD[a,b],
Francis A. Farraye, MD, MSc[a,b,]*

KEYWORDS

- Cervical cancer • Depression • Health maintenance
- Inflammatory bowel disease • Osteoporosis • Prevention
- Screening • Smoking • Vaccine

Recent data suggest that inflammatory bowel disease (IBD) patients do not receive preventive services with the same rigor as other medical patients,[1] partly because their gastroenterologist is often the main care provider for patients with IBD and visits to the primary care physician (PCP) are often infrequent. As the treating gastroenterologist, it is incumbent on us to take a proactive role in the health care needs of our IBD patients, recognizing that we are oftentimes fulfilling both specialty and primary care roles. Although it is crucial to clarify with the patient the limits of your responsibilities and delegate routine health care issues to the PCP, it is even more important to alert the PCP to the unique health maintenance needs of the IBD patient.

VACCINES

IBD patients treated with corticosteroids, immunomodulators, and biologic agents are at increased risk of developing infectious complications because of the immune suppression from these medications. There are multiple case reports of infections including fulminant hepatitis or fatal varicella,[2,3] and some of these diseases are vaccine preventable. Several studies have documented that IBD patients, like other patients on immunosuppressive medications, are inadequately vaccinated.[4] It seems that both primary care clinicians and gastroenterologists are hesitant to take ownership for vaccinating these patients.[5] In a survey study of 108 gastroenterologists, 83% thought that the primary care doctor was responsible for administering

The authors have nothing to disclose.
[a] Section of Gastroenterology, Boston Medical Center, 85 East Concord Street, 7th Floor, Boston, MA 02118, USA
[b] Boston University School of Medicine, Boston, MA, USA
* Corresponding author. Section of Gastroenterology, Boston Medical Center, 85 East Concord Street, 7th Floor, Boston, MA 02118.
E-mail address: francis.farraye@bmc.org

Gastroenterol Clin N Am 41 (2012) 325–337
doi:10.1016/j.gtc.2012.01.006
0889-8553/12/$ – see front matter © 2012 Elsevier Inc. All rights reserved.
gastro.theclinics.com

vaccines.[6] However, in a survey study of family care physicians, only 29% were comfortable making a recommendation for vaccinating their IBD patients.[5]

From a primary care perspective, the immune response to vaccination in IBD patients can be confusing; there remain questions about the appropriate immune response to vaccination in immunosuppressed patients. There are limited data on immune response to vaccines in IBD patients.[7] As such, many of the expert recommendations have been extrapolated from large studies of patients with other chronic immunologic diseases, such as multiple sclerosis, systemic lupus erythematosus, and rheumatoid arthritis.[8-11] Although there are 2 case reports of relapsed ulcerative colitis after influenza vaccine,[12,13] there are 2 larger, controlled studies in 60 and 575 patients evaluating the influenza vaccine in the IBD patient that have demonstrated safety without flare of their IBD.[14,15]

Several studies have demonstrated that IBD patients on a single immunosuppressive medication are able to achieve an adequate immune response. In a study of 36 patients who were receiving azathioprine or 6-mercaptopurine, responses to *Haemophilus influenzae* type B vaccine after 24 weeks of immunomodulator therapy were comparable with controls, suggesting that these patients were able to mount a normal immune response.[16] Similarly, in a study of 64 IBD patients, response to the pneumococcal vaccine was found to be comparable to controls in patients on 1 immunomodulator.[17] However, there seems to be a diminished response to vaccinations in patients on 2 immunosuppressant drugs. In a study of 29 healthy pediatric controls and 51 pediatric IBD patients (all on immunomodulators and/or anti-tumor necrosis factor agents [TNF]), patients on infliximab plus either 6-mercaptopurine, corticosteroids, or methotrexate were more likely to have inadequate response to vaccine: Titers achieved protective level at rate of 0.89 to 1.00 in control group versus 0.33 to 0.85 in IBD group.[18] More recently, in a study of 108 adults with IBD vaccinated with the H1N1 influenza vaccine, immunosuppressed subjects taking 6-mercaptopurine, corticosteroids, azathioprine, or biologic therapy had a lower rate of seroprotection than the nonimmunosuppressed (36% vs 64%).[19] The authors also noted that patients on combination immunosuppression had lower postvaccine titers than those on monotherapy. Similarly, studies in the transplant literature looking at serologic response after vaccination suggest that patients may have a diminished immune response as reflected by diminished antibody titers.[20,21] Although larger trials are required to better understand the immune response to vaccinations in IBD, data suggest that early vaccination before the need to escalate therapy to the use of 2 immunosuppressive agents is perhaps the best way to maximize the appropriate immune response to the various vaccines. In addition to further research on IBD-specific populations, additional studies are also needed to identify the sustainability of the immune response and determine whether subsequent booster doses are needed.

GOALS OF VACCINATION

IBD patients are at risk for the same preventable diseases as the general population, although they often present with more serious complications when on immunosuppressive therapy. Administration of live, attenuated vaccines to immunosuppressed patients is contraindicated, so the timing of vaccinations in IBD patients becomes paramount. The goal of vaccination for individuals with IBD is to utilize the opportune and sometimes short timeframe when their immune suppression is minimal, particularly if immunosuppressive agents are likely to be used in the future.

An expert panel convened by the Crohn and Colitis Foundation of America considered a patient immunosuppressed if they are on corticosteroids (prednisone

>20 mg/d dose equivalent) for 2 or more weeks, or are on treatment dose of 6-mercaptopurine/azathioprine, methotrexate, or biologic agents, and for the 3 months after stopping any of these therapies.[22] Patients with significant protein-calorie malnutrition are also considered immunosuppressed.[22] These patients should not receive live vaccines, most commonly measles, mumps, rubella (MMR), intranasal influenza, varicella, and the herpes zoster vaccines (HZV).

LIVE VACCINES

Administration of live, attenuated vaccines presents unique concerns when a patient is expected to be immunosuppressed in the future.

MMR

MMR is generally given to children. Adults with an unknown vaccine history should have titers checked. If a patient lacks immunity, the vaccine can be administered as long as there is no plan to start immunosuppressive therapy in the subsequent 6 weeks. It is important to note that MMR can be given safely to household contacts of immunosuppressed patients without fear of adverse effect or virus spread.[23]

Varicella

Varicella vaccine is recommended for immunocompetent children and adults with no prior history of varicella infection. For patients who may be candidates for immuno-suppression, a titer should be checked if immune status is unclear. There is no evidence-based data regarding how long to wait after administering the varicella vaccine before safely initiating immunosuppressive therapy. Based on data from the HZV, which contains at least a 10-fold greater titers than the varicella vaccine, waiting at least 4 weeks after varicella or zoster vaccination before initiating immunosuppres-sive therapy is suggested.[24] Like MMR, vaccination of household contacts of immunosuppressed individuals is not contraindicated for varicella. However, if the vaccinated family member develops a vaccine-related rash, the immunosuppressed patient should avoid contact with the affected individual. If a varicella-naive, immu-nocompromised patient is exposed to either a vaccine-related rash or to active varicella, prophylactic immunoglobulin is recommended only for the case of exposure to active varicella.

Varicella-Zoster Virus

Herpes zoster, also called shingles, results from reactivation of latent varicella-zoster virus within the dorsal root ganglia. The clinical course among immunocompetent patients is variable, ranging from a unilateral and painful vesicular rash, to debilitating post-herpetic neuralgia. In the general population, about 1 in 3 people develop zoster or a zoster-related diagnosis during their lifetime. The incidence of zoster is greater, and occurs earlier, in transplant patients, HIV-positive patients, and patients with chronic diseases requiring immunosuppression, such as rheumatoid arthritis, lupus, and IBD. In 1 retrospective study, the risk for zoster was greater in those with Crohn disease compared with ulcerative colitis, and in those receiving immunomodulators and corticosteroids compared with those on mesalazine.[25] The HZV licensed in the United States is a live, attenuated strain of varicella zoster virus, and the same strain used in varicella vaccines. Its minimum potency is 14 times the potency of the single antigen varicella vaccine. It is recommended for individuals age 50 years and older to prevent herpes zoster and/or reduce the severity of complications from zoster infection. In 2008, the US Centers for Disease Control (CDC) in conjunction with the

Advisory Committee on Immunization Practices (ACIP) recommended that patients on low doses of methotrexate (≤0.4 mg/kg/wk), azathioprine (≤3.0 mg/kg/d), or 6-mercaptopurine (≤1.5 mg/kg/d) for treatment of IBD are not considered sufficiently immunosuppressed to create vaccine safety concerns and should not be contraindications for administration of HZV. The CDC/ACIP workgroup recognized that persons with lower levels of immunosuppression are able to tolerate attenuated varicella-zoster virus–based vaccine such that varicella vaccine is recommended for HIV-infected children without prior immunity to varicella-zoster virus. The workgroup also recognized that even persons with a prior history of varicella (ie, the population for which the HZV would be recommended) are at little or no risk of second episodes of varicella, even when becoming profoundly immunosuppressed, because varicella-zoster virus-specific immunity is well-maintained in those patients. For these reasons, the HZV is recommended for persons taking low levels of immunosuppressive agents.[26]

As with the varicella vaccine, there is no clear data to determine the optimal interval between vaccination and initiation of immunosuppressive therapy. There is a risk of disseminated herpes zoster after initiating immunosuppressive therapy, so windows of 1 to 3 months have been suggested.[24,26,27] Household contacts can be immunized, but those who develop a vaccine-related rash should avoid contact with immunocompromised individuals.

INACTIVATED VACCINES

Inactivated vaccines are well tolerated by patient with IBD regardless of their degree of immunosuppression or immune competency. It is also safe for household contacts to receive inactivated vaccines. As noted, however, patients mount a diminished immune response when on dual therapy with an immunomodulator and a biologic agent; therefore, early vaccination remains important.

Influenza

Influenza is available in both a live, intranasal form and an inactivated, intramuscular form. Regardless of the type or number of immunosuppressive medications a patient is taking, it is important to immunize all IBD patients against influenza, because some have an adequate response to the vaccine, and even a partial response may provide some degree of protection. Although some patients may prefer the intranasal administration, it is important to note that the safety and effectiveness of a live, attenuated influenza vaccine has not been established in groups of patients who are at risk for more complications from influenza. IBD patients should therefore receive the intramuscular inactivated vaccine annually.[28]

Tetanus and Diphtheria

Tetanus and diphtheria is recommended every 10 years, with the tetanus, diphtheria, and acellular pertussis given at least once during this period. Any patient with an unclear vaccine history should receive the primary series of tetanus vaccines, which consists of 3 doses. After the initial series, all patients should receive the booster every 10 years. Two studies looking at immune response to the booster have found conflicting results in IBD patients—one suggested impaired humoral response to the booster in IBD,[29,30] whereas the other found normal antitetanus antibody levels. Despite this inconsistency, it is recommended to administer tetanus and diphtheria vaccine to the standard vaccine schedule in all IBD patients.

HPV

HPV is recommended for all females beginning at age 11 or 12 and extending to age 26 years old, including those with a history of genital warts, abnormal Papanicolaou test (Pap), or positive HPV DNA test.[31] In October 2011, the CDC's ACIP voted to expand recommendations to include vaccinating adolescent males age 11 to 12, with catch up doses for males aged 13 to 21 years in an effort to expand protection to more men and women, citing low rates of vaccination among women as the motivation for altering the original recommendations, and attempting to minimize any stigma associated with receiving the vaccine. The new recommendation, however, will not become official until voted on by the CDC and published in their *Morbidity and Mortality Weekly Report*.[32] Female patients with IBD on immunosuppressive agents are at increased risk of cervical dysplasia,[33,34] and as a result the administration of HPV vaccine should be a priority in this group.

Pneumococcal Vaccine

Pneumococcal vaccine is recommended for all IBD patients, regardless of age or immunosuppressive regimen. A 1-time revaccination is recommended after 5 years in patients ages 65 and older and in individuals on immunosuppressive agents. Although it is preferable to administer the vaccine before beginning immunomodulator and/or biologic therapy, even those patients already on immunosuppressants may have some degree of protection.[31]

Hepatitis B

Hepatitis B has been implicated in case reports of fatal liver failure after the initiation of biologic therapy.[35,36] As such, it is now recommended to check hepatitis B serology before starting anti-TNF therapy.[4] In patients who lack immunity, doses should be administered at 0, 2, and 4 to 6 months; postvaccine titers should be checked 1 month after the last dose to ensure an adequate response. Patients on immunosuppressive therapy may not achieve an adequate postvaccine titer, although younger patients seem to have a higher rate of response.[37] Subsequent studies have examined both readministration of the 3-vaccine series using twice the standard dose, or subsequent administration of the combined hepatitis A and B vaccine with similar results: Both seem to be effective in increasing postvaccine titers to adequate levels.[38]

Meningococcal Vaccine

Meningococcal vaccine is recommended for adults who are asplenic or have complement deficiencies, college students living in dormitories, military recruits, and individuals traveling to endemic areas for meningococcal disease. Because many IBD patients are young and otherwise healthy, it is important to remember to vaccinate for meningococcus if appropriate.

HEALTH MAINTENANCE: BEYOND VACCINES
Cervical Cancer Screening

There is a higher prevalence of abnormal Pap smears in women with IBD, and this is associated with treatment with immunomodulators.[33,34,39,40] In 1 study comparing 40 IBD patients who underwent routine cervical cancer screening with a total of 134 Pap smears, the incidence of abnormal Pap in a woman with IBD was 42.5% versus 7% among age-, race-, and parity-matched controls.[34] The authors also noted a significant increase in higher risk cervical cytology in the IBD group, and more abnormalities in Pap smears performed more than 6 months after exposure to an immunosuppressant (odds ratio [OR], 1.5; 95% confidence interval [CI], 1.2–4.1; $P =$ .021).[34] All abnormal tests were associated with either HPV serotype 16 or 18, so it is important to document a current Pap smear to assess for cervical cytology and HPV infection before, or soon after, initiating immunosuppressive therapy. The HPV vaccine is given in 3 doses over a 6-month period, and is indicated for prevention of disease caused by HPV types 16 and 18, which is associated with 70% of cervical cancers, as well as types 6 and, 11 which are associated with genital warts.[34] As above, women with IBD on immunosuppressive agents should be considered for the vaccine, and all women on immunomodulator therapy should undergo annual Pap testing as recommended by the American College of Obstetrics and Gynecology's guidelines.[34,41] In some situations, women with HPV and dysplasia may require discontinuation of their immunomodulators.[33]

Osteoporosis

IBD patients have an increased risk of developing osteoporosis and osteopenia.[42,43] In 1 study of 2035 IBD patients, bone density was performed in 317 patients with osteopenia identified in 48% and osteoporosis in 26%. Further studies have demonstrated that the typical incidence of osteoporosis in IBD has generally been in the range of 10% to 15%.[44,45] It is thought that low bone density in IBD is multifactorial, resulting from vitamin D malabsorption, glucocorticoid use, and the direct effects of systemic inflammation on bone.[44] General risk factors for osteopenia and osteoporosis include age over 60 years, family history, lifestyle and dietary habits, low body mass index, obstetric history, severity of intestinal inflammation, and use of corticosteroids, with the American Gastroenterological Association (AGA) guidelines noting age and glucocorticoid use as the strongest risk factors, so every effort should be made to limit exposure to corticosteroids.[44]

Universal testing of bone density is recommended with 1 or more of the following risk factors: age older than 60, low body mass index, smoking, postmenopausal women, steroid treatment for at least 3 months, repeated courses of steroids, and a history of fractures.[46] In 2003, both the AGA and the American College of Gastroenterology issued guidelines that recommended screening all IBD patients meeting 1 of 5 criteria: Postmenopausal state, ongoing corticosteroid treatment, cumulative prior use of corticosteroids exceeding 3 months, history of low-trauma fractures, and age over 60 years.[44,45,47]

The gold standard for assessing fracture risk is via dual x-ray absorptiometry (DEXA), and results of DEXA scan can be used to guide therapy. Osteopenia is defined as a T-score of -1 to -2.5 on DEXA, and osteoporosis is a T-score below -2.5.

For patients with a T score above -1, recommendations are preventative, and should include calcium and vitamin D supplementation, exercise, smoking cessation, limiting alcohol use, and minimizing corticosteroid use. Patients with osteopenia should also implement these measures, and consider repeat the DEXA in 2 years.[47] Bisphosphonates are recommended for known osteoporosis (T-score < -2.5), history of atraumatic fracture, or failure to withdraw from corticosteroids after 3 months.[47] Finally, if an IBD patient is found to be osteoporotic or sustains a low-trauma fracture, screening for secondary causes of low bone density, such as celiac disease, hypogonadism, and vitamin D deficiency, should be performed.[47]

Colorectal Cancer Screening

Patients with long-standing ulcerative colitis are at an increased risk for developing dysplasia and colorectal carcinoma.[48-52] According to AGA guidelines, all patients, regardless of extent of disease, should undergo a screening colonoscopy a maximum of 8 years after onset of symptoms, with biopsies taken throughout the entire colon to assess the microscopic extent of inflammation. Patients with ulcerative proctitis or proctosigmoiditis are not at increased for IBD-related cancer, and thus may be screened according to average risk recommendations. Patients with extensive or left-sided colitis should begin surveillance 1 to 2 years after initial screening colonoscopy. Crohn disease patients with colitis involving at least one third of the colon should also have these surveillance guidelines applied.

The optimal surveillance intervals have not been clearly defined. After 2 examinations without evidence of dysplasia or cancer, surveillance intervals can be extended to every 1 to 3 years. Although there has been concern that after 20 years of disease, the risk of colorectal cancer increases and perhaps surveillance intervals should be reduced again to every 1 to 2 years, recent data actually suggest that this is not necessary.[48,49] Surveillance intervals can be continued at 1 to 3 years, but should be determined on an individual basis depending on an individual's risk factors. Factors that should prompt more frequent examinations include first-degree relatives with colorectal cancer, ongoing inflammation (either endoscopically or histologically), and anatomic abnormalities such as foreshortened colon, strictures, or multiple inflammatory pseudopolyps.[48,49] Patients with primary sclerosing cholangitis are at increased risk for developing colorectal cancer, and should undergo surveillance at the time of diagnosis and annually thereafter.[48,49]

With respect to obtaining surveillance biopsies throughout the colon, there are no prospective studies looking at the optimal number of specimens to obtain. One study has recommended a minimum of 33 biopsies be taken in patients with pancolitis.[53] Chromoendoscopy has been shown to have higher sensitivity for detecting dysplasia than traditional white light endoscopy, so an alternative to 33 random biopsies is for targeted biopsies to be performed by endoscopists skilled in this technique.[49,52] In general, it is ideal to perform surveillance while disease is in remission; however, surveillance should not be put off if the disease continues to be active.

The British Society of Gastroenterology (BSG) guidelines are similar, but warrant discussion because they address several additional points.[52] The BSG guidelines recommend screening beginning at 10 years after onset of colonic symptoms. Surveillance is then recommended in either 1-, 3-, or 5-year intervals, depending on extent of disease and individual risk factors (primary sclerosing cholangitis or family history prompts more frequent screening). British guidelines favor chromoendoscopy with targeted biopsies, but if this technique is unavailable random biopsies throughout the colon are reasonable. Finally, like the American guidelines, the BSG recommends that if a dysplastic polyp is detected within an area of inflammation and can be removed entirely, it is not necessary to recommend colectomy.

Skin Cancer Screening

Nonmelanoma skin cancers (NMSC) are among the most common malignancies in the United States, and include both squamous cell and basal cell carcinoma.[54] Previous data suggested that there are over 1,000,000 new cases of NMSC per year, although new data estimate as many as 3.5 million cases per year. There is an increased incidence of NMSC in patients after solid organ transplantation on immunosuppressive agents. Several epidemiologic studies have documented an increase in NMSC cases in IBD patients.[55,56] In 1 study from the United States,[56] persistent use of thiopurines (>365 days) was associated with an increased risk of NMSC (OR, 4.27; 95% CI, 3.08–5.92). In patients on anti-TNF agents, the OR was 2.18 (95% CI, 1.07–4.46). The combined use of thiopurines and anti-TNF agents was associated with an even higher risk (OR, 6.75; 95% CI, 2.74–16.65).

There are no specific IBD guidelines for prevention of NMSC, but IBD patients should follow recommendations for the general population, which include sun protection strategies. It should be noted that the United States Preventative Services Task Force (USPSTF) concluded that there was insufficient evidence to recommend universal screening for skin cancer by primary care clinicians or self-examination.[57] Although there are no IBD guidelines for the secondary prevention of skin cancer by performing annual skin examinations, the case can be made that IBD patients on immunomodulators or biologics warrant regular (annual) examinations.

Smoking Cessation

All IBD patients should be encouraged to stop smoking.[58] Smoking cessation is a crucial aspect in the management of Crohn patients that is often overlooked. Individuals who smoke have an increased prevalence of Crohn disease. Crohn disease patients who are smokers have more severe ileal disease, more frequent flares, and an increased need for steroids and immunomodulators, as well as higher rates of surgery. Smoking cessation is associated with a decreased risk of relapses and decreased need for steroids and immunomodulators. The negative effects of smoking are dose dependent, so even a partial decrease in the number of cigarettes smoked daily is beneficial in improving the course of Crohn disease.

Depression Screening

Depression is a common problem that may affect as many as 15% to 35% of individuals with IBD.[59,60] In 1 population-based study, the lifetime risk for major depressive disorder was more than twice as high in the IBD cohort, occurring in more than one quarter of those with IBD.[61] Predisposing factors for the development of depression include the chronic relapsing nature of the disease, as well as some of the medications used as treatment. The American College of Preventive Medicine (ACPM) and the USPSTF recommend screening in all clinical practices that have systems in place to assure accurate diagnosis, effective treatment, and follow-up of depression.[62] The ACPM also cites several studies that have concluded effective screening can be performed with just 2 brief questions[62]:

1. Over the past month, have you felt down, depressed, or hopeless?
2. Over the past month, have you felt little interest or pleasure in doing things?

Although most gastroenterology practices are not equipped for treatment of depression, it is important to recognize the increased risk of depression in IBD patients, screen appropriately, and to refer to mental health or primary care where more definitive diagnosis and treatment can be pursued. Depression is a treatable illness with psychological counseling and/or antidepressant medications.

SUMMARY

Gastroenterologists are in a unique position to make very positive differences in the lives of their IBD patients. We understand that IBD patients do not receive preventive services at the same rate as general medical patients. Because these individuals are at increased risk for complications from preventable diseases, we have a valuable opportunity to protect this population (**Table 1**). Establishing a close working relationship with PCPs can facilitate delivering quality care, but it is important to note that some of these patients rely solely on their GI clinician for the majority of their care. In such a vulnerable population, it is important to be aggressive with vaccine recommendations, monitoring for depression, tobacco cessation, and in

Table 1
Health maintenance by visit

	Check Titers Before Vaccinating	Plan to Administer Regardless of Immunosuppression Status	Administer Only if no Plans to Administer Immunosuppressive Therapy in the Next 4–12 Weeks	Review Screening
Initial visit	Hepatitis A	Tdap	MMR[a]	Cervical cancer
	Hepatitis B	HPV[c]	Varicella[b]	Skin cancer
	MMR[a]	Influenza[d]	Zoster[c]	Colorectal cancer
	Varicella[b]	Pneumococcus		Depression screen
		Hepatitis A		Tobacco cessation
		Hepatitis B		Bone health
		Meningococcus		

	Review Vaccine Status and Update	Vaccinate Only if no Plans to Administer Immunosuppressive Therapy in the Next 4–12 Weeks	Review Screening
Follow-up visits	Td	MMR[a]	Cervical cancer
	HPV[c]	Varicella[b]	Skin cancer
	Influenza[d]	Zoster[c]	Colorectal cancer
	Pneumococcus		Depression screen
	Hepatitis A		Tobacco cessation
	Hepatitis B		Bone Health
	Meningococcus[c]		

Abbreviations: HPV, human papillomavirus; MMR, measles, mumps, rubella; Td/Tdap, tetanus diphtheria, pertussis.

[a] If no history of vaccination against MMR.
[b] If no history of chicken pox or vaccination against varicella.
[c] If applicable based on patient demographics.
[d] Intramuscular inactive vaccine should be administered if immunosuppressed.

performing the appropriate cancer screening examinations. As professional societies and health care system increase their focus on quality measures,[63] incorporating these important issues into routine practice will ultimately result in addressing quality standards; perhaps more important, it should provide our patients with the best individual care possible.

REFERENCES

1. Selby L, Kane S, Wilson J, et al. Receipt of preventive health services by IBD patients is significantly lower than by primary care patients. Inflamm Bowel Dis 2008;14: 253–8.
2. Keene JK, Lowe DK, Grosfeld JL, et al. Disseminated varicella complicating ulcerative colitis. JAMA 1978;239:45–6.
3. Domm S, Cinatl J, Mrowietz U. The impact of treatment with tumour necrosis factor-alpha antagonists on the course of chronic viral infections: a review of the literature. Br J Dermatol 2008;159:1217–28.
4. Melmed GY, Ippoliti AF, Papadakis KA, et al. Patients with inflammatory bowel disease are at risk for vaccine-preventable illnesses. Am J Gastroenterol 2006;101:1834–40.
5. Selby L, Hoellein A, Wilson JF. Are primary care providers uncomfortable providing routine preventive care for inflammatory bowel disease patients? Dig Dis Sci 56:819-24.
6. Wasan SK, Coukos JA, Farraye FA. Vaccinating the inflammatory bowel disease patient: deficiencies in gastroenterologists knowledge. Inflamm Bowel Dis 2011;17: 2536–40.
7. Wasan SK, Baker SE, Skolnik PR, et al. A practical guide to vaccinating the inflammatory bowel disease patient. Am J Gastroenterol 105:1231–8.
8. Del Porto F, Lagana B, Biselli R, et al. Influenza vaccine administration in patients with systemic lupus erythematosus and rheumatoid arthritis. Safety and immunogenicity. Vaccine 2006;24:3217–23.
9. Fomin I, Caspi D, Levy V, et al. Vaccination against influenza in rheumatoid arthritis: the effect of disease modifying drugs, including TNF alpha blockers. Ann Rheum Dis 2006;65:191–4.
10. Kaine JL, Kivitz AJ, Birbara C, et al. Immune responses following administration of influenza and pneumococcal vaccines to patients with rheumatoid arthritis receiving adalimumab. J Rheumatol 2007;34:272–9.
11. Chalmers A, Scheifele D, Patterson C, et al. Immunization of patients with rheumatoid arthritis against influenza: a study of vaccine safety and immunogenicity. J Rheumatol 1994;21:1203–6.
12. Kwon OS, Park YS, Choi JH, et al. [A case of ulcerative colitis relapsed by influenza vaccination]. Korean J Gastroenterol 2007;49:327–30.
13. Fields SW, Baiocco PJ, Korelitz BI. Influenza vaccinations: should they really be encouraged for IBD patients being treated with immunosuppressives? Inflamm Bowel Dis 2009;15:649–51.
14. Debruyn JC, Hilsden R, Fonseca K, et al. Immunogenicity and safety of influenza vaccination in children with inflammatory bowel disease. Inflamm Bowel Dis 2012;18: 25–33.
15. Rahier JF, Papay P, Salleron J, et al. H1N1 vaccines in a large observational cohort of patients with inflammatory bowel disease treated with immunomodulators and biological therapy. Gut 2011;60:456–62.
16. Dotan I, Vigodman S, Malter L, et al. Azathioprine (AZA)/6-mercaptopurine (6MP) therapy has NO significant effect on cellular or humoral immune responses in patients with inflammatory bowel disease. Gastroenterology 2007;132:A51.

17. Melmed GY, Agarwal N, Frenck RW, et al. Immunosuppression impairs response to pneumococcal polysaccharide vaccination in patients with inflammatory bowel disease. Am J Gastroenterol 105:148-54.
18. Mamula P, Markowitz JE, Piccoli DA, et al. Immune response to influenza vaccine in pediatric patients with inflammatory bowel disease. Clin Gastroenterol Hepatol 2007; 5:851–6.
19. Cullen G, Bader C, Korzenik JR, et al. Serological response to the 2009 H1N1 influenza vaccination in patients with inflammatory bowel disease. Gut 2011. [Epub ahead of print].
20. Donati M, Zuckerman M, Dhawan A, et al. Response to varicella immunization in pediatric liver transplant recipients. Transplantation 2000;70:1401–4.
21. Giebink GS, Warkentin PI, Ramsay NK, et al. Titers of antibody to pneumococci in allogeneic bone marrow transplant recipients before and after vaccination with pneumococcal vaccine. J Infect Dis 1986;154:590–6.
22. Sands BE, Cuffari C, Katz J, et al. Guidelines for immunizations in patients with inflammatory bowel disease. Inflamm Bowel Dis 2004;10:677–92.
23. Watson JC, Hadler SC, Dykewicz CA, et al. Measles, mumps, and rubella: vaccine use and strategies for elimination of measles, rubella, and congenital rubella syndrome and control of mumps: recommendations of the Advisory Committee on Immunization Practices (ACIP). MMWR Recomm Rep 1998;47:1–57.
24. Kotton CN. Nailing down the shingles in IBD. Inflamm Bowel Dis 2007;13:1178–9.
25. Gupta G, Lautenbach E, Lewis JD. Incidence and risk factors for herpes zoster among patients with inflammatory bowel disease. Clin Gastroenterol Hepatol 2006;4:1483–90.
26. Harpaz R, Ortega-Sanchez IR, Seward JF. Prevention of herpes zoster: recommendations of the Advisory Committee on Immunization Practices (ACIP). MMWR Recomm Rep 2008;57:1–30.
27. Singh A, Englund K. Q: who should receive the shingles vaccine? Cleve Clin J Med 2009;76:45–8.
28. Fiore AE, Uyeki TM, Broder K, et al. Prevention and control of influenza with vaccines: recommendations of the Advisory Committee on Immunization Practices (ACIP), 2010. MMWR Recomm Rep 59:1–62.
29. Nielsen HJ, Mortensen T, Holten-Andersen M, et al. Increased levels of specific leukocyte- and platelet-derived substances during normal anti-tetanus antibody synthesis in patients with inactive Crohn disease. Scand J Gastroenterol 2001;36: 265–9.
30. Brogan MD, Shanahan F, Oliver M, et al. Defective memory B cell formation in patients with inflammatory bowel disease following tetanus toxoid booster immunization. J Clin Lab Immunol 1987;24:69–74.
31. Recommended adult immunization schedule: United States, 2009*. Ann Intern Med 2009;150:40–4.
32. Mitchell D. ACIP Expands HPV vaccine recommendation to adolescent boys. 2011 [updated 2011]. Available at: http://www.aafp.org/online/en/home/publications/news/news-now/health-of-the-public/20111026acip-hpv-hepb.html. Accessed November 3, 2011.
33. Kane S. Abnormal Pap smears in inflammatory bowel disease. Inflamm Bowel Dis 2008;14:1158–60.
34. Kane S, Khatibi B, Reddy D. Higher incidence of abnormal Pap smears in women with inflammatory bowel disease. Am J Gastroenterol 2008;103:631–6.

35. Esteve M, Saro C, Gonzalez-Huix F, et al. Chronic hepatitis B reactivation following infliximab therapy in Crohn's disease patients: need for primary prophylaxis. Gut 2004;53:1363–5.
36. Montiel PM, Solis JA, Chirinos JA, et al. Hepatitis B virus reactivation during therapy with etanercept in an HBsAg-negative and anti-HBs-positive patient. Liver Int 2008; 28:718–20.
37. Vida Perez L, Gomez Camacho F, Garcia Sanchez V, et al. [Adequate rate of response to hepatitis B virus vaccination in patients with inflammatory bowel disease]. Med Clin (Barc) 2009;132:331–5.
38. Cardell K, Akerlind B, Sallberg M, et al. Excellent response rate to a double dose of the combined hepatitis A and B vaccine in previous nonresponders to hepatitis B vaccine. J Infect Dis 2008;198:299–304.
39. Lees CW, Critchley J, Chee N, et al. Lack of association between cervical dysplasia and IBD: a large case-control study. Inflamm Bowel Dis 2009;15:1621–9.
40. Singh H, Demers AA, Nugent Z, et al. Risk of cervical abnormalities in women with inflammatory bowel disease: a population-based nested case-control study. Gastroenterology 2009;136:451–8.
41. ACOG Practice Bulletin no. 109: Cervical cytology screening. Obstet Gynecol 2009; 114:1409–20.
42. Bernstein CN, Leslie WD, Leboff MS. AGA technical review on osteoporosis in gastrointestinal diseases. Gastroenterology 2003;124:795–841.
43. Lichtenstein GR, Sands BE, Pazianas M. Prevention and treatment of osteoporosis in inflammatory bowel disease. Inflamm Bowel Dis 2006;12:797–813.
44. Etzel JP, Larson MF, Anawalt BD, et al. Assessment and management of low bone density in inflammatory bowel disease and performance of professional society guidelines. Inflamm Bowel Dis 17:2122–9.
45. Kornbluth A, Hayes M, Feldman S, et al. Do guidelines matter? Implementation of the ACG and AGA osteoporosis screening guidelines in inflammatory bowel disease (IBD) patients who meet the guidelines' criteria. Am J Gastroenterol 2006;101:1546–50.
46. Raisz LG. Clinical practice. Screening for osteoporosis. N Engl J Med 2005;353: 164–71.
47. American Gastroenterological Association medical position statement: guidelines on osteoporosis in gastrointestinal diseases. Gastroenterology 2003;124:791–4.
48. Farraye FA, Odze RD, Eaden J, et al. AGA technical review on the diagnosis and management of colorectal neoplasia in inflammatory bowel disease. Gastroenterology 138:746–74.
49. Farraye FA, Odze RD, Eaden J, et al. AGA medical position statement on the diagnosis and management of colorectal neoplasia in inflammatory bowel disease. Gastroenterology 138:738–45.
50. Kornbluth A, Sachar DB. Ulcerative colitis practice guidelines in adults: American College of Gastroenterology, Practice Parameters Committee. Am J Gastroenterol 105:501–23.
51. Ullman T, Odze R, Farraye FA. Diagnosis and management of dysplasia in patients with ulcerative colitis and Crohn's disease of the colon. Inflamm Bowel Dis 2009;15: 630–8.
52. Cairns SR, Scholefield JH, Steele RJ, et al. Guidelines for colorectal cancer screening and surveillance in moderate and high risk groups (update from 2002). Gut 59:666–89.
53. Rubin CE, Haggitt RC, Burmer GC, et al. DNA aneuploidy in colonic biopsies predicts future development of dysplasia in ulcerative colitis. Gastroenterology 1992;103: 1611–20.

54. Long MD, Kappelman MD, Pipkin CA. Nonmelanoma skin cancer in inflammatory bowel disease: a review. Inflamm Bowel Dis 17:1423–7.
55. Long MD, Herfarth HH, Pipkin CA, et al. Increased risk for non-melanoma skin cancer in patients with inflammatory bowel disease. Clin Gastroenterol Hepatol 8:268–74.
56. Peyrin-Biroulet L, Khosrotehrani K, Carrat F, et al. Increased risk for nonmelanoma skin cancers in patients who receive thiopurines for inflammatory bowel disease. Gastroenterology 2011;141:162128.e1–28.e5.
57. Screening for skin cancer: U.S. Preventive Services Task Force recommendation statement. Ann Intern Med 2009;150:188–93.
58. Cosnes J. What is the link between the use of tobacco and IBD? Inflamm Bowel Dis 2008;14(Suppl 2):S14–5.
59. Graff LA, Walker JR, Bernstein CN. Depression and anxiety in inflammatory bowel disease: a review of comorbidity and management. Inflamm Bowel Dis 2009;15:1105–18.
60. Graff LA, Walker JR, Clara I, et al. Stress coping, distress, and health perceptions in inflammatory bowel disease and community controls. Am J Gastroenterol 2009;104:2959–69.
61. Walker JR, Ediger JP, Graff LA, et al. The Manitoba IBD cohort study: a population-based study of the prevalence of lifetime and 12-month anxiety and mood disorders. Am J Gastroenterol 2008;103:1989–97.
62. Nimalasuriya K, Compton MT, Guillory VJ. Screening adults for depression in primary care: A position statement of the American College of Preventive Medicine. J Fam Pract 2009;58:535–8.
63. Kappelman MD, Palmer L, Boyle BM, et al. Quality of care in inflammatory bowel disease: a review and discussion. Inflamm Bowel Dis 16:125–33.

Detecting and Treating *Clostridium Difficile* Infections in Patients with Inflammatory Bowel Disease

Ashwin N. Ananthakrishnan, MD, MPH

KEYWORDS

- Inflammatory bowel disease • *Clostridium difficile*
- Crohn disease • Ulcerative colitis

Clostridium difficile is a Gram-positive anaerobe described as early as 1935 as being a member of the intestinal flora in neonates.[1] It was not until 1978 that it was first described in association with antibiotic-associated pseudomembranous colitis (PMC).[2] *C difficile* infection (CDI) is now the predominant cause of PMC and an important cause of health care–associated diarrhea. The last 2 decades have witnessed several shifts in its epidemiology. In addition to the nearly worldwide increase in its incidence, it has been increasingly recognized as an important cause of diarrhea in the community setting in individuals not previously considered at high risk, including in children, adults with no recent antibiotic or health care exposure, pregnant women, and, more recently, individuals with underlying inflammatory bowel diseases (IBD).[3–8] The similarity in clinical presentation between CDI and an IBD flare but divergent treatment paradigms with directed antibiotic therapy in the case of CDI and escalation of immunosuppression in an IBD flare makes it important for the treating clinician to have a high index of suspicion for CDI in patients with IBD. This review attempts to summarize the changes in CDI epidemiology over the last 2 decades, its growing impact on patients with IBD, diagnostic algorithms, and treatment modalities.

BURDEN OF *C DIFFICILE* INFECTION

There has been a dramatic increase in the occurrence of CDI among hospitals in the United States with a doubling of incidence from 31 in 100,000 population in 1996 to

The author has no relevant financial disclosures or conflicts of interest.
Massachusetts General Hospital, Harvard Medical School, 165 Cambridge Street, 9th Floor, Boston, MA 02114, USA
E-mail address: aananthakrishnan@partners.org

Gastroenterol Clin N Am 41 (2012) 339–353
doi:10.1016/j.gtc.2012.01.003
0889-8553/12/$ – see front matter © 2012 Elsevier Inc. All rights reserved.

61 in 100,000 population in 2003. There were an estimated 348,950 hospitalizations in 2008.[9,10] Studies from other regions such as Quebec, reveal an even steeper increase, with the incidence reaching 156 in 100,000 population in 2003.[11] During the same period, the proportion of patients with severe or complicated CDI also doubled from 7% to 18% with a corresponding increase in mortality.[11] The prevalence of community-acquired CDI (CA-CDI) remains lower than that in hospital-based studies but still significant at 7 to 46 cases per 100,000 population.[12,13] Data from the United Kingdom mandatory reporting and surveillance showed a reduction in CDI incidence by 54% between 2007 and 2010; such a decrease has not yet been shown in the other cohorts.[14]

Paralleling the increase in the non-IBD population, there has been a similar increase in CDI among patients with IBD.[4,15–18] In a study utilizing a national hospitalization database, Ananthakrishnan and coworkers[4] found an increase in the rate of CDI among patients hospitalized with ulcerative colitis (UC) from 24 in 1000 to 39 in 1000 with a significant but less steep increase among patients with Crohn disease (CD; 8 in 1000 to 12 in 1000) from 1998 to 2004.[4] Data from 2007 show that the incidence has continued to increase.[15] An earlier study by Rodemann and colleagues[18] found a similar rate of increase at their tertiary referral center between 1998 and 2004. Specifically, among patients presenting with a disease flare, early reports suggested between 5% and 18% of patients may have superimposed CDI[19–22]; more recent reports have identified rates as high as 47% among adults[23] and 25% to 60% among children.[24 25]

PATHOGENESIS AND VARIANT STRAINS OF *C DIFFICILE*

C difficile is a spore-forming anaerobe that exerts its effect through the formation of toxins, the 2 key toxins being toxins A and B, encoded by the genes *tcdA* and *tcdB,* respectively.[26,27] These cytotoxins act by causing glycosylation of the *rho* and *ras* proteins essential for maintaining cytoskeletal integrity.[26,28] The resultant disruption of the tight junctions leads to loss of epithelial integrity and the consequent watery diarrhea associated with CDI. Initial research suggested toxin A to be the key toxin, and, indeed, early-generation enzyme-linked immunosorbent assay tests for diagnosis of CDI detected toxin A alone. Subsequent human and animal data suggest that toxin B was the dominant toxin[27]; strains that produced toxin A alone but not toxin B were not pathogenic in animal models of CDI. Approximately 10% to 15% of human CDI may be caused by *C difficile* strains producing toxin B alone.[29] A third toxin, the binary toxin, encoded at a distinct locus, has been associated with an increased production of toxins A and B.[27,30] Scanning electron microscopy studies suggest that this binary toxin may be more pathogenic by facilitating adhesion of the clostridia to the intestinal epithelium by enabling actin polymerization and redistribution of microtubules.[31]

Several variant strains of *C difficile* have been described, some of them "hypervirulent" with an association with severe disease. The most prominent of such strains is the BI/NAP1/027 strain that was first identified to be responsible for an epidemic of CDI in Quebec, Canada.[32] This strain has been identified subsequently in several other countries and in association with other regional outbreaks, some of them leading to fatality.[33–35] The BI/NAP1/027 strain produces binary toxin and may have greater adherence to intestinal epithelium. The exact prevalence of this strain in the IBD population is not known, but estimates from other countries have attributed between 25% to 50% of all CDI to this strain, including a majority of the hospital isolates,[33,36] although others have arrived at a lower estimate.[37] A similar prevalence can be estimated to occur in patients with IBD.[38] A second variant strain, the ribotype 078 strain, was initially identified in the

Netherlands and has been associated with severe disease. This strain may be responsible for 8% to 10% of all hospital-acquired CDI.[37,39]

RISK FACTORS FOR CDI
General Risk Factors

Broad-spectrum antibiotic use and health care contact are well recognized as key risk factors for CDI. Historically, as many as 65% to 95% of patients with CDI reported recent use of antibiotics.[40-43] The spectrum of agents associated with CDI spans all antibiotic classes with the risk being greater for broad-spectrum antibiotics and those that lead to greater disruption of the intestinal flora. Clindamycin, cephalosporins, and fluoroquinolones are associated with the greatest excess risk for CDI. Given their widespread use, up to one-third of CDI may be attributable to fluoroquinolone use with a small proportion being attributable to cephalosporins (10%) and clindamycin.[44] The emergence of the BI/NAP/027 appears to be, in part, selected by wide spread use of fluoroquinolones, as the strain is resistant to this class of antibiotics.[44]

Antibiotic use and health care contact are less common risk factors in patients with IBD with between 40% and 60% of IBD patients not reporting recent use of antibiotics.[38,45] Although the majority of CDI-IBD cases have been nosocomially acquired,[46] a sizeable minority of patients acquire CDI outside the health care setting.[18] Thus, lack of traditional risk factors should not preclude considering CDI in the differential diagnosis of patients presenting with an IBD flare. Both age and comorbidity increase risk of CDI.[16] Proton-pump inhibitor use or gastric acid suppression has been variably reported as a risk factor for CDI in non-IBD cohorts[47] but appears to be uncommon in patients with IBD.[24,38,48]

In addition to these extrinsic factors, host immune response plays a key role in CDI pathogenesis. Individuals who are able to mount a strong antitoxin antibody response are more likely to remain asymptomatic or colonized with *C difficile*, whereas those with lower levels of antitoxin antibody are more likely to develop symptomatic disease.[27,49]

IBD-Specific Risk Factors

Several IBD-specific factors increase the risk for CDI, the most important being immunosuppression. Maintenance immunosuppression confers a 2-fold increase in the risk for CDI[17] (odds ratio [OR], 2.58; 95% confidence interval [CI], 1.28–5.12).[17,38] Colonic disease is also a risk factor for CDI (OR, 3.12; 95% CI, 1.28–5.12) with several studies reporting higher rates of CDI in those with UC compared with those with CD.[4, 6,17,50] Severity and extent of colonic inflammation may also modulate CDI risk with a greater risk of CDI in patients with pancolitis compared with those with limited distal disease.[24,50]

CLINICAL FEATURES

The clinical symptoms associated with CDI are often indistinguishable from an IBD flare and include diarrhea, sometimes watery, with or without the presence of overt bleeding. There may be associated abdominal pain, cramping, or tenesmus. Physical examination may find abdominal tenderness; rebound or guarding is a sign of severe colitis. Fever and leukocytosis are seen with both CDI and an IBD flare. Markers of severe CDI include renal dysfunction, markedly elevated white blood cell count, or an increased serum lactate level.[51-53] Diarrhea may not be universally seen in severe disease, as 20% of patients may have concomitant ileus.[51] Radiologic evaluation is useful to establish ileus and also aids in the diagnosis of toxic megacolon in patients with severe disease. Although a plain x-ray may suffice in many patients, a computed tomography scan is more sensitive for early disease. None of these features are specific for *C difficile* and may not aid in differentiating CDI from an IBD flare. However, patients with previously known limited or distal colonic disease now showing pancolonic thickening should raise suspicion for superimposed CDI. The classic colonoscopic appearance of CDI is the pseudomembrane, which histologically comprises exudates and debris on a base of mucosal denudation ("volcano" lesion).[54,55] However, this finding has been found uncommonly in patients with underlying IBD.[17,38,56] In a multicenter study of hospitalized CDI-IBD patients, Ben-Horin and colleagues[56] identified pseudomembranes in 12 of 93 patients (13%) who underwent a lower endoscopy; the only factor independently associated with pseudomembranes was the presence of fever. Nevertheless, in patients who do not yield a positive diagnosis using noninvasive stool testing, a limited sigmoidoscopy allows to (1) evaluate for the presence or absence of pseudomembranes; (2) assess for the endoscopic severity of disease, including presence of deep ulcers, which has prognostic significance; (3) to obtain biopsies to rule out cytomegalovirus infection; and (4) to obtain stool aspirate for *C difficile* testing.

IMPACT OF *C DIFFICILE* INFECTION ON COURSE OF IBD

Single-center and multicenter studies have consistently demonstrated the significant adverse impact of CDI on patients with IBD.[4,5,15–17,23,45] Compared with non-IBD controls, patients with IBD in whom CDI developed have 4-fold greater mortality and are 6 times more likely to require bowel surgery.[4] They also had a substantially longer hospital stay and an excess $11,406 in adjusted hospitalization charges.[4] Compared with those with IBD alone, patients with both CDI and IBD had 6-fold greater in-hospital mortality and a 2-fold increase in emergency gastrointestinal surgery or colectomy.[46] Between 20% and 45% of IBD patients hospitalized with CDI may require colectomy, with the common indications being refractory disease or toxic complications.[17,23] Ananthakrishnan and colleagues[15] examined temporal changes in the excess morbidity associated with CDI in patients with IBD and found that there was a nonsignificant increase in the excess mortality risk associated with CDI between 1998 and 2007 ($P = .15$) but the odds of colectomy compared with non-CDI controls significantly increased over the same time period ($P = .03$).

There are few reports examining if CDI has an impact on the natural history of disease beyond the acute episode. Jodorkovsky and coworkers[23] found a higher rate of UC-related emergency room visits or hospitalizations 1 year after the initial episode of CDI with a 2-fold increase in the rate of colectomy. Jen and colleagues,[46] using data from the National Health Service in England found a nearly 6-fold excess mortality at 30 days and 365 days after the initial hospitalization for CDI.[46] Chiplunker and colleagues[57] identified a mean increase in 0.89 hospitalizations per patient in the year after CDI with more than half the patients requiring escalation of maintenance therapy for their IBD (one-quarter of the CDI-IBD cohort required new initiation or escalation of biologic therapy).[57]

SPECIAL SITUATIONS RELATED TO CDI IN IBD PATIENTS
Healthy Carriage

Not all patients with *C difficile* have overt infection. Between 1% and 4% of healthy adults may be colonized with *C difficile* with a much higher rate among neonates (hypothesized to be because of a lack of intestinal epithelial receptors for *C difficile* toxin). In a study by Clayton and coworkers,[58] the rate of asymptomatic carriage in adults with IBD on aminosalicylate therapy was greater (8%) than that among healthy volunteers; whether the same extends to patients on immunosuppression is unclear.[58]

Pouchitis

Patients with an ileal pouch anal anastomosis frequently require antibiotics for treatment of acute ileal pouch anal anastomosis, predisposing them to the development of CDI. In one series of 115 patients with IPAA, *C difficile* toxin was identified in 21 patients (19%).[59] Risk factors for CDI of the pouch included male sex and prior history of left-sided colitis.[59] Thus, a diagnosis of CDI should be entertained in patients with refractory or recurrent pouchitis, particularly if unresponsive to standard antibiotic therapy.

Enteritis

Patients with a colectomy and ileostomy are not excluded from risk of CDI and can get *C difficile* enteritis.[60] Lundeen and colleagues[61] reported a series of 6 patients with *C difficile* enteritis who presented with high-volume ileostomy output, fever, and ileus. All patients in this series responded to a combination of metronidazole and vancomycin although the morbidity and mortality rate have been high in other case series.[60,62–66] CDI can also involve segments of diverted bowel; such infection responds to topical vancomycin.

DIAGNOSIS OF *C DIFFICILE* INFECTION

The diagnosis of CDI depends on demonstrating the toxin or a toxigenic strain in the diarrheal stool of the suspected patient. Testing formed stool samples has limited value and should be avoided. The most commonly used test is the enzyme immunoassay (EIA) directed against both toxins A and B (**Table 1**).[41,43,55,67–69] The performance of this test has varied widely in different settings with an estimated sensitivity of 63% to 94% and a specificity of 75% to 100%.[69] More relevant measures of test performance in the clinical setting are the positive (PPV) and negative predictive values (NPV). At low CDI prevalence, the PPV for a single stool EIA is low at 52% to 70% with a high NPV. The performance improves at higher CDI prevalence, however, with a still substantial rate of false-negative test results.[69] Testing repeat stool samples has yielded few additional cases in the non-IBD population and may not be cost effective.[70,71] Nevertheless, in the right clinical setting, testing multiple samples may improve the yield; such a practice has been adopted in some patients with IBD.[17] In those with a high index of suspicion, one might consider repeating with a different diagnostic test.[41] Another recently available test is the real-time polymerase chain reaction that detects the toxigenic genes. This test has a significantly greater sensitivity and specificity than the EIA with a similar turnaround time.[69] Its performance specifically in the IBD population has not been determined.

The gold standard for the diagnosis of CDI is the toxigenic culture or the cell-culture cytotoxicity assay, a 2-step test consisting of culturing *C difficile* from diarrheal stool followed by demonstration of the toxin-mediated cytopathic effect after 24 to 48 hours of inoculation.[41,55,68,69] A simpler test with a high NPV is the EIA against the *C difficile* common antigen (glutamate dehydrogenase). The PPV of this test is low and requires that a positive test be followed by a second, confirmatory antitoxin EIA. However, a negative test result has a high NPV in ruling out CDI and can avoid the need for the more expensive antitoxin EIA.[68,69] Such a 2-step testing strategy has been proposed but has not yet been widely adopted.

Table 1
Diagnostic testing for *Clostridium difficile* infection

Test	Comment
Diagnostic tests	
EIA – Toxin A or EIA Toxin A/B	Relatively inexpensive, fast turnaround time, suboptimal sensitivity
Polymerase chain reaction – Toxin B gene	Rapid, sensitive
Cell culture cytotoxicity assay	Sensitive, relatively long turnaround time, technically complex
Anaerobic culture	Sensitive, relatively long turnaround time
Supportive tests	
Fecal leukocytes	Not specific, cannot differentiate between CDI and IBD flare
White blood cell count, serum creatinine, serum albumin	Useful in assessing severity of disease, no role in diagnosis
Plain abdominal x-ray	Can detect toxic megacolon or free perforation. Less sensitive to demonstrate colitis. Cannot differentiate CDI from IBD flare.
Computed tomography abdomen	Sensitive in demonstrating colitis. Cannot differentiate CDI from IBD flare. Can detect toxic megacolon or free perforation.
Sigmoidoscopy/colonoscopy	May demonstrate pseudomembranes (uncommon in IBD patients). Allows for assessment of severity of disease and to obtain biopsies to rule out cytomegalovirus infection.

TREATMENT OF *C DIFFICILE* INFECTION

General measures in the treatment of all patients with CDI include cessation of the offending antibiotic, if possible, or switching to an agent with a narrower spectrum of action (**Table 2**). Such measures have been successful in the treatment of a small proportion of patients with mild CDI[38]; however, specific directed therapy against CDI is required in the majority of patients with IBD. Specific trials for the treatment of IBD patients with CDI are lacking; management algorithms for such patients are extrapolated from the non-IBD patients. Other general measures include avoiding antimotility drugs or agents with anticholinergic activity.

Choice of First-Line Therapy

Until recently, oral vancomycin was the only agent approved by the US Food and Drug Administration for the treatment of CDI. Fidaxomicin, a first-in-class macrocyclic antibiotic has also recently received US Food and Drug Administration approval for the treatment of CDI. Metronidazole remains most commonly used and is typically given at a dose of 500 mg orally every 8 hours or 250 mg every 6 hours.[68] Oral vancomycin may be used in doses ranging from 125 to 500 mg every 6 hours with comparable efficacy among the different dosing regimens.[68,72] Intravenous vancomycin has no effect against *C difficile* owing to poor luminal concentration. The duration of treatment with either antibiotic is 10 to 14 days. The ratio of colonic luminal

Table 2	
Suggested treatment of *Clostridium difficile* infection in patients with IBD	
Clinical Scenario	**Treatment Option**
Initial episode, mild	☐ Oral metronidazole 500 mg every 8 hours or 250 mg every 6 hours ☐ Continue current immunosuppression
Initial episode, severe	☐ Oral vancomycin 250–500 mg every 6 hours ☐ Consider adding intravenous metronidazole 500 mg every 8 hours in patients with ileus or severe disease ☐ Other potential adjunctive therapies include tigecycline, fidaxomicin, intravenous immunoglobulin, fecal bacteriotherapy
Recurrent episode	☐ Prolonged course of oral vancomycin with gradual taper over 4–6 weeks ☐ Two-week course of oral vancomycin followed by 4–6 weeks of rifaximin 200–400 mg every 8 hours ☐ Fidaxomicin 200 mg (oral) twice a day ☐ Other potential therapies include fecal bacteriotherapy and intravenous immunoglobulin
Refractory disease	☐ Oral vancomycin 500 mg every 6 hours AND intravenous metronidazole 500 mg every 8 hours ☐ Consider supplementing oral vancomycin with vancomycin retention enemas ☐ Early surgical consultation

Supportive care common to all patients include cessation of offending antibiotic (where possible) or switching to narrow-spectrum antibiotics and avoiding antimotility agents. Consider minimizing initiation of new immunosuppressants (particularly steroids) or escalation of immunosuppressive therapy in the setting of untreated *C difficile* infection.

concentration to minimum inhibitory concentration for *C difficile* is higher for vancomycin than metronidazole, although both agents achieve luminal concentration well above the minimum inhibitory concentration. Metronidazole is less expensive than vancomycin but may also not be tolerated because of metallic taste, gastrointestinal side effects, and risk of neuropathy with long-term use. Vancomycin has the theoretical risk of increasing the spread of vancomycin-resistant enterococci. The high cost of oral vancomycin ($300–$600 per course compared with $20 for metronidazole) may be offset by the oral administration of the generic intravenous formulation for hospitalized patients (estimated cost $45). Early randomized trials from the 1980s and 1990s showed comparable efficacy of both metronidazole and vancomycin.[73,74] However, more recent data have raised concern regarding lower treatment efficacy and a higher recurrence rate with metronidazole.[75–78] In a landmark trial, Zar and colleagues[79] compared the efficacy of both drugs stratified by severity of CDI. Severe CDI was defined by the presence of pseudomembranes, intensive care unit admission, or any 2 of the following: fever, leukocytosis, hypoalbuminemia, or age greater than 60 years. For mild disease, both metronidazole and vancomycin had similar efficacy (98% vs 90%, $P = .36$). However, vancomycin had significantly greater clinical cure rates in those with severe disease (97% vs 76%, $P = .02$).[79] A second trial comparing the 2 agents also included a third arm consisting of tolevamer, a binding resin.[80] Similar to the Zar trial, vancomycin was similar to metronidazole for mild or moderate disease but more efficacious in those with severe disease.[80] There are no similar studies evaluating drug efficacy stratified by disease severity in patients with IBD. Given the greater morbidity and mortality noted with CDI in patients with IBD, it is reasonable to infer IBD patients requiring hospitalization for CDI as having "severe" disease and using oral vancomycin as the first line in such patients. In patients with milder IBD or ambulatory patients, oral metronidazole may be an appropriate first-line option.

A recent study published in abstract form compared the performance of oral vancomycin, metronidazole, or combination therapy with both metronidazole and vancomycin in the treatment of CDI.[81] Although the study did not comment on rates of clinical cure, the rate of recurrent CDI was greater in those who received vancomycin alone compared with the 2 other groups. However, the nonrandom allocation of treatment, lack of treatment efficacy as a primary endpoint, and potential confounding by disease severity limits the generalizability of those results. Nevertheless, a combination of intravenous metronidazole and oral vancomycin may have a role in the treatment of patients with severe CDI and ileus who may not achieve adequate colonic luminal concentration of vancomycin.

Two recent phase 3 trials compared the efficacy of vancomycin (125 mg 4 times daily) with that of fidaxomicin, a novel macrocyclic antibiotic (200 mg twice daily) over a 10-day treatment period. In this noninferiority trial comprising 629 patients, the rate of clinical cure was similar in both treatment groups (88% fidaxomicin vs 86% vancomycin).[80] However, the rate of recurrent CDI was significantly lower in the fidaxomicin arm (15%) compared with the vancomycin arm (25%), an effect likely caused by less disruption of the intestinal flora by fidaxomicin.[80] However, this advantage was not seen in patients infected with the BI/NAP/027 strain. Experience with this antibiotic in patients with IBD is limited; however, it promises to be an effective alternative, particularly in patients with recurrent disease or those at high risk for recurrence. Other agents that have shown efficacy in the treatment of CDI include rifaximin (90% efficacy in a single open-label trial), teicoplanin (not available in the United States), nitazoxanide, fusidic acid, bacitracin, and binding resins, such as cholestyramine and colestipol. Data on the efficacy of these agents in IBD patients is lacking.

Immunosuppression in Patients with CDI

One challenge in the treatment of CDI in patients with IBD is the management of immunosuppression. It is well recognized that immunosuppression increases risk of CDI and may predispose to adverse outcomes. However, symptoms of a disease flare are indistinguishable from that of CDI, and, in many cases, the 2 may coexist. A multicenter study by Ben-Horin and coworkers[82] examined the outcomes of CDI-IBD patients treated with antibiotics (AB) alone compared with those who received antibiotics in combination with immunomodulator (AB-IM) therapy. The composite primary endpoint of death, colectomy, toxic megacolon, or respiratory failure was more common in the AB-IM cohort; treatment with 2 or 3 immunomodulators substantially increased the likelihood of the primary outcome (OR, 17; 95% CI, 3–91). As evidenced by the wide confidence interval, the number of patients in each subgroup was small. Moreover, the nonrandom allocation to treatment arms raises concern regarding confounding by severity. Extrapolating data from opportunistic infections, it is reasonable to conclude that one must avoid escalation of immuno-suppression in the setting of untreated CDI. In particular, the dose of steroids should be minimized where possible. However, in a significant proportion of the cases, it may be necessary to avoid combination treatment with both antibiotics and immunosuppressive agents.[83]

Management of Refractory Disease and the Role of Surgery

Despite optimal medical therapy, a significant proportion of patients with CDI-IBD remain refractory. An inflamed colon may increase luminal concentration of intravenous metronidazole, which is a useful adjunct to oral vancomycin in those with severe colitis or coexisting ileus). Vancomycin can also be administered via a nasoenteric tube or directly into the colon through a retention enema. Careful rectal administration of 500 mg of vancomycin mixed in 100 mL of saline every 4 to 12 hours through a Foley catheter placed in the rectum (after insufflation of the balloon) has been effective in some patients.[84] Tigecycline is an alternate intravenous antibiotic (50 mg twice daily) that has been used in patients with severe disease with good efficacy.[85] Small case series have reported successful treatment of severe or recurrent CDI with the use of intravenous immunoglobulin (single dose of 150–400 mg/kg).[86] Rates of failure with this therapy remain high, reflecting the severity of disease in this cohort.

Early surgical consultation is essential in patients with refractory or severe CDI, as late surgery has been associated with substantial morbidity and mortality. Factors predicting severe disease requiring surgery include marked leukocytosis ($>15,000/$ mm^3), elevated serum lactate level, or underlying IBD.[51,52] The treatment of choice is a subtotal colectomy with end-ileostomy. Segmental resection or hemicolectomy is associated with a high mortality and is not preferred. A recent study published in abstract form described 34 patients with severe CDI (non-IBD) who underwent a temporary loop ileostomy with intraoperative lavage with 8 L of PEG-3350/electrolyte solution and intracolonic administration of vancomycin, 500 mg every 8 hours.[87] The mortality rate in this cohort was 21% (compared with 47% in historical controls) with 24 of 27 survivors retaining their colon (and 10 of 18 having their ileostomy reversed at 6 months).

MANAGEMENT OF RECURRENT DISEASE

The rate of recurrence after the first episode of CDI is between 6% and 33% and remains a management challenge. The rate of recurrence can increase to 65% after the first recurrence.[88] Continuation of the offending antibiotic or gastric acid suppressive therapy increases the likelihood of recurrence as does older age and lower antitoxin antibody levels.[89] Retreatment with metronidazole may be an option in those with a mild first recurrence of CDI.[68] Multiple episodes of recurrent disease merits the use of oral vancomycin (or potentially fidaxomicin).[68] The dose administration of vancomycin is similar to that used for the primary episode; a prolonged taper over 6 to 8 weeks with gradual decrease of the dose from 125 mg 4 times daily to 125 mg every third day has been useful in treating recurrent disease.[88,90] Rifaximin (400–1200 mg/d) has also been effective in treating recurrent CDI,[91] including in the IBD population.[92] Probiotics, particularly *Sacharomyces boulardii*, may be useful as adjunctive agents in preventing or treating recurrent disease, although there is lack of sufficient high-quality data supporting their use in this setting.[93] One strategy for preemptive prevention of recurrent disease is to continue treatment for the primary CDI episode for 7 to 10 days after cessation of the course of treatment with the offending antibiotic agent. Oral vancomycin may be the preferred strategy in such settings owing to low luminal concentration of metronidazole in the noninflamed colon. Given the association of recurrent disease with low antitoxin antibody levels, one promising strategy has been the administration of intravenous immunoglobulin[94] or, more recently, monoclonal antibodies against toxins A and B.[95] In a phase 2 randomized, controlled trial by Lowy and coworkers[95] the rate of recurrent CDI was lower in patients who received a single intravenous infusion of the monoclonal antibody (7%) compared with placebo (25%). The most effective treatment for recurrent disease is fecal transplant with resolution of infection in nearly all patients treated with this modality. A randomized trial of this modality is ongoing (FECAL trial),[96] but lower patient and physician acceptability continues to limit its use. Considerable research is also ongoing toward the development of active and passive vaccination strategies against *C difficile.*[14,49] Phase 2 trials of candidate vaccines are ongoing; such approaches, if effective, can have significant potential in preventing morbidity, mortality, and health care expenditure.

INFECTION CONTROL

Within a health care institution, adequate infection control measures are essential to prevent interperson spread of *C difficile,* as the spores are resistant to environmental degradation and can persist for several months. Quaternary ammonium-based cleaning solutions are not effective in eradicating *C difficile* spores. Hypochlorite-based solutions are more effective and should be preferred for environmental decontaminant.[68,97] Careful and thorough soap-and-water hand washing is essential to prevent transmission via health care workers; alcohol-based hand gels are not effective in eradicating spores.[68,97] Hospitalized patients with suspected or proven CDI should be placed in contact isolation with required use of gowns and gloves. Standard infection control policies are sufficient in endoscopy units.

GAPS IN RESEARCH

There are several areas of knowledge deficit in the management of CDI among patients with IBD. Prospective studies adjusting for severity of underlying IBD and CDI are essential to estimate the excess risk of CDI in patients with IBD; accurate determination of the morbidity and mortality burden as well as determining predictors of severe disease and poor patient outcome are imperative. Treatment trials of existing agents stratifying by disease severity are essential to inform the appropriate treatment algorithm. There is also need to detail risk factors for community-acquired CDI in IBD patients, as this promises to be a growing at-risk group. Significant advances in genetics have revolutionized our understanding of IBD pathogenesis; whether such underlying defects in innate or adaptive immunity or intestinal barrier function also predispose the IBD patient to the development of CDI or severe disease has not been studied. Another area that merits examination is whether the impact of CDI on IBD is restricted to the acute infection episode or if there is a more long-term modification of natural history of disease.

SUMMARY

The prevalence of CDI in patients with IBD has increased over the last decade. The excess morbidity and mortality associated with CDI appears to be greater in patients with IBD than in those without preexisting bowel disease. The risk factors for CDI in IBD and non-IBD populations appear similar; unique IBD-related risk factors are use of maintenance immunosuppression and extent and severity of prior colitis. Nevertheless, a significant proportion of CDI-IBD patients may have the disease without traditional risk factors (ie, antibiotic use, recent hospitalization). The absence of such risk factors must not preclude considering CDI in the differential diagnosis of IBD patients presenting with a disease flare. Vancomycin and metronidazole appear to have similar efficacy with vancomycin being the preferred agent for severe disease. Early surgical consultation is key for improving outcomes of patients with severe disease. Several gaps in research exist; prospective multicenter cohorts of CDI-IBD are essential to improve our understanding of the impact of CDI on IBD patients and define appropriate therapeutic regimens to improve patient outcomes.

REFERENCES

1. Bartlett JG. Historical perspectives on studies of Clostridium difficile and C. difficile infection. Clin Infect Dis 2008;46 (Suppl 1):S4–11.
2. Bartlett JG, Chang TW, Gurwith M, et al. Antibiotic-associated pseudomembranous colitis due to toxin-producing clostridia. N Engl J Med 1978;298:531–4.
3. Ananthakrishnan AN, Issa M, Binion DG. Clostridium difficile and inflammatory bowel disease. Gastroenterol Clin North Am 2009;38:711–28.
4. Ananthakrishnan AN, McGinley EL, Binion DG. Excess hospitalisation burden associated with Clostridium difficile in patients with inflammatory bowel disease. Gut 2008;57:205–10.
5. Goodhand JR, Alazawi W, Rampton DS. Systematic review: Clostridium difficile and inflammatory bowel disease. Aliment Pharmacol Ther 2011;33:428–41.
6. Pituch H. Clostridium difficile is no longer just a nosocomial infection or an infection of adults. Int J Antimicrob Agents 2009;33 (Suppl 1):S42–5.
7. Freeman J, Bauer MP, Baines SD, et al. The changing epidemiology of Clostridium difficile infections.Clin Microbiol Rev 2010;23:529–49.
8. Kim J, Smathers SA, Prasad P, et al. Epidemiological features of Clostridium difficile-associated disease among inpatients at children's hospitals in the United States, 2001–2006. Pediatrics 2008;122:1266–70.
9. Ananthakrishnan AN. Clostridium difficile infection: epidemiology, risk factors and management. Nat Rev Gastroenterol Hepatol 2011;8:17–26.
10. McDonald LC, Owings M, Jernigan DB. Clostridium difficile infection in patients discharged from US short-stay hospitals, 1996-2003. Emerg Infect Dis 2006;12:409–15.
11. Pepin J, Valiquette L, Alary ME, et al. Clostridium difficile-associated diarrhea in a region of Quebec from 1991 to 2003: a changing pattern of disease severity. CMAJ 2004;171:466–72.
12. Kuijper EJ, Coignard B, Tull P. Emergence of Clostridium difficile-associated disease in North America and Europe. Clin Microbiol Infect 2006;12 (Suppl 6):2–18.
13. Kutty PK, Woods CW, Sena AC, et al. Risk factors for and estimated incidence of community-associated Clostridium difficile infection, North Carolina, USA. Emerg Infect Dis 2010;16:197–204.
14. O'Donoghue C, Kyne L. Update on Clostridium difficile infection. Curr Opin Gastroenterol 2011;27:38–47.
15. Ananthakrishnan AN, McGinley EL, Saeian K, et al. Temporal trends in disease outcomes related to Clostridium difficile infection in patients with inflammatory bowel disease. Inflamm Bowel Dis 2011;17:976–83.
16. Nguyen GC, Kaplan GG, Harris ML, et al. A national survey of the prevalence and impact of Clostridium difficile infection among hospitalized inflammatory bowel disease patients. Am J Gastroenterol 2008;103:1443–50.
17. Issa M, Vijayapal A, Graham MB, et al. Impact of Clostridium difficile on inflammatory bowel disease. Clin Gastroenterol Hepatol 2007;5:345–51.
18. Rodemann JF, Dubberke ER, Reske KA, et al. Incidence of Clostridium difficile infection in inflammatory bowel disease. Clin Gastroenterol Hepatol 2007;5:339–44.
19. Bolton RP, Sherriff RJ, Read AE. Clostridium difficile associated diarrhoea: a role in inflammatory bowel disease? Lancet 1980;1:383–4.
20. Gryboski JD. Clostridium difficile in inflammatory bowel disease relapse. J Pediatr Gastroenterol Nutr 1991;13:39–41.

21. Meyer AM, Ramzan NN, Loftus EV Jr, et al. The diagnostic yield of stool pathogen studies during relapses of inflammatory bowel disease. J Clin Gastroenterol 2004;38: 772–5.
22. Mylonaki M, Langmead L, Pantes A, et al. Enteric infection in relapse of inflammatory bowel disease: importance of microbiological examination of stool. Eur J Gastroenterol Hepatol 2004;16:775–8.
23. Jodorkovsky D, Young Y, Abreu MT. Clinical outcomes of patients with ulcerative colitis and co-existing Clostridium difficile infection. Dig Dis Sci 2010;55:415–20
24. Pascarella F, Martinelli M, Miele E, et al. Impact of Clostridium difficile infection on pediatric inflammatory bowel disease. J Pediatr 2009;154:854–8.
25. Wultanska D, Banaszkiewicz A, Radzikowski A, et al. Clostridium difficile infection in Polish pediatric outpatients with inflammatory bowel disease. Eur J Clin Microbiol Infect Dis 2010;29:1265–70.
26. Voth DE, Ballard JD. Clostridium difficile toxins: mechanism of action and role in disease. Clin Microbiol Rev 2005;18:247–63.
27. Rupnik M, Wilcox MH, Gerding DN. Clostridium difficile infection: new developments in epidemiology and pathogenesis. Nat Rev Microbiol 2009;7:526–36.
28. Giesemann T, Egerer M, Jank T, et al. Processing of Clostridium difficile toxins. J Med Microbiol 2008;57:690–6.
29. Drudy D, Harnedy N, Fanning S, et al. Isolation and characterisation of toxin A-negative, toxin B-positive Clostridium difficile in Dublin, Ireland. Clin Microbiol Infect 2007;13:298–304.
30. Rupnik M, Grabnar M, Geric B. Binary toxin producing Clostridium difficile strains. Anaerobe 2003;9:289–94.
31. Schwan C, Stecher B, Tzivelekidis T, et al. Clostridium difficile toxin CDT induces formation of microtubule-based protrusions and increases adherence of bacteria. PLoS Pathog 2009;5:e1000626.
32. Pepin J, Valiquette L, Cossette B. Mortality attributable to nosocomial Clostridium difficile-associated disease during an epidemic caused by a hypervirulent strain in Quebec. CMAJ 2005;173:1037–42.
33. Clements AC, Magalhaes RJ, Tatem AJ, et al. Clostridium difficile PCR ribotype 027: assessing the risks of further worldwide spread. Lancet Infect Dis 2010;10:395–404.
34. Loo VG, Poirier L, Miller MA, et al. A predominantly clonal multi-institutional outbreak of Clostridium difficile-associated diarrhea with high morbidity and mortality. N Engl J Med 2005;353:2442–9.
35. McDonald LC, Killgore GE, Thompson A, et al. An epidemic, toxin gene-variant strain of Clostridium difficile. N Engl J Med 2005;353:2433–41.
36. Bauer MP, Notermans DW, van Benthem BH, et al. Final results of the first pan-European Clostridium difficile infection survey, In 20th European Congress of Clinical Microbiology and Infectious Diseases (ECCMID), 10-13 April, 2010, Vienna, Austria 2010.
37. Bauer MP, Notermans DW, van Benthem BH, et al. Clostridium difficile infection in Europe: a hospital-based survey. Lancet 2011;377:63–73.
38. Bossuyt P, Verhaegen J, Van Assche G, et al. Increasing incidence of Clostridium difficile-associated diarrhea in inflammatory bowel disease. J Crohns Colitis 2009;3:4–7.
39. Goorhuis A, Bakker D, Corver J, et al. Emergence of Clostridium difficile infection due to a new hypervirulent strain, polymerase chain reaction ribotype 078. Clin Infect Dis 2008;47:1162–70.
40. Owens RC Jr, Donskey CJ, Gaynes RP, et al. Antimicrobial-associated risk factors for Clostridium difficile infection. Clin Infect Dis 2008;46 (Suppl 1):S19–31.

41. Kelly CP. A 76-year-old man with recurrent Clostridium difficile-associated diarrhea: review of C. difficile infection. JAMA 2009;301:954–62.
42. Bartlett JG. Clinical practice. Antibiotic-associated diarrhea. N Engl J Med 2002;346: 334–9.
43. Bartlett JG, Gerding DN. Clinical recognition and diagnosis of Clostridium difficile infection. Clin Infect Dis 2008;46 (Suppl 1):S12–8.
44. Pepin J, Saheb N, Coulombe MA, et al. Emergence of fluoroquinolones as the predominant risk factor for Clostridium difficile-associated diarrhea: a cohort study during an epidemic in Quebec. Clin Infect Dis 2005;41:1254–60.
45. Issa M, Ananthakrishnan AN, Binion DG. Clostridium difficile and inflammatory bowel disease. Inflamm Bowel Dis 2008;14:1432–42.
46. Jen MH, Saxena S, Bottle A, et al. Increased health burden associated with Clostridium difficile diarrhoea in patients with inflammatory bowel disease. Aliment Pharmacol Ther 2011;33:1322–31.
47. Dial S, Alrasadi K, Manoukian C, et al. Risk of Clostridium difficile diarrhea among hospital inpatients prescribed proton pump inhibitors: cohort and case-control studies. CMAJ 2004;171:33–8.
48. Arif M, Weber LR, Knox JF, et al. Patterns of proton pump inhibitor use in Inflammatory Bowel disease and concomitant risk of Clostridium difficile infection. Gastroenterology 2007;132:A513.
49. Kelly CP, Kyne L. The host immune response to Clostridium difficile. J Med Microbiol 2011;60(Pt 8):1070–9.
50. Powell N, Jung SE, Krishnan B. Clostridium difficile infection and inflammatory bowel disease: a marker for disease extent? Gut 2008;57:1183–4; author reply 1184.
51. Butala P, Divino CM. Surgical aspects of fulminant Clostridium difficile colitis. Am J Surg 2010;200:131–5.
52. Greenstein AJ, Byrn JC, Zhang LP, et al. Risk factors for the development of fulminant Clostridium difficile colitis. Surgery 2008;143:623–9.
53. Henrich TJ, Krakower D, Bitton A, et al. Clinical risk factors for severe Clostridium difficile-associated disease. Emerg Infect Dis 2009;15:415–22.
54. Fekety R, Shah AB. Diagnosis and treatment of Clostridium difficile colitis. JAMA 1993;269:71–5.
55. Kelly CP, LaMont JT. Clostridium difficile infection. Annu Rev Med 1998;49:375–90.
56. Ben-Horin S, Margalit M, Bossuyt P, et al. Prevalence and clinical impact of endoscopic pseudomembranes in patients with inflammatory bowel disease and Clostridium difficile infection. J Crohns Colitis 2010;4:194–8.
57. Chiplunker A, Ananthakrishnan AN, Beaulieu DB, et al. Long-term impact of Clostridium difficile on inflammatory bowel disease. Gastroenterology 2009;136 (Suppl 1): S1145.
58. Clayton EM, Rea MC, Shanahan F, et al. The vexed relationship between Clostridium difficile and inflammatory bowel disease: an assessment of carriage in an outpatient setting among patients in remission. Am J Gastroenterol 2009;104:1162–9.
59. Shen BO, Jiang ZD, Fazio VW, et al. Clostridium difficile infection in patients with ileal pouch-anal anastomosis. Clin Gastroenterol Hepatol 2008;6:782–8.
60. Kim JH, Muder RR. Clostridium difficile enteritis: a review and pooled analysis of the cases. Anaerobe 2011;17:52–5.
61. Lundeen SJ, Otterson MF, Binion DG, et al. Clostridium difficile enteritis: an early postoperative complication in inflammatory bowel disease patients after colectomy. J Gastrointest Surg 2007;11:138–42.
62. Causey MW, Spencer MP, Steele SR. Clostridium difficile enteritis after colectomy. Am Surg 2009;75:1203–6.

63. Lavallee C, Laufer B, Pepin J, et al. Fatal Clostridium difficile enteritis caused by the BI/NAP1/027 strain: a case series of ileal C. difficile infections. Clin Microbiol Infect 2009;15:1093–9.
64. Miller DL, Sedlack JD, Holt RW. Perforation complicating rifampin-associated pseudomembranous enteritis. Arch Surg 1989;124:1082.
65. Vesoulis Z, Williams G, Matthews B. Pseudomembranous enteritis after proctocolectomy: report of a case. Dis Colon Rectum 2000;43:551–4.
66. Yee HF Jr, Brown RS Jr, Ostroff JW. Fatal Clostridium difficile enteritis after total abdominal colectomy. J Clin Gastroenterol 1996;22:45–7.
67. McFarland LV. Renewed interest in a difficult disease: Clostridium difficile infections—epidemiology and current treatment strategies. Curr Opin Gastroenterol 2009;25:24–35.
68. Cohen SH, Gerding DN, Johnson S, et al. Clinical practice guidelines for Clostridium difficile infection in adults: 2010 update by the society for healthcare epidemiology of America (SHEA) and the infectious diseases society of America (IDSA). Infect Control Hosp Epidemiol 2010;31:431–55.
69. Crobach MJ, Dekkers OM, Wilcox MH, et al. European Society of Clinical Microbiology and Infectious Diseases (ESCMID): data review and recommendations for diagnosing Clostridium difficile-infection (CDI). Clin Microbiol Infect 2009;15:1053–66.
70. Deshpande A, Pasupuleti V, Patel P, et al. Repeat stool testing to diagnose Clostridium difficile infection using enzyme immunoassay does not increase diagnostic yield. Clin Gastroenterol Hepatol 2011;9:665–9, e1.
71. Nemat H, Khan R, Ashraf MS, et al. Diagnostic value of repeated enzyme immunoassays in Clostridium difficile infection. Am J Gastroenterol 2009;104:2035–41.
72. Fekety R, Silva J, Kauffman C, et al. Treatment of antibiotic-associated Clostridium difficile colitis with oral vancomycin: comparison of two dosage regimens. Am J Med 1989;86:15–9.
73. Teasley DG, Gerding DN, Olson MM, et al. Prospective randomised trial of metronidazole versus vancomycin for Clostridium-difficile-associated diarrhoea and colitis. Lancet 1983;2:1043–6.
74. Wenisch C, Parschalk B, Hasenhundl M, et al. Comparison of vancomycin, teicoplanin, metronidazole, and fusidic acid for the treatment of Clostridium difficile-associated diarrhea. Clin Infect Dis 1996;22:813–8.
75. Pepin J, Alary ME, Valiquette L, et al. Increasing risk of relapse after treatment of Clostridium difficile colitis in Quebec, Canada. Clin Infect Dis 2005;40:1591–7.
76. Musher DM, Aslam S, Logan N, et al. Relatively poor outcome after treatment of Clostridium difficile colitis with metronidazole. Clin Infect Dis 2005;40:1586–90.
77. Aslam S, Hamill RJ, Musher DM. Treatment of Clostridium difficile-associated disease: old therapies and new strategies. Lancet Infect Dis 2005;5:549–57.
78. Leffler DA, Lamont JT. Treatment of Clostridium difficile-associated disease. Gastroenterology 2009;136:1899–912.
79. Zar FA, Bakkanagari SR, Moorthi KM, et al. A comparison of vancomycin and metronidazole for the treatment of Clostridium difficile-associated diarrhea, stratified by disease severity. Clin Infect Dis 2007;45:302–7.
80. Louie T. Results of a phase III trial comparing tolveamer, vancomycin and metronidazole in Clostridium difficile-associated diarrhea (CDAD). Program and abstracts of the 47th Interscience Conference on Antimicrobial Agents and Chemotherapy (Washington DC). Herndon (VA): ASM Press, 2007 [abstract k-4259].
81. Libot A, Issa M, Zadvornova Y, et al. Initial vancomycin monotherapy is associated with higher rates of subsequent Clostridium difficile Infection in inflammatory bowel disease population. Chicago (IL) Digestive Disease Week; 2011 [abstract # 992].

82. Ben-Horin S, Margalit M, Bossuyt P, et al. Combination immunomodulator and antibiotic treatment in patients with inflammatory bowel disease and clostridium difficile infection. Clin Gastroenterol Hepatol 2009;7:981–7.
83. Yanai H, Nguyen GC, Yun L, et al. Practice of gastroenterologists in treating flaring inflammatory bowel disease patients with clostridium difficile: Antibiotics alone or combined antibiotics/immunomodulators? Inflamm Bowel Dis 2011;17:1540–6.
84. Gerding DN, Muto CA, Owens RC Jr. Treatment of Clostridium difficile infection. Clin Infect Dis 2008;46 (Suppl 1):S32–42.
85. Herpers BL, Vlaminckx B, Burkhardt O, et al. Intravenous tigecycline as adjunctive or alternative therapy for severe refractory Clostridium difficile infection. Clin Infect Dis 2009;48:1732–5.
86. Abougergi MS, Broor A, Cui W, et al. Intravenous immunoglobulin for the treatment of severe Clostridium difficile colitis: an observational study and review of the literature. J Hosp Med 2010;5:E1–9.
87. Zuckerbraun B, Alverdy J, Simmons RL. Minimally invasive temporary loop ileostomy, colonic lavage, and intracolonic antegrade vancomycin for severe complicated clostridium difficile disease. In: American Surgical Association 131st Annual Meeting. Boca Raton (FL) 2011.
88. Johnson S. Recurrent Clostridium difficile infection: a review of risk factors, treatments, and outcomes. J Infect 2009;58:403–10.
89. Garey KW, Sethi S, Yadav Y, et al. Meta-analysis to assess risk factors for recurrent Clostridium difficile infection. J Hosp Infect 2008;70:298–304.
90. McFarland LV, Elmer GW, Surawicz CM. Breaking the cycle: treatment strategies for 163 cases of recurrent Clostridium difficile disease. Am J Gastroenterol 2002;97: 1769–75.
91. Johnson S, Schriever C, Patel U, et al. Rifaximin Redux: treatment of recurrent Clostridium difficile infections with rifaximin immediately post-vancomycin treatment. Anaerobe 2009;15:290–1.
92. Issa M, Weber LR, Brandenburg H, et al. Rifaximin and treatment of recurrent Clostridium difficile infection in patients with inflammatory bowel disease. Am J Gastroenterol 2006;101:S469.
93. McFarland LV. Meta-analysis of probiotics for the prevention of antibiotic associated diarrhea and the treatment of Clostridium difficile disease. Am J Gastroenterol 2006;101:812–22.
94. Wilcox MH. Descriptive study of intravenous immunoglobulin for the treatment of recurrent Clostridium difficile diarrhoea. J Antimicrob Chemother 2004;53:882–4.
95. Lowy I, Molrine DC, Leav BA, et al. Treatment with monoclonal antibodies against Clostridium difficile toxins. N Engl J Med 2010;362:197–205.
96. van Nood E, Speelman P, Kuijper EJ, et al. Struggling with recurrent Clostridium difficile infections: is donor faeces the solution? Euro Surveill 2009;14.
97. Gerding DN, Muto CA, Owens RC Jr. Measures to control and prevent Clostridium difficile infection. Clin Infect Dis 2008;46 (Suppl 1):S43–9.

Evaluating Pouch Problems

Yue Li, MD[a,b], Bo Shen, MD[b],*

KEYWORDS

- Complications • Inflammatory bowel disease • Ulcerative colitis
- Crohn disease • Ileal pouch-anal anastomosis

INTRODUCTION AND CLASSIFICATION OF COMPLICATIONS OF ILEAL POUCH

Approximately 20% to 30% of patients with ulcerative colitis (UC) eventually require surgery for failure of medical therapy or development of neoplasia.[1] Restorative proctocolectomy with ileal pouch-anal anastomosis (IPAA), initially described in 1978, has become the surgical treatment of choice for the majority of patients with UC who require proctocolectomy.[2] Pouch configuration with two (J), three (S), or four (W) loops of small intestine has been performed, and the J pouch has become the most commonly used one.[3] The normal configurations of the J and S pouch are illustrated in **Figs. 1** and **2**. The IPAA procedure preserves intestinal continuity, substantially decreases the risk for dysplasia, and improves health-related quality of life.[4] However, adverse sequelae related to the ileal pouch occur frequently. Recognition and proper diagnosis of those conditions are key for maintaining a healthy pouch and prolonging pouch survival.

Early complications are common after restorative proctocolectomy. The most frequent are bowel obstruction, pouch bleeding, pelvic and wound sepsis. Late complications include stricture of the anastomosis, fistula and abscess, reduced fertility,[5,6] and pouchitis.[7] Of these complications, pouchitis is the most frequent. The majority of nonmechanical pouch-related complications can be addressed without surgical intervention. However, pouch failure does occur. Pouch failure is defined as the need for permanent diversion, with or without pouch excision or revision. The reported cumulative incidence of pouch failure ranged from 4% to 10%.[8-11] A metaanalysis of 43 studies of 9317 patients showed that pouch failure rate after IPAA increases proportionally to the length of follow-up: from 6.8% with a median follow-up period of 37 months to 8.5% after more than 60 months.[11] The most common causes for pouch failure are pelvic sepsis,[12,13] chronic refractory pouchitis, Crohn disease (CD) of the pouch,[9,14,15] and pouch fistula or sinus.[16]

Based on published studies as well as the authors' clinical experience in the unique subspecialty Pouchitis Clinic at the Cleveland Clinic, the authors proposed a

[a] Department of Gastroenterology, Peking Union Medical College Hospital, Beijing, China
[b] Digestive Disease Institute, The Cleveland Clinic Foundation, 9500 Euclid Avenue, Cleveland, OH 44195, USA
* Corresponding author.
E-mail address: shenb@ccf.org

Gastroenterol Clin N Am 41 (2012) 355–378
doi:10.1016/j.gtc.2012.01.013
0889-8553/12/$ – see front matter © 2012 Elsevier Inc. All rights reserved.

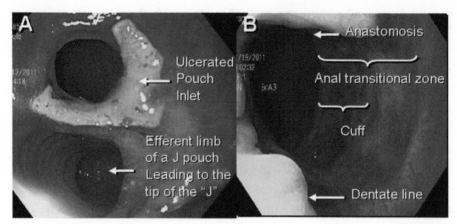

Fig. 1. (*A*) Endoscopic landmarks of the proximal part of a J pouch. An owl's eye anatomy with the pouch inlet and the opening of afferent limb. (*B*) Endoscopic landmarks of distal part of a J pouch.

classification system of pouch-related complications in 2008 (**Box 1**).[17] The complications are classified into mechanical, inflammatory, functional, neoplastic, and metabolic conditions related to the pouch by suspected underlying pathophysiologic condition. In this article, the authors provide an update for evaluation of ileal pouch disorders.

Surgical and Mechanical Complications

Surgical or mechanical complications are those adverse sequelae that are caused mainly by factors related to the surgery; these include anastomotic leaks, pelvic sepsis and abscess, pouch sinuses and fistulae, strictures, afferent limb syndrome and efferent limb syndrome, infertility,[5,6] portal vein thrombi,[18,19] pouch prolapse,[20]

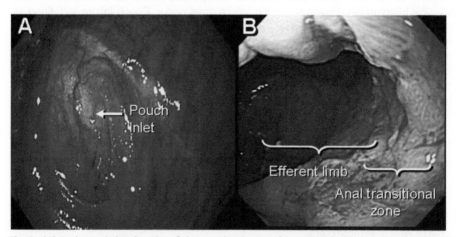

Fig. 2. (*A*) Endoscopic landmarks of the proximal part of an S pouch. Notice the absence of the owls' eye anatomy seen in the J pouch. (*B*) Endoscopic landmarks of the distal part of an S pouch. Notice the long segment between the pouch body and anal transitional zone (efferent limb of the S pouch).

Box 1
Classification of ileal pouch disorders and associated complications

Surgical and mechanical

- Anastomotic leaks
- Pelvic/perianal sepsis and abscess
- Pouch sinuses
- Pouch fistulae
- Strictures
- Afferent limb and efferent limb syndromes
- Infertility and sexual dysfunction
- Portal vein system thrombi
- Pouch prolapse, twisted pouch, pouch bleeding, sphincter injury or dysfunction, pouchocele

Inflammatory and infectious

- Pouchitis
- Cuffitis
- Crohn disease of the pouch
- Proximal small bowel bacterial overgrowth
- Inflammatory polyps

Functional

- Irritable pouch syndrome
- Anismus
- Pseudoobstruction or megapouch
- "Pouchalgia fugax"

Dysplastic and neoplastic

- Dysplasia or adenocarcinoma of the pouch or anal transitional zone
- Squamous cell cancer at the anal transitional zone
- Lymphoma

Systemic and metabolic

- Anemia from chronic disease or iron or vitamin B_{12} deficiency
- Bone loss
- Vitamin D deficiency
- Nephrolithiasis
- Celiac disease

and pouch twist.[21] Anastomotic leak is defined as anastomotic separation leading to exodus of pouch luminal content. The most common location of an anastomotic leak is at the pouch-anal anastomosis followed by the tip of the "J", and the body of the pouch along the staple line[22,23] (**Fig. 3**). Pelvic sepsis is defined as any infective process present in the peripouch area or at the true pelvis distal to the pelvic inlet,[12] whereas pelvic abscess is a collection of purulent exudates without demonstrable anastomotic leaks. Pouch sinus, which is typically a later presentation of an initial anastomotic leak, is defined as a blind tract that may lead to abscess cavity (**Fig. 4**). Pouch fistula (**Fig. 5**) is defined as an abnormal passage from one epithelial surface (ie, the ileal pouch) to another epithelial surface (eg, vagina, bladder, or skin). Afferent limb syndrome is defined as distal small bowel obstruction caused by an acute angulation, prolapse, or intussusceptions of the afferent limb at the junction to the pouch (**Fig. 6**).[17,24] Efferent limb syndrome typically occurs in patients with an S

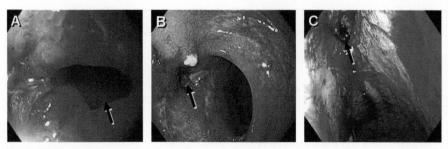

Fig. 3. Pouch leaks (*arrows*). Leaks at the tip of "J" (*A*), at the midpouch along suture line (*B*) and at the anastomosis (*C*).

pouch with a dysfunctional or excessively long efferent limb, which partially obstructs the outlet of the pouch (**Fig. 7**).[25] Other surgery-related complications include pouchocele and pouch mucosal or full-thickness prolapse (**Fig. 8**), anal sphincter injury or dysfunction, adhesions, small bowel obstruction, pouch and small bowel herniation or intussusceptions, twisted pouch, and incisional hernia.[26]

Inflammatory Disorders

Pouchitis is the most common long-term complication in patients with IPAA. The reported cumulative frequency rate of pouchitis 10 to 11 years after IPAA surgery for UC ranges from 23% to 46%.[4,27] Furthermore, it is commonly recognized that the incidence of pouchitis increases proportionally to the length of follow-up; approximately 50% of patients after IPAA for UC will develop at least one episode of pouchitis.[28] The cause and pathogenesis of pouchitis are unknown. It is speculated that pouchitis is an abnormal mucosal immune response to altered commensal bacterial flora in the reservoir causing acute or chronic inflammation.[8,29–31] Reported risk factors for pouchitis (**Box 2**) include genetic polymorphisms of interleukin-1-receptor antagonist[32–34] and NOD2/CARD15[35,36]; noncarrier status of tumor-necrosis factor allele 2[33]; extensive UC[4,37,38]; the presence of backwash ileitis[37]; precolectomy thrombocytosis[39–41]; preoperative corticosteroid use[40,42]; extraintestinal manifestations,

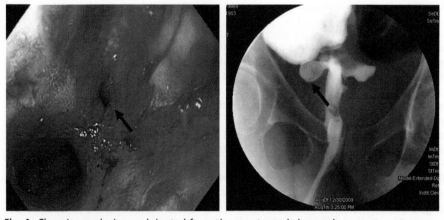

Fig. 4. Chronic pouch sinus originated from the anastomosis (*arrows*).

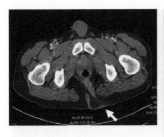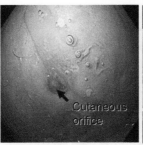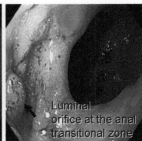

Fig. 5. Perianal fistula in a pouch patient (*arrows*).

especially the presence of concurrent primary sclerosing cholangitis (PSC) or arthralgia or arthropathy[38,40,42–44]; seropositive perinuclear antineutrophil cytoplasmic antibodies (p-ANCA)[45,46] or anti-CBir1 flagellin[4]; being a nonsmoker[40,47,48]; S pouch reconstruction[42]; the use of nonsteroidal antiinflammatory drugs (NSAIDs)[38,48]; and the presence of concurrent autoimmune disorders.[49]

In patients with a stapled pouch–anal anastomosis, in order to allow transanal insertion of the stapler head, it is normally necessary to leave a 1- to 2-cm strip of the rectal columnar cuff, which is at risk for developing symptomatic inflammation (cuffitis) or dysplasia.[50,51] Cuffitis typically represents a recurrence of UC in the residual mucosa. However, other disease processes may also contribute to the development of cuffitis, such as CD and ischemia.[52] In a study of 61 consecutive symptomatic patients with IPAA, 7% had cuffitis.[53] Bleeding ranging from blood on tissue paper to frank blood or blood clots was significantly more common in cuffitis than in pouchitis. Cuffitis may represent an underrecognized disease with limited data in literature. No standardized diagnostic criteria have been proposed.

An intriguing inflammatory disorder is CD-like condition of the pouch. CD of the pouch can occur after IPAA, which is intentionally performed in a selected group of patients with

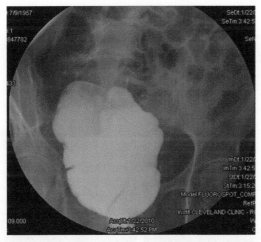

Fig. 6. Afferent limb syndrome. Water-soluble contrasted enema could not reach the afferent limb because of sharp angulation of bowel lumen at the pouch inlet.

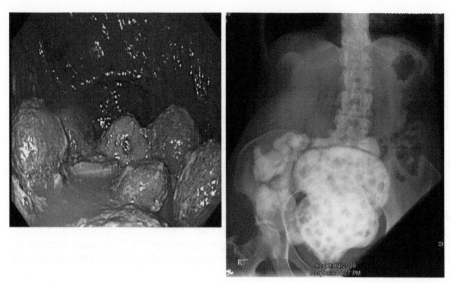

Fig. 7. Efferent limb syndrome in a patient with S pouch. Outlet angulation causing obstruction and retained fecal bezoars.

Crohn colitis without small intestinal or perianal diseases.[54] CD is also unexpectedly found in proctocolectomy specimens in patients with a preoperative diagnosis of UC or colonic inflammatory bowel disease unclassified (IBDU). However, a majority of patients with CD of the pouch were considered to develop the disease de novo. The reported cumulative frequencies of CD of the pouch range from 2.7% to 13%.[55–62] Clinically, CD of the pouch can be classified into inflammatory, fibrostenotic, or fistulizing phenotypes.[17,63] Diagnosis of CD of the pouch often needs a combined assessment of symptom, endoscopy, histology, radiography, and sometimes examination under anesthesia.[63]

Other inflammatory disorders related to the pouch include proximal small bowel bacterial overgrowth and inflammatory polyps. Polyps in the pouch and anal

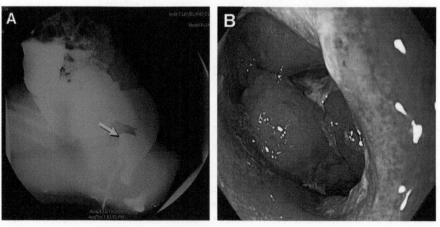

Fig. 8. Anterior pouchocele (*A, arrow*) and distal pouch prolapse (*B*).

Box 2
Reported risk factors of pouchitis

Genetic

- Interleukin-1-receptor antagonist
- NOD2/CARD15
- Noncarrier status of tumor-necrosis factor allele 2

Preoperative disease distribution

- Extensive ulcerative colitis
- Presence of backwash ileitis
- Disease proximal to splenic flexure

Demographic

- Age at operation
- Age at diagnosis
- Nonsmoker

Surgical

- S-pouch reconstruction
- Two-stage instead of three-stage operation

Laboratory

- Precolectomy thrombocytosis
- Seropositive perinuclear antineutrophil cytoplasmic antibodies (p-ANCA)
- Seropositive anti-CBir1 flagellin

Extraintestinal manifestations

- Presence of concurrent primary sclerosing cholangitis
- Presence of concurrent arthralgia or arthropathy
- Presence of concurrent autoimmune disorders

Medication

- Preoperative corticosteroid use
- Use of NSAIDs after pouch construction

---

transitional zone (ATZ) mucosa are more common in patients with IPAA for familial adenomatous polyposis than patients with UC.[64–68] Inflammatory polyps in underlying UC patients are typically detected on the background of pouchitis, cuffitis, or CD.[68] Endoscopic polypectomy with concomitant medical therapy is recommended for large, non-CAP (>10 mm in size) and/or symptomatic (the ones causing obstruction or bleeding) polyps for the eradication of dysplasia or symptom relief.[68]

Functional Disorders of the Ileal Pouch

Irritable pouch syndrome (IPS) is a functional disorder in patients with IPAA.[53] It is a diagnosis of exclusion based on the presence of increased frequency of bowel movements with a change in stool consistency, abdominal pain, and perianal or pelvic discomfort in the absence of endoscopic, radiographic, or histologic abnormalities.[53] Patients with anismus, with characteristic paradoxical contractions on pouch-anal manometry, present with dyschezia (**Fig. 9**). Anismus can be classified as primary (in the absence of mechanical or inflammatory conditions of the distal pouch or ATZ) and secondary (due to mechanical or inflammatory conditions, such as distal pouch

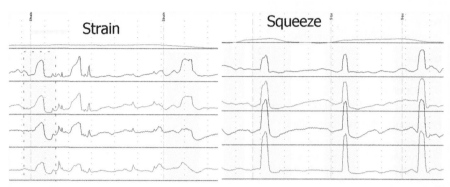

Fig. 9. Anismus with paradoxical contractions on pouch-anal manometry.

stricture, cuffitis, and perianal fistula). Some patients, particularly men, may present with periodic sharp and lightning-type pain at the distal pouch, a condition termed *pouchalgia fugax*. Pseudoobstruction with megapouch can also occur after IPAA (**Fig. 10**).

Neoplasia

Proctocolectomy with IPAA substantially reduces, but does not completely abolish, the risk for UC-associated dysplasia or cancer. As of 2011, a total of 77 patients with pouch dysplasia and 50 with pouch cancer have been reported.[69] In a large cohort study from the authors' group, they reported that the cumulative incidence for pouch cancer at 5, 10, 15, 20, and 25 years was 0.2%, 0.4%, 0.8%, 2.4%, and 3.4%, respectively.[70] Pooled prevalence of dysplasia in the pouch body seems

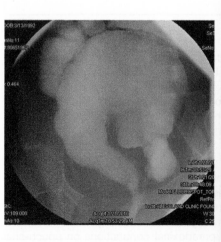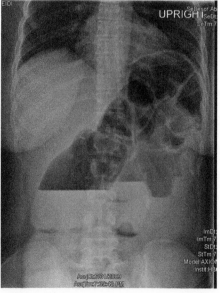

Fig. 10. Pseudoobstruction and megapouch in two patients.

higher than that in the ATZ; however, pouch adenocarcinoma has been discovered more often in ATZ (64%) than in the pouch body (19%).[69] Patients with a longer duration of UC (irrespective of duration of IPAA),[71] a preoperative or intraoperative diagnosis of dysplasia or cancer from underlying UC,[72–74] the presence of pancolitis with backwash ileitis,[75,76] villous atrophy of the pouch mucosa or histologic type C mucosa (pouch mucosa with persistent severe atrophy),[77–79] chronic pouchitis,[71,75] or PSC [71,80] are at higher risk for dysplasia or cancer in the pouch or ATZ. In our historical cohort study, the main risk for pouch neoplasia is the presence of UC-associated dysplasia or cancer in colon before colecomy.[70] Routine surveillance pouchoscopy annually is recommended for patients at risk.

Metabolic and Systemic Complications

Systemic complications such as iron deficiency anemia and bone loss are frequently observed post-IPAA. The prevalence of anemia has been reported to be 17% among ileal pouch patients with underlying UC and 26% in patients with familial adenomatous polyposis.[81] Low bone mineral density was found in 26% in the spine and 19% in the femoral neck of IPAA patients.[82] The pathophysiologic cause for anemia and bone loss may be multifactorial. All the following factors can contribute to anemia: poor oral iron intake, inadequate iron absorption, chronic inflammation, overt or obscure gastrointestinal bleeding, vitamin B_{12} malabsorption, and malignancy. Bone loss is associated with low body mass index, advanced age, inflammation activity, nonuse of daily calcium supplement, and villous atrophy of the pouch mucosa.[82,83] The authors also anecdotally notice that nephrolithiasis are common in patients with IPAA Vitamin D deficiency was also found to be common in pouch patients.[84]

CLINICAL EVALUATION
Symptoms and Signs

Patients with diseased pouches can have a variety of clinical presentations. However, symptoms are nonspecific and commonly not sufficiently distinctive for a definitive diagnosis.[85] Increased stool frequency, urgency, hematochezia, abdominal pain, and perianal pain are the most common symptoms.[86] Dyschezia or incomplete evacuation can be seen in anismus, afferent/efferent limb syndrome, and dysfunctional megapouch. Nausea, vomiting, and bloating could signify small bowel obstruction, pouch strictures, or afferent/efferent limb syndromes. Patients with fistula, drainage, and perianal pain should be evaluated for CD of the pouch, postoperative leaks, sinus, or abscess.[17] Gas, incontinence, nocturnal symptoms, and liquid stools are rarely noted in the normal pouch in patients with an intact anal sphincter.[87] Of note, constitutional symptoms such as fever, chills, and weight loss are uncommon in patients with conventional pouchitis.

Although symptoms are not typically diagnostic for specific complications of IPAA, bleeding is almost exclusively seen in cuffitis.[87] Patients with presacral sinus or abscess may present with characteristic pain at the distal tail bone. Patients with pouch-vaginal fistula typically present with continuous or intermittent vaginal discharge of air and/or stool or recurrent vaginitis. Patients with pouch-vesicular fistula may present with frequent refractory urinary tract infection. The diagnosis of pouch problems may not be static. For example, a patient may have typical pouchitis at one point and may present with characteristics of CD of the pouch later. Hence, periodic diagnostic endoscopy combined with symptom assessment and histologic evaluation are important in differentiating the causes of pouch problems.[85]

Extraintestinal manifestations such as erythema nodosum and arthralgia can occur in patients with healthy or diseased pouches. In fact, patients with extraintestinal manifestations may have a higher risk for developing pouchitis. Patients with concurrent PSC may present with liver-associated signs or symptoms such as icterus and jaundice. Patients with PSC are at higher risk for chronic pouchitis as well as enteritis. We postulate that PSC-associated pouchitis/enteritis may represent a unique form for disease entity of IPAA.[88]

Detailed physical examination may yield clues for diagnosis and differential diagnosis of ileal pouch disorders. Special attention should be paid to the previous ileostomy site, surgical incision area in the abdomen (for trigger point pain, hernia, or wound infection), and perianal area (for abscess, fistula, skin tags, prolapse, hemorrhoids, dermatitis).

ENDOSCOPIC EVALUATION
Diagnosis

Endoscopic evaluation is valuable for the diagnosis and differential diagnosis of inflammatory and mechanical pouch disorders.[89] A gastroscope is preferred because of its flexibility and smaller caliber. The common endoscopic features shared by pouchitis, CD of the pouch, and cuffitis at different segments of IPAA include erythema, nodularity, increased granularity, loss of vascular pattern, hemorrhage, mucous exudates, friability, ulcers, and erosions, which are all listed in the Pouchitis Disease Activity Index (PDAI) instrument (**Table 1**). Endoscopy helps to assess the prepouch ileum, pouch body, and rectal cuff or ATZ for signs of CD of the pouch and cuffitis. Cuffitis occurs specifically in patients with a stapled IPAA with a retained rectal cuff. The presence of isolated, afferent limb ulcers should raise the suspicion of CD of the pouch, NSAID-related pouchitis,[90] or ischemia.[91] Pouch ischemia may specifically present with asymmetric distribution of pouch inflammation, particularly with half of the pouch inflamed and the other half noninflamed, which usually has a sharp demarcation between the two parts along the suture line.[91] Occasionally pseudomembrane may be observed in patients with Clostridium difficile pouchitis. Therefore, the absence of pseudomembranes under endoscopy does not exclude C difficile infection (CDI) in suspected patients with an ileal pouch. Endoscopy is also useful for the diagnosis of IPS, because IPS is currently a diagnosis of exclusion.[85]

Dysplasia Surveillance

Pouch endoscopy is the main tool to detect pouch neoplasia. Endoscopy with surveillance biopsy is recommended annually in high-risk pouch patients, such as patients after 10 years of UC diagnosis, with a preoperative diagnosis of UC-associated neoplasia, in addition to those who have chronic inflammatory conditions of the pouch, family history of colorectal cancer, or concomitant PSC.[69] Although there is no consensus on where and how endoscopic biopsy should be performed, four to six pieces need be taken from the ATZ for surveillance. Dysplasia or cancer lesions are often harbored in the underlying inflammation of the pouch or ATZ; this condition can present as flat mucosa, ulcerated lesions, or masslike lesions. Large (>1-cm) polypoid lesions of the pouch or ATZ should be removed endoscopically because of potential possibility to be neoplastic (8.7%, 2 of 23).[68] Pouch dysplasia or cancer may have no endoscopically visible lesions.[70] Therefore, blind biopsy of normal or abnormal ATZ mucosa is advocated in high-risk patients. New techniques, such as high-magnification chromoscopic pouchoscopy, have been reported to permit more accurate anatomical localization of the residual rectal mucosa and ATZ in vivo and permit improved biopsy accuracy.[92] Imaging enhanced endoscopy, such as narrow band imaging and confocal microscopy, may also be considered for detecting dysplasia in pouch patients.

Table 1	
The pouchitis disease activity index	
Criteria	**Score**
Clinical	
Stool frequency	
Usual postoperative stool frequency	0
1–2 stools/d >postoperative usual	1
3 or more stools/d >postoperative usual	2
Rectal bleeding	
None or rare	0
Present daily	1
Fecal urgency or abdominal cramps	
None	0
Occasional	1
Usual	2
Fever (temperature >37.8°C)	
Absent	0
Present	1
Endoscopic inflammation	
Edema	1
Granularity	1
Friability	1
Loss of vascular pattern	1
Mucous exudate	1
Ulceration	1
Acute histologic inflammation	
Polymorphic nuclear leukocyte infiltration	
Mild	1
Moderate + crypt abscess	2
Severe + crypt abscess	3
Ulceration per low-power field (mean)	
<25%	1
25%–50%	2
>50%	3

From Sandborn WJ, Tremaine WJ, Batts KP, et al. Pouchitis after ileal pouch-anal anastomosis: a Pouchitis Disease Activity Index. Mayo Clin Proc 1994;69:409–15.

Therapeutic Pouch Endoscopy

Pouch endoscopy can treat certain structural diseases of the pouch, such as endoscopic balloon dilatation of pouch inlet or outlet strictures, even the angulated and tight strictures.[93,94] Recently, Doppler ultrasound–guided endoscopic needle knife stricturoplasty for refractory anastomotic stricture has been first introduced by the authors.[95] In addition to treatment for strictures, successful endoscopic needle knife treatment of presacral sinus at the anastomosis was also reported by the authors' group.[96] Based on the (B.S.) own experience, healing of the anastomotic sinus may succeed in half of selected patients. With the development of novel therapeutic instruments, the authors believe that more surgery-related complications could be treated endoscopically.

LABORATORY EVALUATION

Laboratory tests are usually performed for the following purposes: (1) investigation of risk factors associated with cause, pathogenesis, and prognosis of pouch disorders; (2) assessment of disease activity, diagnosis, and differential diagnosis between inflammatory and noninflammatory pouch disorders; (3) microbiological evaluation to identify superimposed infection from pathogens; and (4) evaluation of metabolic and systemic adverse sequelae associated with IPAA.[97]

Laboratory Tests in Assessing Risk Factors and Implication in Pathogenesis

Immunogenotypic markers have been studied extensively in pouchitis. Dysregulated cytokine production including interleukin-1β (IL-1β), tumor necrosis factor-α (TNF-α), and abnormalities in endogenous inhibitors of these cytokines such as IL-1 receptor antagonist and soluble TNF-α receptors, have been reported in pouchitis.[98–100] Polymorphisms of TNF-α have been also investigated as a risk factor for pouchitis.[33] Carriage of the TNF-α allele2 was found to be inversely associated with pouchitis.[33] Polymorphisms of NOD2 (nucleotide binding oligomerization domain-2)/CARD15 (caspase recruitment domain family member-15), which are associated with ileal CD, have a higher prevalence in patients with pouchitis.[35] However, these genetic tests are not routinely performed in patients suspected of having ileal pouch disorders.

The IBD-associated serology markers, such as perinuclear antineutrophil cytoplasmic antibody (pANCA), have been investigated in patients with pouchitis or CD of the pouch. In prospective studies, both pANCA and anti-CBir1 expression were found to be associated with pouchitis.[45,101,102] Anti-*Saccharomyces cerevisiae* antibodies (ASCA) are antibodies directed against a cell wall component of the yeast, *S cerevisiae*. Preoperative presence of ASCA immunoglobulin (Ig) A antibodies in patients with UC may have a higher risk of developing CD of the pouch after IPAA surgery.[103] Patients with positive ASCA may also be at an increased risk for the development of fistulas postoperatively.[104] Some of these antimicrobial antibodies were reported to be associated with chronic pouchitis and CD-like complications of the pouch.[102]

Laboratory Tests for Assessment of Disease Activity and Diagnosis of Ileal Pouch Problems

Erythrocyte sedimentation rate (ESR), a nonspecific marker of inflammation, has been studied as a marker of pouchitis. In reported studies, ESR was found to correlate with the PDAI score[105] and episodes of pouchitis.[106] C-reactive protein (CRP) has also been evaluated as a marker of pouchitis disease activity. A significant correlation was observed between CRP and the PDAI score.[105] Elevated CRP levels might be useful to monitor the degree of inflammatory activity in a pouch noninvasively. However, the CRP level as a snapshot had a limited role in distinction between a healthy and diseased pouch based on longitudinal clinical and endoscopic evaluation.[106] In a separate study from the authors' center, false-positive celiac serology was discovered to be common in patients with IPAA, and it might be associated with chronic antibiotic-refractory pouchitis.[107] Therefore, in the authors' clinical practice, they routinely screen for celiac disease,[90] along with other autoimmune markers (such as antimicrosomal antibodies[108] in the subgroup of patients with chronic pouchitis, because it may coexist and contribute to worsening symptoms in IPAA patients.

Fecal inflammatory markers may closely reflect the presence of intestinal inflammation. Fecal pyruvate kinase, calprotectin, and lactoferrin are being investigated to assess the correlation with pouchitis and PDAI scores.[109–113] Recently, sensitivity, specificity, positive predictive value, and negative predictive value for fecal calprotectin concentration (>300 µg/g) to detect recurrent pouchitis were reported to be 57%, 92%, 67%, and 89%, respectively.[111] Fecal lactoferrin assay as an initial evaluation may be more cost effective for the diagnosis of pouchitis than routine pouchoscopy with biopsy.[114] These simple laboratory tests may be cost-effective for evaluating pouchitis and may be used as an adjunct first-line modality to pouch endoscopy.

Microbiological Evaluation

Microbiota play a key role in the initiation and exacerbation of pouch inflammation. Attempts have been made to identify the culprit pathogens for inflammatory conditions of the pouch. Stool bacterial culture and sensitivity tests are not a part of routine clinical practice but may have some value in identifying sensitive bacteria in the treatment antibiotic-refractory pouchitis.[115] A recent study reported fecal coliform sensitivity analysis to successfully identify effective antibiotic therapy for patients with antibiotic-resistant pouchitis.[115]

CDI can occur in patients who have undergone a colectomy; it has been recently recognized in patients with an IPAA, particularly in those with chronic antibiotic-refractory pouchitis.[90,116,117] Although patients with C difficile can be healthy carriers, fulminant or even lethal CDI can occur in pouch patients.[118] CDI should be excluded in pouch patients with active symptoms with or without endoscopic findings of pouchitis or other pouch disorders.[97] There has been a wide range of reported sensitivities in enzyme immunoassay-based C difficile toxin assays. At present, polymerase chain reaction (PCR) testing seems to be the only single, rapid test method available with a high sensitivity and specificity for directly detecting virulent C difficile.[119,120] Practicing clinicians should have a high index of suspicion of CDI in managing patients with pouch disorders.

Cytomegalovirus (CMV) infection in patients with IPAA was also recognized as a cause that may superimpose inflammation of the pouch reservoir, even if most reported patients were immunocompetent.[90,121–124] Patients who presented as chronic pouchitis refractory to antibiotics and those who have systemic symptoms, such as general malaise and fever, should be suspected of and tested for CMV infection. In the authors' clinical practice, pouch endoscopy with the biopsy for immunohistochemistry as well as CMV DNA by PCR in the blood is often useful for detecting CMV infection.

Laboratory Tests for Evaluations of Systemic Adverse Sequelae Associated With IPAA

The IPAA procedure with or without inflammatory complications can be associated with various systemic and metabolic conditions, such as anemia, vitamin B_{12} deficiency, and bone loss.[17] Early identification and diagnosis of these conditions would help in administering appropriate further evaluation and therapeutic intervention. Hemoglobin and hematocrit are critical for patients with IPAA, because anemia is present in 17% of IPAA patients with underlying UC.[81] Bone metabolism can be assessed by measuring serum levels of parathyroid hormone, osteocalcin, 25-hydroxyvitamin D_3, calcium, alkaline phosphatase, and urinary N-telopeptide cross-linked of type I collagen in patients with IPAA. In the authors' previous study, abnormal liver function tests (LFTs) were observed in 17.4% of pouch patients. The presence of coexisting autoimmune disorders, family history of IBD, extensive colitis before colectomy, the presence of PSC, and a high body mass index were found to be risk factors for any abnormal LFTs. Patients with the previously mentioned risk factors need to have LFTs as a part of their routine evaluation.[125]

HISTOLOGY

Histology evaluation is an important component for the evaluation of pouch disorders. Histologic activity evaluation for pouchitis has been proposed as a part of the PDAI.[126] However, inflammation graded by histology does not correlate with patients' symptoms or endoscopy inflammation scores.[85] Hence, histology has a limited role in grading pouch inflammation. Furthermore, the authors' group has shown that pouch endoscopy without biopsy was the most cost-effective approach in the diagnosis of pouchitis.[127] Subsequently, the authors proposed the modified Pouchitis Disease Activity Index (mPDAI) with omission of endoscopic biopsy and histology from the standard PDAI[126] (see **Table 1**), offering similar sensitivity and specificity for patients with acute or acute relapsing pouchitis.[128]

Histologic evaluation, however, is helpful to identify causes of secondary pouchitis and is useful for differential diagnosis.[90] Villous blunting and mononuclear cell infiltration in the lamina propria may represent normal adaptive changes of the ileal pouch mucosa to fecal stasis. Neutrophil and eosinophil infiltrations and mucosal ulceration are nonspecific histologic features and are found in pouchitis as well as CD of the pouch and cuffitis.[87] Although specific for CD, characteristic noncaseating granulomas are rarely detected in patients with CD of the pouch. Pyloric gland metaplasia, more often seen in CD, was also detected in pouchitis or cuffitis.[87] In addition, transmural inflammation, which is considered as a hallmark of CD, is seen in both CD of the pouch and chronic antibiotic-refractory pouchitis.[129] In a recent study from the authors' group, hemosiderin and hematoidin pigment deposits were more commonly detected in patients with ischemic pouchitis. In addition, pyloric gland metaplasia, a histologic feature of chronic mucosal inflammation, was absent in ischemic pouchitis.[91] Pouch CMV infection has specific histopathologic features on conventional hematoxylin and eosin staining, including the characteristic mononuclear cells with viral inclusion bodies, which are two- to fourfold larger than the surrounding normal cells and often present as a characteristic owl's eye appearance. Immunostaining for CMV antigen using monoclonal antibodies may increase the detection rate of CMV infection in patients with pouchitis.[123] More recently, the authors' group has described a new disease entity: IgG4-associated pouchitis, with the following features: a persistent high serum IgG4 and symptomatic response to oral budesonide therapy; mucosal biopsy showed lymphoplasmacytic infiltrates with abundant IgG4-positive plasma cells in the pouch body and to a much lesser degree of the afferent limb.[130]

Another important role of histology would be the evaluation for dysplasia and neoplasia. IBD-associated dysplasia in biopsy and resection specimens can be graded as no dysplasia, indefinite for dysplasia, low grade dysplasia (LGD), and high grade dysplasia (HGD). Accurate grading of dysplasia is often challenging, because confounding factors such as underlying mucosal inflammation may lead to wide interobserver variation among pathologists.[131] Therefore, consensus signing out for patients with any grade of dysplasia is strongly advocated.[132] Pouch adenocarcinoma is often of mucinous and poorly differentiated type with poor prognosis.[69] Invasive cancer at the time of diagnosis is common. Synchronous dysplasia (LGD and HGD) is frequently present around cancer.[69]

ABDOMINAL IMAGING

There are several imaging diagnostic modalities commonly used for evaluating pouch problems, including contrast pouchography or gastrograffin enema (GGE), computerized tomography enterography (CTE), and abdominal/pelvic magnetic resonance imaging (MRI). Abdominal imaging modalities offer complementary information to pouch endoscopy, which is the first-line and most commonly used diagnostic tool. Each imaging modality has some specificity in evaluating certain kinds of pouch complications.

Water-Soluble Contrast Enemas

A water-contrasted pouchography, in other words, soluble contrast enema, GGE, is useful in evaluating concurrent abnormalities of the pouch, particularly strictures, sinus, afferent or efferent limb syndromes, and prolapse.[87] Soluble contrast enemas can also help detect the leaks.[133] For patients suspected of subtle fistulae, the sensitivity of pouchography was reported to be low, due to the notion that transrectal contrast material often follows the path of least resistance within the bowel lumen rather than opacifying the fistula.[134,135]

CT Enterography

CT currently is a widely acknowledged method to assess pouch-anal anastomosis-related septic complications.[134] CTE is a good tool in investigating small bowel involvement when CD is suspected after pouch surgery. For evaluating pouch inlet, outlet, and distal small bowel strictures, CTE, however, was shown to be of low accuracy.[135] In addition, the sensitivity for CTE to depict fistulae was reported to be as low as 33% to 33.3%.[134,135] In our personal experience, contrasted CTE might be helpful in discriminating causes of pouchitis. For example, mucosal hyperenhancement on CTE, which is one of the leading features of inflammatory pouch, was seldom seen in patients with ischemic pouchitis.[91] CTE or CT of the pelvis is not an ideal diagnostic modality to evaluate the perianal or distal pouch structures, such as abscess, sinus, or fistula. In addition, the findings of inflammation and stricture on CTE are not necessarily correlated with endoscopic findings. A combined assessment is important to improve the diagnostic accuracy.[135]

MRI

Pelvic MRI, in contrast to CT, has been reported to have excellent accuracy for diagnosing extraluminal disease such as abscess and fistulae.[135,136] In particular, MRI is an excellent modality to delineate extent and complexity of perianal or distal pouch fistulae. Furthermore, MRI has also been shown to be helpful for diagnosing mucosal disease as well as transmural disease.[137] However, MRI has a poor performance in detecting short pouch sinus.[135]

Combination of these imaging modalities may increase the accuracy for the detection of different structural abnormalities of the pouch. For patients suspected to have obstructive abnormalities of the proximal pouch or afferent limb, CTE and GGE can be performed before or after pouch endoscopy to provide additional guidance for endoscopic therapy. For patients who have symptoms or endoscopic findings of suspected fistulae or sinus, pelvis MRI and GGE should be considered.[135]

EXAMINATION UNDER ANESTHESIA

Examination under anesthesia (EUA) is performed when a patient cannot be adequately examined without sedation or general anesthesia (eg, for reasons of physical or psychological discomfort) or to provide information that will help guide a subsequent surgical procedure. The goals of EUA could be summarized as follows: (1) to seek clues for confirm size and locations of structural abnormalities, particularly for sinuses, fistulas, and leaks; (2) to seek decisions on further surgical intervention, such as redo pouch or performing permanent ileostomy; (3) to allow examination of patients and use of examination techniques that were not previously possible because of patients' discomfort; (5) provide specific treatment, such as debridement of sinus tract. Although there are scant data on EUA in evaluating pouch problems, it is reported that for evaluating Crohn perianal fistulas, combined EUA with MRI will increase the diagnostic accuracy to 100% in non-pouch patients.[138] Accurate diagnosis of CD of the pouch needs a combined assessment of endoscopy, histology, radiography, and EUA.[63] More recently, an unusual cause of anal pain, as a result of the anastomotic staples that had migrated into the highly sensitive anoderm below the dentate line, has been revealed and resolved by EUA.[139] EUA plus debridement of the sinus tract is found to be useful in patients with anastomotic sinuses after IPAA.[140] In addition, from the authors' experience, multidisciplinary approach including surgeons, endoscopists, and physicians is advocated during EUA.

MOTILITY AND FUNCTIONAL ASSESSMENT

Functional pouch disorders can be evaluated by barium defecography, MRI defecography, and pouch manometry with balloon expulsion.[141,142] The barostat technique is commonly used to study biomechanical features and visceral sensitivity of ileal pouches under normal physiologic conditions.[143–145] The authors' group used this barostat technique to demonstrate visceral hypersensitivity in patients with IPS.[146]

Functional assessment also includes the evaluation of health-related quality of life (QOL). The three-item Cleveland Global Quality of Life (CGQL, scale 0–1.0, with 1.0

Table 2	
Management of ileal pouch disorders	
Classification	**Management**
Surgical and mechanical	
Anastomotic leaks/sinuses/fistulae	Surgery/endoscopy
Pelvic sepsis and abscess	Drainage/surgery
Strictures	Endoscopic balloon dilation/endoscopic needle knife stricturoplasty/surgery
Pouch prolapse, twisted pouch, pouch bleeding, sphincter injury or dysfunction	Surgery
Inflammatory and infectious	
Pouchitis	Antibiotics/5-aminosalicylate/corticosteroid agents/immunomodulators/biologics
Cuffitis	
Crohn disease of the pouch	
Functional	
Irritable pouch syndrome	Biofeedback
Dysplastic and neoplastic	
Dysplasia or cancer of the pouch	Surgery/chemotherapy/radiotherapy
Systemic and metabolic	
Anemia/bone loss/vitamin B_{12} deficiency	Supplement treatment

being the best), and 34-item Irritable Bowel Syndrome–Quality of Life (IBS-QOL, scale 34–170, with 34 being the best) designed for patients with functional bowel disorders have been validated to assess the health-related QOL in patients with IPAA.[87,147]

TREATMENTS

Accurate diagnosis of pouch problems, identification of underlying cause or pathogenesis, and a multidisciplinary approach are necessary for successful management of patients with pouch disorders. Treatments of pouch disorders are composed of two major parts: medication and intervention; the latter includes both endoscopic and surgical interventions. Here, a brief introduction of appropriate management to pouch problems based on classification is shown in **Table 2**.

SUMMARY

IPAA is a technically demanding procedure that requires appropriate skills and expertise. Adverse sequelae of IPAA are common. Accurate diagnosis and classification of pouch disorders and associated complications are important for proper management and prognosis. Based on presenting symptoms, appropriate and combined diagnostic modalities should apply. A multidisciplinary approach involving gastroenterologists, colorectal surgeons, gastrointestinal pathologists, and gastrointestinal radiologists is advocated for diagnosis and treatment of pouch disorders.

REFERENCES

1. Cosnes J, Gower-Rousseau C, Seksik P, et al. Epidemiology and natural history of inflammatory bowel diseases. Gastroenterology 2011;140:1785–94.
2. Parks AG, Nicholls RJ. Proctocolectomy without ileostomy for ulcerative colitis. Br Med J 1978;2:85–8.
3. Sagar PM, Taylor BA. Pelvic ileal reservoirs: the options. Br J Surg 1994;81:325–32.
4. Fazio VW, Ziv Y, Church JM, et al. Ileal pouch-anal anastomoses complications and function in 1005 patients. Ann Surg 1995;222:120–7.
5. Olsen KO, Joelsson M, Laurberg S, et al. Fertility after ileal pouch-anal anastomosis in women with ulcerative colitis. Br J Surg 1999;86:493–5.
6. Rajaratnam SG, Eglinton TW, Hider P, et al. Impact of ileal pouch-anal anastomosis on female fertility: meta-analysis and systematic review. Int J Colorectal Dis 2011; 26:1365–74.
7. Hahnloser D, Pemberton JH, Wolff BG, et al. Results at up to 20 years after ileal pouch-anal anastomosis for chronic ulcerative colitis. Br J Surg 2007;94:333–40.
8. Sandborn WJ. Pouchitis following ileal pouch-anal anastomosis: definition, pathogenesis, and treatment. Gastroenterology 1994;107:1856–60.
9. Tulchinsky H, Hawley PR, Nicholls J. Long-term failure after restorative proctocolectomy for ulcerative colitis. Ann Surg 2003;238:229–34.
10. Belliveau P, Trudel J, Vasilevsky CA, et al. Ileoanal anastomosis with reservoirs: complications and long-term results. Can J Surg 1999;42:345–52.
11. Hueting WE, Buskens E, van der Tweel I, et al. Results and complications after ileal pouch anal anastomosis: a meta-analysis of 43 observational studies comprising 9,317 patients. Dig Surg 2005;22:69–79.
12. Sagap I, Remzi FH, Hammel JP, et al. Factors associated with failure in managing pelvic sepsis after ileal pouch-anal anastomosis (IPAA)–a multivariate analysis. Surgery 2006;140:691–703 [discussion: 703–4].
13. Prudhomme M, Dehni N, Dozois RR, et al. Causes and outcomes of pouch excision after restorative proctocolectomy. Br J Surg 2006;93:82–6.

14. Sagar PM, Dozois RR, Wolff BG. Long-term results of ileal pouch-anal anastomosis in patients with Crohn's disease. Dis Colon Rectum 1996;39:893–8.

15. Grobler SP, Hosie KB, Affie E, et al. Outcome of restorative proctocolectomy when the diagnosis is suggestive of Crohn's disease. Gut 1993;34:1384–8.

16. Lepisto A, Luukkonen P, Jarvinen HJ. Cumulative failure rate of ileal pouch-anal anastomosis and quality of life after failure. Dis Colon Rectum 2002;45:1289–94.

17. Shen B, Remzi FH, Lavery IC, et al. A proposed classification of ileal pouch disorders and associated complications after restorative proctocolectomy. Clin Gastroenterol Hepatol 2008;6:145–58 [quiz: 124].

18. Bernstein CN, Blanchard JF, Houston DS, et al. The incidence of deep venous thrombosis and pulmonary embolism among patients with inflammatory bowel disease: a population-based cohort study. Thromb Haemost 2001;85:430–4.

19. Remzi FH, Fazio VW, Oncel M, et al. Portal vein thrombi after restorative proctocolectomy. Surgery 2002;132:655–61 [discussion: 661–2].

20. Ehsan M, Isler JT, Kimmins MH, et al. Prevalence and management of prolapse of the ileoanal pouch. Dis Colon Rectum 2004;47:885–8.

21. Swarnkar K, Hopper N, Ryder J, et al. 3 years follow-up of a twisted ileoanal pouch. Colorectal Dis 2004;6:133–4.

22. Paye F, Penna C, Chiche L, et al. Pouch-related fistula following restorative proctocolectomy. Br J Surg 1996;83:1574–7.

23. Rossi HL, Brand MI, Saclarides TJ. Anal complications after restorative proctocolectomy (J-pouch). Am Surg 2002;68:628–30.

24. Kirat HT, Kiran RP, Remzi FH, et al. Diagnosis and management of afferent limb syndrome in patients with ileal pouch-anal anastomosis. Inflamm Bowel Dis 2011; 17:1287–90.

25. Baixauli J, Delaney CP, Wu JS, et al. Functional outcome and quality of life after repeat ileal pouch-anal anastomosis for complications of ileoanal surgery. Dis Colon Rectum 2004;47:2–11.

26. Kmiot WA, Keighley MR. Intussusception presenting as ileal reservoir ischaemia following restorative proctocolectomy. Br J Surg 1989;76:148.

27. Stocchi L, Pemberton JH. Pouch and pouchitis. Gastroenterol Clin North Am 2001;30:223–41.

28. Ferrante M, Declerck S, De Hertogh G, et al. Outcome after proctocolectomy with ileal pouch-anal anastomosis for ulcerative colitis. Inflamm Bowel Dis 2008;14:20–8.

29. Gionchetti P, Rizzello F, Helwig U, et al. Prophylaxis of pouchitis onset with probiotic therapy: a double-blind, placebo-controlled trial. Gastroenterology 2003;124: 1202–9.

30. Gionchetti P, Rizzello F, Venturi A, et al. Oral bacteriotherapy as maintenance treatment in patients with chronic pouchitis: a double-blind, placebo-controlled trial. Gastroenterology 2000;119:305–9.

31. Mimura T, Rizzello F, Helwig U, et al. Once daily high dose probiotic therapy (VSL#3) for maintaining remission in recurrent or refractory pouchitis. Gut 2004;53:108–14.

32. Carter MJ, Di Giovine FS, Cox A, et al. The interleukin 1 receptor antagonist gene allele 2 as a predictor of pouchitis following colectomy and IPAA in ulcerative colitis. Gastroenterology 2001;121:805–11.

33. Aisenberg J, Legnani PE, Nilubol N, et al. Are pANCA, ASCA, or cytokine gene polymorphisms associated with pouchitis? Long-term follow-up in 102 ulcerative colitis patients. Am J Gastroenterol 2004;99:432–41.

34. Brett PM, Yasuda N, Yiannakou JY, et al. Genetic and immunological markers in pouchitis. Eur J Gastroenterol Hepatol 1996;8:951–5.

35. Meier CB, Hegazi RA, Aisenberg J, et al. Innate immune receptor genetic polymorphisms in pouchitis: is CARD15 a susceptibility factor? Inflamm Bowel Dis 2005;11: 965–71.
36. Sehgal R, Berg A, Hegarty JP, et al. NOD2/CARD15 mutations correlate with severe pouchitis after ileal pouch-anal anastomosis. Dis Colon Rectum 2010;53:1487–94.
37. Schmidt CM, Lazenby AJ, Hendrickson RJ, et al. Preoperative terminal ileal and colonic resection histopathology predicts risk of pouchitis in patients after ileoanal pull-through procedure. Ann Surg 1998;227:654–62 [discussion: 663–5].
38. Achkar JP, Al-Haddad M, Lashner B, et al. Differentiating risk factors for acute and chronic pouchitis. Clin Gastroenterol Hepatol 2005;3:60–6.
39. Okon A, Dubinsky M, Vasiliauskas EA, et al. Elevated platelet count before ileal pouch-anal anastomosis for ulcerative colitis is associated with the development of chronic pouchitis. Am Surg 2005;71:821–6.
40. Fleshner P, Ippoliti A, Dubinsky M, et al. A prospective multivariate analysis of clinical factors associated with pouchitis after ileal pouch-anal anastomosis. Clin Gastroenterol Hepatol 2007;5:952–8 [quiz: 887].
41. Lian L, Fazio VW, Lavery IC, et al. Evaluation of association between precolectomy thrombocytosis and the occurrence of inflammatory pouch disorders. Dis Colon Rectum 2009;52:1912–8.
42. Lipman JM, Kiran RP, Shen B, et al. Perioperative factors during ileal pouch-anal anastomosis predict pouchitis. Dis Colon Rectum 2011;54:311–7.
43. Penna C, Dozois R, Tremaine W, et al. Pouchitis after ileal pouch-anal anastomosis for ulcerative colitis occurs with increased frequency in patients with associated primary sclerosing cholangitis. Gut 1996;38:234–9.
44. Hata K, Watanabe T, Shinozaki M, et al. Patients with extraintestinal manifestations have a higher risk of developing pouchitis in ulcerative colitis: multivariate analysis. Scand J Gastroenterol 2003;38:1055–8.
45. Fleshner PR, Vasiliauskas EA, Kam LY, et al. High level perinuclear antineutrophil cytoplasmic antibody (pANCA) in ulcerative colitis patients before colectomy predicts the development of chronic pouchitis after ileal pouch-anal anastomosis. Gut 2001;49:671–7.
46. Kuisma J, Jarvinen H, Kahri A, et al. Factors associated with disease activity of pouchitis after surgery for ulcerative colitis. Scand J Gastroenterol 2004;39:544–8.
47. Merrett MN, Mortensen N, Kettlewell M, et al. Smoking may prevent pouchitis in patients with restorative proctocolectomy for ulcerative colitis. Gut 1996;38:362–4.
48. Shen B, Fazio VW, Remzi FH, et al. Risk factors for diseases of ileal pouch-anal anastomosis after restorative proctocolectomy for ulcerative colitis. Clin Gastroenterol Hepatol 2006;4:81–9 [quiz: 2–3].
49. Shen B, Remzi FH, Nutter B, et al. Association between immune-associated disorders and adverse outcomes of ileal pouch-anal anastomosis. Am J Gastroenterol 2009;104:655–64.
50. Shen B, Lashner BA, Bennett AE, et al. Treatment of rectal cuff inflammation (cuffitis) in patients with ulcerative colitis following restorative proctocolectomy and ileal pouch-anal anastomosis. Am J Gastroenterol 2004;99:1527–31.
51. Thompson-Fawcett MW, Mortensen NJ, Warren BF. "Cuffitis" and inflammatory changes in the columnar cuff, anal transitional zone, and ileal reservoir after stapled pouch-anal anastomosis. Dis Colon Rectum 1999;42:348–55.
52. Shen B, Liu X. De novo collagenous cuffitis. Inflamm Bowel Dis 2011;17:1249–50.
53. Shen B, Achkar JP, Lashner BA, et al. Irritable pouch syndrome: a new category of diagnosis for symptomatic patients with ileal pouch-anal anastomosis. Am J Gastroenterol 2002;97:972–7.

54. Panis Y, Poupard B, Nemeth J, et al. Ileal pouch/anal anastomosis for Crohn's disease. Lancet 1996;347:854–7.
55. Keighley MR. The final diagnosis in pouch patients for presumed ulcerative colitis may change to Crohn's disease: patients should be warned of the consequences. Acta Chir Iugosl 2000;47:27–31.
56. Peyregne V, Francois Y, Gilly FN, et al. Outcome of ileal pouch after secondary diagnosis of Crohn's disease. Int J Colorectal Dis 2000;15:49–53.
57. Goldstein NS, Sanford WW, Bodzin JH. Crohn's-like complications in patients with ulcerative colitis after total proctocolectomy and ileal pouch-anal anastomosis. Am J Surg Pathol 1997;21:1343–53.
58. Deutsch AA, McLeod RS, Cullen J, et al. Results of the pelvic-pouch procedure in patients with Crohn's disease. Dis Colon Rectum 1991;34:475–7.
59. Yu CS, Pemberton JH, Larson D. Ileal pouch-anal anastomosis in patients with indeterminate colitis: long-term results. Dis Colon Rectum 2000;43:1487–96.
60. Neilly P, Neill ME, Hill GL. Restorative proctocolectomy with ileal pouch-anal anastomosis in 203 patients: the Auckland experience. Aust N Z J Surg 1999;69:22–7.
61. Gemlo BT, Wong WD, Rothenberger DA, et al. Ileal pouch-anal anastomosis. Patterns of failure. Arch Surg 1992;127:784–6 [discussion: 787].
62. Hartley JE, Fazio VW, Remzi FH, et al. Analysis of the outcome of ileal pouch-anal anastomosis in patients with Crohn's disease. Dis Colon Rectum 2004;47:1808–15.
63. Shen B. Crohn's disease of the ileal pouch: reality, diagnosis, and management. Inflamm Bowel Dis 2009;15:284–94.
64. van Duijvendijk P, Vasen HF, Bertario L, et al. Cumulative risk of developing polyps or malignancy at the ileal pouch-anal anastomosis in patients with familial adenomatous polyposis. J Gastrointest Surg 1999;3:325–30.
65. Thompson-Fawcett MW, Marcus VA, Redston M, et al. Adenomatous polyps develop commonly in the ileal pouch of patients with familial adenomatous polyposis. Dis Colon Rectum 2001;44:347–53.
66. Tysk C, Schnurer LB, Wickbom G. Obstructing inflammatory fibroid polyp in pelvic ileal reservoir after restorative proctocolectomy in ulcerative colitis. Report of a case. Dis Colon Rectum 1994;37:1034–7.
67. Widgren S, Cox JN. Inflammatory fibroid polyp in a continent ileo-anal pouch after colectomy for ulcerative colitis–case report. Pathol Res Pract 1997;193:643–7 [discussion: 649–52].
68. Schaus BJ, Fazio VW, Remzi FH, et al. Clinical features of ileal pouch polyps in patients with underlying ulcerative colitis. Dis Colon Rectum 2007;50:832–8.
69. Liu ZX, Kiran RP, Bennett AE, et al. Diagnosis and management of dysplasia and cancer of the ileal pouch in patients with underlying inflammatory bowel disease. Cancer 2011;117:3081–92.
70. Kariv R, Remzi FH, Lian L, et al. Preoperative colorectal neoplasia increases risk for pouch neoplasia in patients with restorative proctocolectomy. Gastroenterology 2010;139:806–12, 812.e1–2.
71. Das P, Johnson MW, Tekkis PP, et al. Risk of dysplasia and adenocarcinoma following restorative proctocolectomy for ulcerative colitis. Colorectal Dis 2007;9:15–27.
72. Ziv Y, Fazio VW, Sirimarco MT, et al. Incidence, risk factors, and treatment of dysplasia in the anal transitional zone after ileal pouch-anal anastomosis. Dis Colon Rectum 1994;37:1281–5.
73. Remzi FH, Fazio VW, Delaney CP, et al. Dysplasia of the anal transitional zone after ileal pouch-anal anastomosis: results of prospective evaluation after a minimum of ten years. Dis Colon Rectum 2003;46:6–13.

74. Lee SW, Sonoda T, Milsom JW. Three cases of adenocarcinoma following restorative proctocolectomy with hand-sewn anastomosis for ulcerative colitis: a review of reported cases in the literature. Colorectal Dis 2005;7:591–7.

75. Thompson-Fawcett MW, Marcus V, Redston M, et al. Risk of dysplasia in long-term ileal pouches and pouches with chronic pouchitis. Gastroenterology 2001;121:275–81.

76. Heuschen UA, Hinz U, Allemeyer EH, et al. Backwash ileitis is strongly associated with colorectal carcinoma in ulcerative colitis. Gastroenterology 2001;120: 841–7.

77. Veress B, Reinholt FP, Lindquist K, et al. Long-term histomorphological surveillance of the pelvic ileal pouch: dysplasia develops in a subgroup of patients. Gastroenterology 1995;109:1090–7.

78. Gullberg K, Stahlberg D, Liljeqvist L, et al. Neoplastic transformation of the pelvic pouch mucosa in patients with ulcerative colitis. Gastroenterology 1997;112:1487–92.

79. Freeman H. Dysplasia-associated polypoid mucosal lesion in a pelvic pouch after restorative proctocolectomy for ulcerative colitis. Can J Gastroenterol 2001;15: 485–8.

80. Rahman M, Desmond P, Mortensen N, et al. The clinical impact of primary sclerosing cholangitis in patients with an ileal pouch-anal anastomosis for ulcerative colitis. Int J Colorectal Dis 2011;26:553–9.

81. Oikonomou IK, Fazio VW, Remzi FH, et al. Risk factors for anemia in patients with ileal pouch-anal anastomosis. Dis Colon Rectum 2007;50:69–74.

82. Kuisma J, Luukkonen P, Jarvinen H, et al. Risk of osteopenia after proctocolectomy and ileal pouch-anal anastomosis for ulcerative colitis. Scand J Gastroenterol 2002;37:171–6.

83. Shen B, Remzi FH, Oikonomou IK, et al. Risk factors for low bone mass in patients with ulcerative colitis following ileal pouch-anal anastomosis. Am J Gastroenterol 2009;104:639–46.

84. Miller HL, Farraye FA, Coukos J, et al. Vitamin D deficiency and insufficiency are common in ulcerative colitis patients after ileal pouch-anal anastomosis. Inflamm Bowel Dis 2012. [Epub ahead of print].

85. Shen B, Achkar JP, Lashner BA, et al. Endoscopic and histologic evaluation together with symptom assessment are required to diagnose pouchitis. Gastroenterology 2001;121:261–7.

86. Lohmuller JL, Pemberton JH, Dozois RR, et al. Pouchitis and extraintestinal manifestations of inflammatory bowel disease after ileal pouch-anal anastomosis. Ann Surg 1990;211:622–7 [discussion: 627–9].

87. Shen B, Fazio VW, Remzi FH, et al. Comprehensive evaluation of inflammatory and noninflammatory sequelae of ileal pouch-anal anastomoses. Am J Gastroenterol 2005;100:93–101.

88. Wasmuth HH, Trano G, Endreseth BH, et al. Primary sclerosing cholangitis and extraintestinal manifestations in patients with ulcerative colitis and ileal pouch-anal anastomosis. J Gastrointest Surg 2010;14:1099–104.

89. McLaughlin SD, Clark SK, Thomas-Gibson S, et al. Guide to endoscopy of the ileo-anal pouch following restorative proctocolectomy with ileal pouch-anal anastomosis; indications, technique, and management of common findings. Inflamm Bowel Dis 2009;15:1256–63.

90. Navaneethan U, Shen B. Secondary pouchitis: those with identifiable etiopathogenetic or triggering factors. Am J Gastroenterol 2010;105:51–64.

91. Shen B, Plesec TP, Remer E, et al. Asymmetric endoscopic inflammation of the ileal pouch: a sign of ischemic pouchitis? Inflamm Bowel Dis 2010;16:836–46.

92. Hurlstone DP, Shorthouse AJ, Cross SS, et al. High-magnification chromoscopic pouchoscopy: a novel in vivo technique for surveillance of the anal transition zone and columnar cuff following ileal pouch-anal anastomosis. Tech Coloproctol 2004; 8:173–8 [discussion: 178].

93. Shen B, Fazio VW, Remzi FH, et al. Endoscopic balloon dilation of ileal pouch strictures. Am J Gastroenterol 2004;99:2340–7.

94. Obusez EC, Lian L, Oberc A, et al. Multimedia article. Successful endoscopic wire-guided balloon dilatation of angulated and tight ileal pouch strictures without fluoroscopy. Surg Endosc 2011;25:1306.

95. Li Y, Shen B. Doppler ultrasound-guided endoscopic needle-knife treatment of an anastomostic stricture following subtotal colectomy. Endoscopy 2011;43(Suppl 2 UCTN):E343.

96. Lian L, Geisler D, Shen B. Endoscopic needle knife treatment of chronic presacral sinus at the anastomosis at an ileal pouch-anal anastomosis. Endoscopy 2010; 42(Suppl 2):E14.

97. Navaneethan U, Shen B. Laboratory tests for patients with ileal pouch-anal anastomosis: clinical utility in predicting, diagnosing, and monitoring pouch disorders. Am J Gastroenterol 2009;104:2606–15.

98. Goldberg PA, Herbst F, Beckett CG, et al. Leucocyte typing, cytokine expression, and epithelial turnover in the ileal pouch in patients with ulcerative colitis and familial adenomatous polyposis. Gut 1996;38:549–53.

99. Stallmach A, Schafer F, Hoffmann S, et al. Increased state of activation of CD4 positive T cells and elevated interferon gamma production in pouchitis. Gut 1998; 43:499–505.

100. Thomas PD, Forbes A, Nicholls RJ, et al. Altered expression of the lymphocyte activation markers CD30 and CD27 in patients with pouchitis. Scand J Gastroenterol 2001;36:258–64.

101. Fleshner P, Ippoliti A, Dubinsky M, et al. Both preoperative perinuclear antineutrophil cytoplasmic antibody and anti-CBir1 expression in ulcerative colitis patients influence pouchitis development after ileal pouch-anal anastomosis. Clin Gastroenterol Hepatol 2008;6:561–8.

102. Tyler AD, Milgrom R, Xu W, et al. Anti-microbial antibodies are associated with a Crohn's disease-like phenotype following ileal pouch-anal anastomosis. Clin Gastroenterol Hepatol 2011. [Epub ahead of print].

103. Melmed GY, Fleshner PR, Bardakcioglu O, et al. Family history and serology predict Crohn's disease after ileal pouch-anal anastomosis for ulcerative colitis. Dis Colon Rectum 2008;51:100–8.

104. Dendrinos KG, Becker JM, Stucchi AF, et al. Anti-Saccharomyces cerevisiae antibodies are associated with the development of postoperative fistulas following ileal pouch-anal anastomosis. J Gastrointest Surg 2006;10:1060–4.

105. M'Koma AE. Serum biochemical evaluation of patients with functional pouches ten to 20 years after restorative proctocolectomy. Int J Colorectal Dis 2006;21: 711–20.

106. Lu H, Lian L, Navaneethan U, et al. Clinical utility of C-reactive protein in patients with ileal pouch anal anastomosis. Inflamm Bowel Dis 2010;16:1678–84.

107. Lian L, Remzi FH, Kiran RP, et al. Clinical implication of false-positive celiac serology in patients with ileal pouch. Dis Colon Rectum 2010;53:1446–51.

108. Navaneethan U, Venkatesh PG, Manilich E, et al. Prevalence and clinical implications of positive serum anti-microsomal antibodies in symptomatic patients with ileal pouches. J Gastrointest Surg 2011;15:1577–82.

109. Walkowiak J, Banasiewicz T, Krokowicz P, et al. Fecal pyruvate kinase (M2-PK): a new predictor for inflammation and severity of pouchitis. Scand J Gastroenterol 2005;40:1493–4.

110. Johnson MW, Maestranzi S, Duffy AM, et al. Faecal calprotectin: a noninvasive diagnostic tool and marker of severity in pouchitis. Eur J Gastroenterol Hepatol 2008;20:174–9.

111. Pakarinen MP, Koivusalo A, Natunen J, et al. Fecal calprotectin mirrors inflammation of the distal ileum and bowel function after restorative proctocolectomy for pediatric-onset ulcerative colitis. Inflamm Bowel Dis 2010;16:482–6.

112. Parsi MA, Shen B, Achkar JP, et al. Fecal lactoferrin for diagnosis of symptomatic patients with ileal pouch-anal anastomosis. Gastroenterology 2004;126:1280–6.

113. Lim M, Gonsalves S, Thekkinkattil D, et al. The assessment of a rapid noninvasive immunochromatographic assay test for fecal lactoferrin in patients with suspected inflammation of the ileal pouch. Dis Colon Rectum 2008;51:96–9.

114. Parsi MA, Ellis JJ, Lashner BA. Cost-effectiveness of quantitative fecal lactoferrin assay for diagnosis of symptomatic patients with ileal pouch-anal anastomosis. J Clin Gastroenterol 2008;42:799–805.

115. McLaughlin SD, Clark SK, Shafi S, et al. Fecal coliform testing to identify effective antibiotic therapies for patients with antibiotic-resistant pouchitis. Clin Gastroenterol Hepatol 2009;7:545–8.

116. Shen B, Goldblum JR, Hull TL, et al. Clostridium difficile-associated pouchitis. Dig Dis Sci 2006;51:2361–4.

117. Shen BO, Jiang ZD, Fazio VW, et al. Clostridium difficile infection in patients with ileal pouch-anal anastomosis. Clin Gastroenterol Hepatol 2008;6:782–8.

118. Shen B, Remzi FH, Fazio VW. Fulminant Clostridium difficile-associated pouchitis with a fatal outcome. Nat Rev Gastroenterol Hepatol 2009;6:492–5.

119. Cohen SH, Gerding DN, Johnson S, et al. Clinical practice guidelines for Clostridium difficile infection in adults: 2010 update by the society for healthcare epidemiology of America (SHEA) and the infectious diseases society of America (IDSA). Infect Control Hosp Epidemiol 2010;31:431–55.

120. Peterson LR, Mehta MS, Patel PA, et al. Laboratory testing for Clostridium difficile infection: light at the end of the tunnel. Am J Clin Pathol 2011;136:372–80.

121. Moonka D, Furth EE, MacDermott RP, et al. Pouchitis associated with primary cytomegalovirus infection. Am J Gastroenterol 1998;93:264–6.

122. Munoz-Juarez M, Pemberton JH, Sandborn WJ, et al. Misdiagnosis of specific cytomegalovirus infection of the ileoanal pouch as refractory idiopathic chronic pouchitis: report of two cases. Dis Colon Rectum 1999;42:117–20.

123. Casadesus D, Tani T, Wakai T, et al. Possible role of human cytomegalovirus in pouchitis after proctocolectomy with ileal pouch-anal anastomosis in patients with ulcerative colitis. World J Gastroenterol 2007;13:1085–9.

124. He X, Bennett AE, Lian L, et al. Recurrent cytomegalovirus infection in ileal pouch-anal anastomosis for ulcerative colitis. Inflamm Bowel Dis 2010;16:903–4.

125. Navaneethan U, Remzi FH, Nutter B, et al. Risk factors for abnormal liver function tests in patients with ileal pouch-anal anastomosis for underlying inflammatory bowel disease. Am J Gastroenterol 2009;104:2467–75.

126. Sandborn WJ, Tremaine WJ, Batts KP, et al. Pouchitis after ileal pouch-anal anastomosis: a Pouchitis Disease Activity Index. Mayo Clin Proc 1994;69:409–15.

127. Shen B, Shermock KM, Fazio VW, et al. A cost-effectiveness analysis of diagnostic strategies for symptomatic patients with ileal pouch-anal anastomosis. Am J Gastroenterol 2003;98:2460–7.

128. Shen B, Achkar J, Connor JT, et al. Modified pouchitis disease activity index. Dis Colon Rectum 2003;46:748–53.

129. Liu ZX, Deroche T, Remzi FH, et al. Transmural inflammation is not pathognomonic for Crohn's disease of the pouch. Surg Endosc 2011;25:3509–17.

130. Shen B, Bennett AE, Navaneethan U. IgG4-associated pouchitis. Inflamm Bowel Dis 2011;17:1247–8.

131. Odze RD, Goldblum J, Noffsinger A, et al. Interobserver variability in the diagnosis of ulcerative colitis-associated dysplasia by telepathology. Mod Pathol 2002; 15:379–86.

132. Itzkowitz SH, Present DH, Crohn's and Colitis Foundation of America Colon Cancer in IBD Study Group. Consensus conference: colorectal cancer screening and surveillance in inflammatory bowel disease. Inflamm Bowel Dis 2005;11:314–21.

133. Hrung JM, Levine MS, Rombeau JL, et al. Total proctocolectomy and ileoanal pouch: the role of contrast studies for evaluating postoperative leaks. Abdom Imaging 1998;23:375–9.

134. Thoeni RF, Fell SC, Engelstad B, et al. Ileoanal pouches: comparison of CT, scintigraphy, and contrast enemas for diagnosing postsurgical complications. AJR Am J Roentgenol 1990;154:73–8.

135. Tang L, Cai H, Moore L, et al. Evaluation of endoscopic and imaging modalities in the diagnosis of structural disorders of the ileal pouch. Inflamm Bowel Dis 2010;16: 1526–31.

136. Libicher M, Scharf J, Wunsch A, et al. MRI of pouch-related fistulas in ulcerative colitis after restorative proctocolectomy. J Comput Assist Tomogr 1998;22:664–8.

137. Nadgir RN, Soto JA, Dendrinos K, et al. MRI of complicated pouchitis. AJR Am J Roentgenol 2006;187:W386–91.

138. Schwartz DA, Wiersema MJ, Dudiak KM, et al. A comparison of endoscopic ultrasound, magnetic resonance imaging, and exam under anesthesia for evaluation of Crohn's perianal fistulas. Gastroenterology 2001;121:1064–72.

139. Merchea A, Dozois EJ. An unusual cause of anal pain following ileal pouch-anal anastomosis. Tech Coloproctol 2011. [Epub ahead of print].

140. Akbari RP, Madoff RD, Parker SC, et al. Anastomotic sinuses after ileoanal pouch construction: incidence, management, and outcome. Dis Colon Rectum 2009;52: 452–5.

141. Navaneethan U, Shen B. Diagnosis and management of pouchitis and ileoanal pouch dysfunction. Curr Gastroenterol Rep 2010;12:485–94.

142. Selvaggi F, Cuocolo A, Giuliani A, et al. The role of scintigraphic defecography in the assessment of bowel function after restorative proctocolectomy for ulcerative colitis. Int J Colorectal Dis 2006;21:448–52.

143. Steens J, Penning C, Bemelman WA, et al. Comparison of ileoanal pouch and rectal function measured by barostat. Dig Dis Sci 2001;46:731–8.

144. Steens J, Bemelman WA, Meijerink WJ, et al. Ileoanal pouch function is related to postprandial pouch tone. Br J Surg 2001;88:1492–7.

145. Steens J, Penning C, Brussee J, et al. Prospective evaluation of ileoanal pouch characteristics measured by barostat. Dis Colon Rectum 2002;45:1295–303.

146. Shen B, Sanmiguel C, Bennett AE, et al. Irritable pouch syndrome is characterized by visceral hypersensitivity. Inflamm Bowel Dis 2011;17:994–1002.

147. Fazio VW, O'Riordain MG, Lavery IC, et al. Long-term functional outcome and quality of life after stapled restorative proctocolectomy. Ann Surg 1999;230: 575–84 [discussion: 584–6].

The Evaluation and Treatment of Crohn Perianal Fistulae: EUA, EUS, MRI, and Other Imaging Modalities

Paul E. Wise, MD[a], David A. Schwartz, MD[b],*

KEYWORDS

- Crohn disease • EUS • Examination under anesthesia (EUA)
- Imaging • MRI • Perianal fistulae • Setons

Perianal fistula, defined as an abnormal communication between the anal canal or lower rectum and the perianal or perineal skin, is among the more morbid manifestations of Crohn disease (CD). The development of a perianal fistula is usually accompanied by pain, fever, and purulent drainage, and may even be associated with fecal incontinence. The exact etiology of perianal fistulae in CD remains unclear,[1] but it signifies a more aggressive and refractory disease phenotype.[2] As a result, patients with fistulizing CD generally experience a lower quality of life than CD patients without perianal involvement.[3,4]

Nearly one quarter of all patients with CD develop a perianal fistula, with fistulae being more common in patients with involvement of the rectum.[5–7] Before the introduction of biologic agents, most fistulae required some surgical intervention, with more than one third of patients developing recurrent fistulae.[5]

The introduction of antitumor necrosis factor (TNF)-α antibodies has given clinicians the most efficacious medication to date for treating perianal fistulae. Induction studies using infliximab at weeks 0, 2, and 6 for active CD perianal fistulae resulted in cessation of drainage of all the fistulae present in 55% of patients who were randomized to the 5 mg/kg dose compared with only 13% of those who received placebo ($P = .001$).[8] However, fistulae usually start to drain again if the anti–TNF-α medication is discontinued.[9] Studies looking at maintaining cessation of fistula

[a] Department of Surgery, Section of Surgical Sciences, Vanderbilt University Medical Center, 1211 21st Avenue South, Nashville, TN 37232-0252, USA
[b] Inflammatory Bowel Disease Clinic, Division of Gastroenterology, Hepatology and Nutrition, Department of Medicine, Vanderbilt University Medical Center, Suite 220, 1211 21st Avenue South, Nashville, TN 37232-0252, USA
* Corresponding address.
E-mail address: David.A.Schwartz@Vanderbilt.Edu

Gastroenterol Clin N Am 41 (2012) 379–391
doi:10.1016/j.gtc.2012.01.009
0889-8553/12/$ – see front matter © 2012 Elsevier Inc. All rights reserved.

drainage utilizing the 3 anti–TNF-α agents currently available (infliximab, adalimumab, and certolizumab) for CD have yielded similar results with about 36% to 39% of patients able to maintain cessation of drainage over a 26- to 54-week study.[9–11]

Several factors likely contribute to the low maintenance rates of fistula healing. Perhaps the 3 most significant factors contributing to the high fistula recurrence rates after initiating anti–TNF-α medications are (1) not utilizing surgical intervention to maximize the effect of the medications, (2) failure to initially identify all of the fistulae or abscesses present and thus the lack of control of fistula healing when using anti–TNF-α agents, and (3) the premature removal of setons before a fistula is completely healed.

The body's natural tendency is to try to close the external cutaneous opening of the fistula. This process is accelerated when utilizing anti–TNF-α agents. When this occurs, an abscess and/or secondary or tertiary fistula branch can develop. Indeed, the Present and ACCENT 2 studies with infliximab showed that the rate of abscess formation was high with use of the anti–TNF-α agents (11% and 15%, respectively).[8,9]

Two retrospective studies showed that the durable fistula healing rate could be improved by establishing drainage and controlling fistula healing before beginning medical treatment. In the study by Regueiro and colleagues,[12] patients in whom an examination under anesthesia (EUA) with seton placement and abscess drainage was performed were significantly less likely to have a recurrence of their fistula compared with those who never had surgical drainage established (44% vs. 79%).[12] Similarly, in the series reported by Topstad and co-authors,[13] the authors demonstrated a 69% complete fistula healing rate in a small number of patients treated with combination surgical and medical therapy.

Correctly identifying all of the fistulae or abscesses present can be problematic with digital rectal examination or even during EUA in these patients because of the induration and scarring that can be present in association with the perianal disease. In 1 study, the accuracy of digital rectal examination in defining fistula anatomy when done by an experienced surgeon was estimated to be only 62%.[14] Similarly, around 10% of fistulae are misclassified by EUA alone, resulting in the need for repeat surgical intervention in those patients in whom the fistula was incorrectly assessed.[1]

Last, although the fistulae usually stop draining within 6 to 12 weeks of initiating anti–TNF-α therapy, inflammatory activity persists for weeks to months within the middle portion of the fistula tract. Relying on physical examination alone to determine fistula activity inaccurately assesses the patient's progress, resulting in premature removal of setons or inappropriate changes in medical therapy. Studies using both ultrasonography and magnetic resonance imaging (MRI) have demonstrated persistent fistula activity in nearly all patients even after the third dose in the infliximab induction sequence.[15–17]

Studies have demonstrated that missing occult tracts can result in recurrent fistulae, abscesses, and/or convert a simple fistula into a complex fistulizing process.[18,19] If the fistulizing process becomes complex, the chance for healing is greatly reduced.[12,18,20] To prevent development of a complex fistula and increase the chance of closure, it is important to optimize the tools available to assess the perianal pathology. Therefore, treatment should begin with correctly assessing disease activity and perianal anatomy as well as establishing drainage and providing control of the fistula, even before starting medical treatment. Ideally this can be accomplished through the use of imaging and by working closely with surgical colleagues (**Fig. 1**). The purpose of this article is to review the different imaging modalities available for the assessment of perianal CD as well as the various operative techniques and treatment that can be utilized in these patients. In the future, larger (and thus more

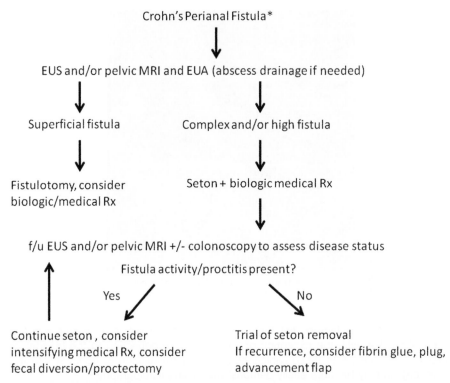

Fig. 1. Algorithm for the treatment of a patient with perianal Crohn fistulae. EUA, examination under anesthesia; EUS, endorectal ultrasonography; MRI, magnetic resonance imaging. *Assumes patient has undergone complete history and physical examination and colonoscopy with or without CT enterography. See text for details of surgical options.

adequately powered), multicenter trials are needed to help guide the optimal management strategies of these complex patients.

IMAGING MODALITIES FOR INITIAL EVALUATION
Fistulography

Fistulography involves inserting a small catheter into the external fistula opening and injecting a small amount of radiopaque contrast material into the tract and imaging the fistula using fluoroscopy. There are several major limitations to this modality. First and most important, fistulograms are not able to directly visualize the sphincter complex; thus, one has to infer the fistula's anatomy in relation to the pelvic musculature. In addition, fistula tracts can be missed owing to the inability of contrast to fill extensions from the primary track, either from inadequate filling or from debris within the track. Fistulography can also be very uncomfortable for the patient and can be difficult technically for the radiologist to even access the tracts at times.

Studies assessing the use of fistulography have found its accuracy to range from 16% to 50%.[21,22] In 1 representative study, the results from fistulography were compared with operative findings in 25 patients.[22] Accuracy was 16%, with a false-positive rate of 12%. This study also showed the false-positive results resulted in unnecessary complications in some patients.

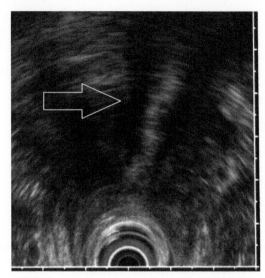

Fig. 2. Rectal EUS showing large trans-sphincteric fistula anteriorly (*arrow*).

Because of these factors, fistulography is not widely used in assessment of CD perianal fistulae, with the exception of times when a connection to the bladder or vagina is suspected. In these clinical scenarios, extravasation of contrast into the other organs may be more easily demonstrated using fistulography.

Axial Computed Tomography

Computed tomography (CT) has been widely used for the evaluation of perianal fistulae. The main factor limiting CT's accuracy for perianal fistulae is its poor spatial resolution in the pelvis, although it is better than that of fistulography. In addition, because the tissue characteristics are very similar, it can be difficult to differentiate between a fistula tract and inflammation using CT imaging. In a small, prospective study of 25 patients, CT was compared with rectal endosonography using a 5-MHz radial probe. The gold standard in this study was either operative findings or clinical course. They found endosonography to be more accurate than CT (82% vs. 24%).[23] CT is primarily used for the assessment of abscesses, fluid collections, or other pathology higher in the pelvis or abdomen than for assessment of the perianal tracts themselves.

Endoscopic Ultrasonography

Rectal endoscopic ultrasonography (EUS) involves inserting either a rigid or flexible radial probe into the distal rectum and anal canal while the patient lies in the left lateral position. Using this modality, fistulae appear as hypoechoic round or oval structures, but can be internally hyperechoic if there is air or gas in the fistula (**Fig. 2**). An abscess usually appears as an anechoic or hypoechoic mass in the perianal tissues. Some clinicians also inject hydrogen peroxide into the cutaneous fistula opening to enhance the identification of the fistula tract on EUS. The hydrogen peroxide creates bubbles that appear hyperechoic and thus make the fistula easier to identify. In Vanderbilt University Medical Center's experience (D.S.'s personal experience) with imaging of CD perianal fistulae (usually with a 7.5-MHz radial scanning ultrasound probe), EUS can usually demonstrate air within a fistula without the addition of hydrogen peroxide. If air is not seen initially, the identification of the tract can be facilitated by applying gentle pressure to visualize the air bubbles moving in the tract, thus making hydrogen peroxide instillation rarely necessary.

The accuracy of ultrasonography in the evaluation of perianal disease has been demonstrated in several studies.[23–36] Most of these studies have utilized a blind, rigid, transrectal probe. There have been 3 prospective, blinded studies using a flexible echoendoscope in the evaluation of perianal disease. One of these studies compared EUS to CT in 25 patients with suspected perianal CD.[23] EUS was conducted using a 5-MHz radial scanning scope. Results were compared with findings at surgery and/or clinical course. EUS was found to be more accurate than CT in the evaluation of perianal fistulae (82% vs. 24%).

The other 2 studies compared EUS to MRI in a group of patients with perianal CD. In a pilot study by Orsoni and associates,[35] rectal EUS, pelvic MRI, and EUA were compared in 22 patients with CD perianal fistulae. Rectal EUS was found to be the most sensitive modality for imaging CD perianal fistulae. The agreement for fistulae with rectal EUS and pelvic MRI when compared with the surgical findings was 82% and 50%, respectively. Rectal EUS in this study was performed with only a 7-MHz linear scanning probe. A similar study by Schwartz and colleagues[36] (see below) comparing EUS to MRI found both to be equally accurate in the assessment of CD perianal fistulae (91% vs. 87%).

Transperineal Ultrasonography

Transperineal ultrasonography is performed by placing the ultrasound transducer directly on the perineum with the probe directly outside of the anus. To examine the fistula and gain a detailed image, the transducer can be placed above any external fistula openings and moved following any fistula up to their internal origin. Several small studies have shown this imaging may be comparable to pelvic MRI and rectal EUS, and that it can provide an accurate assessment of the perianal anatomy with a sensitivity of more than 85%.[37,38] This may be particularly useful in patients with significant anal stenosis preventing passage of an EUS probe or endoanal coil for MRI.

MRI

MRI and EUS have become the imaging modalities of choice for the assessment of CD perianal fistulae. Most centers now use a dedicated external pelvic phased-array coil to achieve the best images in these patients. Most studies in the literature have utilized a 1.0- to 1.5-Tesla coil with accuracies for assessing the pretreatment fistula anatomy of around 80% to 90%.[36,39–42]

Several studies have compared the accuracy of MRI with EUS in the initial evaluation of CD perianal fistulae.[34–36,40] There has been a wide range of differences in outcomes, largely secondary to variations in the equipment utilized in these studies, patient selection, and operator experience. In a representative study of 34 patients with CD perianal fistulae undergoing EUS, MRI and EUA for initial fistula evaluation, the accuracy for EUS, MRI, and EUA was 91%, 87%, and 91%, respectively.[36] In addition, when any 2 modalities were combined, accuracy increased to 100%. Therefore, both imaging modalities (MRI or EUS) have been shown to be accurate in the initial assessment of patients with CD perianal fistulae. The choice of which modality to use largely depends on local institutional expertise.

The use of MRI has been shown to impact patient care related to perianal fistulae. In a representative, prospective study of 56 patients with perianal fistulae (CD and non-CD), the results of the preoperative MRI was withheld from the surgeon initially and then provided once the procedure was finished, allowing the surgeon to revise their initial operation with the new information.[43] The preoperative MRI provided additional information that led to changes in the surgical plan in 21% of the patients. However, if a patient had CD-related fistulae, then the benefit of MRI increased to 40%. Similarly, in study of 71 patients with recurrent perianal fistulae, utilizing the MRI findings to guide surgical treatment reduced the risk of further fistula recurrence by 75% ($P = .008$).[44] In cases where the surgical findings disagreed with the results of MRI, the rate of fistula recurrence was 52%, and the MRI predicted the site of recurrence in all of the cases.

MRI OR EUS TO GUIDE THERAPY AND MONITOR RESPONSE TO THERAPY

Some imaging modalities available for initial assessment of perianal fistulae in CD can also be used to assess the longitudinal response to anti–TNF-α agents or other therapeutic interventions. Several studies utilizing EUS or MRI have shown persistent fistula inflammatory activity even after the fistula stops draining or is no longer symptomatic.[16,17,45–47] This inflammation on these imaging modalities suggests that making treatment decisions based on physical examination or evidence of fistula drainage alone may lead to a higher risk of recurrence or other bad outcomes.

Several investigators have looked at using either EUS or MRI to monitor fistula healing and/or guide treatment. In 1 retrospective study of 21 patients with CD perianal fistulae, the patients were treated according to a treatment protocol of serial EUS examinations. Surgical and medical therapy was tailored to the results of the EUS findings with seton placement and incision and drainage procedures performed when appropriate. Follow-up EUS examinations guided when to remove setons and/or when to stop infliximab or antibiotics. The median follow-up was 68 weeks (range, 35–101). No abscesses developed in any patient. Eighteen of 21 patients (86%) had complete drainage cessation initially, and 16 of 21 (76%) had long-term cessation of drainage. Eleven (52%) had no persistent fistula activity on EUS, and 7 maintained fistula closure after stopping infliximab and antibiotics; the other 4 continued infliximab for their mucosal disease. This study showed that EUS-guided surgical and medical treatment with the use of infliximab had high short- and long-term fistula response rates.

A small, randomized, prospective study of the benefit of EUS monitoring of fistula healing showed a benefit to the use of EUS guidance in these patients as well. One of 5 (20%) in the control group and 4 of 5 (80%) in the EUS group had complete cessation of drainage.[11] In this small study, EUS guidance for combination medical and surgical therapy in perianal CD seemed to improve outcomes.

Similarly, MRI monitoring of fistula healing has also been shown to be beneficial.[4,48,49] In a prospective study of 34 patients with CD perianal fistulae, MRI was done at 6, 12, and 18 months to monitor fistula healing while the patients were on therapy.[4] Those with persistent fistula activity on MRI had their medical therapy increased (e.g., increasing adalimumab to 40 mg weekly). This converted all of the nonresponders to responders by week 52. Therefore, longitudinal surveillance of perianal fistulae with either MRI or EUS seems to improve outcomes for patients with perianal CD by impacting their treatment regimen(s).

SURGICAL EVALUATION AND INTERVENTIONS
EUA

Examination of the perianal tissues and perineum of CD patients with fistulae can often be limited owing to patient discomfort or distorted anatomy. Performing that evaluation in the operating room in the form of an EUA allows for a more thorough examination of the external pathology as well as the anal canal and rectum (facilitated by anoscopy and/or proctoscopy). This is performed with the assistance of anesthesia (whether general anesthesia or monitored sedation) and local anesthetic agents (eg, lidocaine or bupivacaine) to relax patients and their sphincter complex, thus improving visualization of the internal and external pathology associated with the fistula tracts. The fistula tract and its relationship to the sphincter complex can be determined with passage of narrow, malleable probes through the external and/or internal openings of the fistula (and these can be used to guide seton placement as well). If the tracts are more complex, thus making their course through the perianal tissues and sphincters unclear, or the internal opening of the fistula cannot be identified, dilute hydrogen peroxide (usually mixed 50:50 with water or saline) and/or methylene blue (or other contrast agents) can improve the accuracy and effectiveness of the EUA when injected through the external opening. Although EUA has long been considered the gold standard for the assessment of perianal Crohn, as noted, its accuracy is in the 90% range when compared with MRI and EUS.[36,50–52] EUS (with or without hydrogen peroxide) can also be performed at the time of an EUA to guide the assessment and any planned interventions, but there are no data as to whether this improves the effectiveness of the EUA. The clear benefit of EUA over the imaging modalities described is that further interventions can be performed at the time of EUA that can actually treat the perianal CD, including facilitating fistula and/or abscess drainage.

Incision and Drainage and Fistulotomy

The goal of operative procedures for any perianal fistula is to cure the fistula while preserving continence.[53] The initial goal of surgical interventions for perianal CD fistulae and abscesses is to control perineal sepsis through the use of drainage with the placement of draining setons and/or drains, respectively, all while minimizing injury to the anal sphincter complex and trying to avoid large incisions that may not heal well in patients with CD. At the time of the EUA, if an abscess is found (or if it is known to be present preoperatively based on imaging), incision and drainage is performed by making a cruciate incision over the abscess and placing packing, which is removed the next day after which irrigations are used to facilitate ongoing drainage. A "less invasive" but very effective approach is to make a small incision in the skin over the abscess through which a small draining catheter may be placed.[54] The catheter can be left in place as long as needed to allow for continued drainage.

Fistulotomy involves unroofing the skin and other tissues overlying the fistula tract from the external to internal opening, often using the malleable probe through the tract to guide the incision. This is typically reserved for patients with very simple, superficial fistulae or ones that do not involve a significant portion of the anal sphincters (ie, superficial, low trans-sphincteric, or low intersphincteric fistulae). This has been shown to be effective in small retrospective series to treat the fistula (with 80%–100% healing rates) with minimal continence issues, but the patients must be well-selected to optimize outcomes, especially having no evidence of active proctitis because of the fear of poor healing and higher recurrence risk.[50,55,56]

Seton Placement

A seton is a suture or plastic/rubber band or string that is placed through the fistula tract (often guided by the malleable probe at the time of EUA; **Fig. 3**). This helps to maintain drainage from the tract by keeping the external fistula opening patent while allowing any cavities or larger aspects of the tract to narrow by healing around the

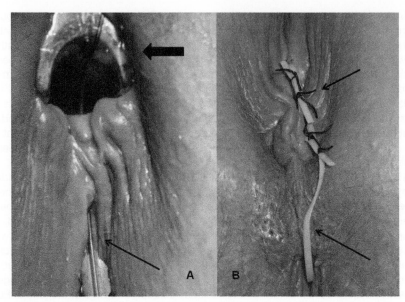

Fig. 3. (*A*) Examination under anesthesia with anoscope (*thick arrow*) in the anal canal with a malleable probe (*thin arrow*) placed into the external opening and out of the internal opening of the fistula. (*B*) Setons in place (*thin arrows*) through 2 fistulae tracts anteriorly and posteriorly.

seton. This is as opposed to "cutting" setons, which are contraindicated in CD patients. Draining setons are the fistula treatment of choice for those patients with active proctitis, more complex fistulae, or fistulae that involve a significant portion of the anal sphincter (ie, high trans-sphincteric, suprasphincteric, or extrasphincteric fistulae). Setons minimize the risk of incontinence when compared with fistulotomy.

As described, outcomes to medical therapy are improved when setons are used in combination with medical therapy for CD to treat perianal fistulae, especially by minimizing abscess formation by preventing closure of the external opening of the tract that occurs with treatment. Unfortunately, even with the setons in place, abscesses can still occur.[57] Initial fistula healing rates with setons in combination with medical therapy is approximately 47% to 79%.[12,13,56] Long-term success of the combination therapy is in the 30% to 40% range, however, especially if medical therapy is not successful in healing any active proctitis.

Fibrin Glue/Sealants and Fibrin Plugs

Fibrin sealants or "glue" are injected into the fistula tract (after initial drainage with a seton for ≥6 weeks) to create a plug, which allows subsequent tissue ingrowth to close the fistula. The procedure is straightforward, causes little to no pain or alterations to continence, can be repeated if necessary, and does not preclude future surgical options in the event the sealant fails. The sealants have been effective in 0% to 57% of perianal CD fistulae, but these data are from subsets of small, retrospective studies (and 1 prospective study in CD patients) with variable follow-up and definitions of healing.[58–61] Although there is little downside to utilizing fibrin sealants for perianal CD fistulae, the cost, poor success rates, and lack of reimbursement from payers has led to its decline in its use in the last decade.

A variety of biosynthetic plugs have also been used for fistulae (being placed through the fistula tract after initial drainage with ≥6 weeks of a seton) and have shown impressive success in complex cryptoglandular fistulae in the earliest retrospective trials, but subsequent enthusiasm and successes have not persisted.[53] Much like fibrin sealants, the fistula plugs are well-tolerated, relatively easily placed, do not preclude other future surgical options, and can be repeated if needed. Small studies have shown early success rates from 26% to 86% with varying follow-up and definitions of healing.[58,62–64] Much like fibrin sealants, however, any initial excitement about plugs in CD has also waned, and many payers will not cover their placement.

Ligation of the Intersphincteric Fistula Tract

The ligation of the intersphincteric fistula tract (LIFT) procedure was first described in 2007 for the treatment of trans-sphincteric fistulae,[65] and involves (after initial seton drainage for ≥6 weeks) dissection between the internal and external sphincter complexes with division and oversewing of the internal aspect of the tract and debridement of the external tract. This has been shown to result in incontinence rates of less than 2% with studies having been performed in complex cryptoglandular disease with 57% to 82% success rates but no studies in CD patients.[66,67] One study combining the LIFT procedure with placement of a biosynthetic graft in the intersphincteric plane ("BioLIFT") included 4 CD patients with success in fistula healing in all 4.[68] Further studies are necessary before the LIFT procedure in any form can be recommended in the setting of CD perianal fistulae.

Endorectal Advancement Flap

Endorectal advancement flaps involve creating a flap or "tongue" of mucosa, submucosa, and (occasionally) a portion of the muscular wall of the rectum from around the internal opening of the fistula and into the lower rectum. The internal opening of the fistula is excised from the distal flap, and the flap is anastomosed to the distal dissection plane to cover the area of the former internal opening and create a "neodentate line," with or without oversewing of the underlying tract. This procedure is usually reserved for CD patients without proctitis and only after initial, less invasive options have failed. The success of this procedure in cryptoglandular disease is in the 80% range.[53,69] The success in CD based on a systematic review of more than 2000 patients (a small subset having CD) is 64.0% (range, 33.3%–92.9%) with incontinence rates of 9.4% (range, 0%–29%).[69] Initial flap failure does not preclude performing a repeat advancement flap.

Fecal Diversion or Proctectomy

Fecal diversion (with a loop ileostomy or [rarely] an end sigmoid colostomy) or proctectomy is reserved for patients with perianal CD refractory to other interventions. Diverting the fecal stream seems to facilitate fistula healing by diminishing the source of infection and facilitating medical and surgical therapy in treating any active proctitis or fistulae. Those patients with perianal CD and fecal diversion have been shown to have equivalent or better quality of life than those CD patients with perianal disease without diversion.[3] Unfortunately, most patients with "temporary" diversion are unable to have their fecal continuity restored, and those that do have the stoma reversed have a high recurrence rate of symptoms.[70] Between 10% and 31% of patients with perianal CD eventually require proctectomy or permanent diversion.[56,70,71] The risks of permanent stoma are increased in patients who require temporary diversion, have more complex perianal disease, have had prior rectal resection, or who have issues with incontinence.[71]

SUMMARY

Perianal fistulizing disease is a common complication of CD that requires a multidisciplinary collaboration between gastroenterology, surgery, and radiology professionals for successful assessment and treatment. Optimal success comes from a combined medical and surgical approach to treat the fistulizing disease (see **Fig. 1**). Unfortunately, even with a variety of surgical options, a subset of patients require permanent fecal diversion and/or proctectomy to successfully treat their disease. Further studies (likely requiring large, multicenter trials) of novel medical and surgical treatments are still warranted to formulate optimal management of this complex condition.

REFERENCES

1. Ingle SB, Loftus EV Jr. The natural history of perianal Crohn's disease. Dig Liver Dis 2007;39:963–9.
2. Beaugerie L, Seksik P, Nion-Larmurier I, et al. Predictors of Crohn's disease. Gastroenterology 2006;130:650–6.
3. Kasparek MS, Glatzle J, Temeltcheva T, et al. Long-term quality of life in patients with Crohn's disease and perianal fistulas: influence of fecal diversion. Dis Colon Rectum 2007;50:2067–74.
4. Ng SC, Plamondon S, Gupta A, et al. Prospective assessment of the effect on quality of life of anti-tumour necrosis factor therapy for perineal Crohn's fistulas. Aliment Pharmacol Ther 2009;30:757–66.
5. Schwartz DA, Loftus EV Jr, Tremaine WJ, et al. The natural history of fistulizing Crohn's disease in Olmsted County, Minnesota. Gastroenterology 2002;122:875-80.
6. Hellers G, Bergstrand O, Ewerth S, et al. Occurrence and outcome after primary treatment of anal fistulae in Crohn's disease. Gut 1980;21:525–7.
7. Tang LY, Rawsthorne P, Bernstein CN. Are perineal and luminal fistulas associated in Crohn's disease? A population-based study. Clin Gastroenterol Hepatol 2006;4: 1130–4.
8. Present DH, Rutgeerts P, Targan S, et al. Infliximab for the treatment of fistulas in patients with Crohn's disease. N Engl J Med 1999;340:1398–405.
9. Sands B, Van Deventer S, Bernstein C. Long-term treatment of fistulizing Crohn's disease: Response to infliximab in ACCENT II trials through 54 weeks. Gastroenterology 2002;122:A81.
10. Colombel JF, Schwartz DA, Sandborn WJ, et al. Adalimumab for the treatment of fistulas in patients with Crohn's disease. Gut 2009;58:940–8.
11. Schreiber S, Lawrance IC, Thomsen OO, et al. Randomised clinical trial: certolizumab pegol for fistulas in Crohn's disease: subgroup results from a placebo-controlled study. Aliment Pharmacol Ther 2010;33:185–93.
12. Regueiro M, Mardini H. Treatment of perianal fistulizing Crohn's disease with infliximab alone or as an adjunct to exam under anesthesia with seton placement. Inflamm Bowel Dis 2003;9:98–103.
13. Topstad DR, Panaccione R, Heine JA, et al. Combined seton placement, infliximab infusion, and maintenance immunosuppressives improve healing rate in fistulizing anorectal Crohn's disease: a single center experience. Dis Colon Rectum 2003;46: 577–83.
14. Van Beers B, Grandin C, Kartheuser A, et al. MRI of complicated anal fistulae: comparison with digital examination. J Comput Assist Tomogr 1994;18:87–90.

15. Van Assche G, Vanbeckevoort D, Bielen D, et al. Magnetic resonance imaging of the effects of infliximab on perianal fistulizing Crohn's disease. Am J Gastroenterol 2003;98:332–9.
16. Rasul I, Wilson S, Cohen Z, et al. Infliximab therapy for Crohn's disease fistulae: Discordance between perianal ultrasound findings and clinical response. Gastroenterology 2001;120:A619.
17. van Bodegraven AA, Sloots CE, Felt-Bersma RJ, et al. Endosonographic evidence of persistence of Crohn's disease-associated fistulas after infliximab treatment, irrespective of clinical response. Dis Colon Rectum 2002;45:39–45.
18. Makowiec F, Jehle EC, Becker HD, et al. Perianal abscess in Crohn's disease. Dis Colon Rectum 1997;40:443–50.
19. Williamson PR, Hellinger MD, Larach SW, et al. Twenty-year review of the surgical management of perianal Crohn's disease. Dis Colon Rectum 1995;38:389–92.
20. Bayer I, Gordon PH. Selected operative management of fistula-in-ano in Crohn's disease. Dis Colon Rectum 1994;37:760–5.
21. Weisman RI, Orsay CP, Pearl RK, et al. The role of fistulography in fistula-in-ano. Report of five cases. Dis Colon Rectum 1991;34:181–4.
22. Kuijpers HC, Schulpen T. Fistulography for fistula-in-ano. Is it useful? Dis Colon Rectum 1985;28:103–4.
23. Schratter-Sehn AU, Lochs H, Vogelsang H, et al. Endoscopic ultrasonography versus computed tomography in the differential diagnosis of perianorectal complications in Crohn's disease. Endoscopy 1993;25:582–6.
24. Law PJ, Talbot RW, Bartram CI, et al. Anal endosonography in the evaluation of perianal sepsis and fistula in ano. Br J Surg 1989;76:752–5.
25. Deen K, Williams J, Hutchinson R, et al. Fistulas in ano: endoanal ultrasonographic assessment assists decision making for surgery. Gut 1994;35:391–4.
26. Cheong DM, Nogueras JJ, Wexner SD, et al. Anal endosonography for recurrent anal fistulas: image enhancement with hydrogen peroxide. Dis Colon Rectum 1993;36: 1158–60.
27. Poen AC, Felt-Bersma RJ, Eijsbouts QA, et al. Hydrogen peroxide-enhanced transanal ultrasound in the assessment of fistula-in-ano. Dis Colon Rectum 1998;41: 1147–52.
28. Mouaaouy E, Tolksdorf A, Starlinger M, et al. Endoskopische sonographie des anorektums bei entzundlichen enddarmerkrankungen. Z Gastroenterolo 1992;30: 486–94.
29. Tio TL, Mulder CJ, Wijers OB, et al. Endosonography of peri-anal and peri-colorectal fistula and/or abscess in Crohn's disease. Gastrointest Endosc 1990;36:331–6.
30. Van Outryve MJ, Pelckmans PA, Michielsen PP, et al. Value of transrectal ultrasonography in Crohn's disease. Gastroenterology 1991;101:1171–7.
31. Solomon MJ. Fistulae and abscesses in symptomatic perianal Crohn's disease. Int J Colorectal Dis 1996;11:222–6.
32. Mulder C, Tio T, Tytgat G. Transrectal ultrasonography in the assessment of perianal fistula and/or abscess in Crohn's disease. Gastroenterology 1988;94:A313.
33. Lunniss PJ, Barker PG, Sultan AH, et al. Magnetic resonance imaging of fistula-in-ano. Dis Colon Rectum 1994;37:708–18.
34. Hussain SM, Stoker J, Schouten WR, et al. Fistula in ano: endoanal sonography versus endoanal MR imaging in classification. Radiology 1996;200:475–81.
35. Orsoni P, Barthet M, Portier F, et al. Prospective comparison of endosonography, magnetic resonance imaging and surgical findings in anorectal fistula and abscess complicating Crohn's disease. Br J Surg 1999;86:360–4.

36. Schwartz DA, Wiersema MJ, Dudiak KM, et al. A comparison of endoscopic ultra-sound, magnetic resonance imaging, and exam under anesthesia for evaluation of Crohn's perianal fistulas. Gastroenterology 2001;121:1064–72.

37. Maconi G, Ardizzone S, Greco S, et al. Transperineal ultrasound in the detection of perianal and rectovaginal fistulae in Crohn's disease. Am J Gastroenterol 2007;102: 2214–9.

38. Stewart LK, McGee J, Wilson SR. Transperineal and transvaginal sonography of perianal inflammatory disease. AJR Am J Roentgenol 2001;177:627–32.

39. Spencer JA, Chapple K, Wilson D, et al. Outcome after surgery for perianal fistula: predictive value of MR imaging. AJR Am J Roentgenol 1998;171:403–6.

40. Buchanan GN, Halligan S, Bartram CI, et al. Clinical examination, endosonography, and MR imaging in preoperative assessment of fistula in ano: comparison with outcome-based reference standard. Radiology 2004;233:674–81.

41. Maier AG, Funovics MA, Kreuzer SH, et al. Evaluation of perianal sepsis: comparison of anal endosonography and magnetic resonance imaging. J Magn Reson Imaging 2001;14:254–60.

42. Al-Khawari HA, Gupta R, Sinan TS, et al. Role of magnetic resonance imaging in the assessment of perianal fistulas. Med Princ Pract 2005;14:46–52.

43. Beets-Tan RG, Beets GL, van der Hoop AG, et al. Preoperative MR imaging of anal fistulas: Does it really help the surgeon? Radiology 2001;218:75–84.

44. Buchanan G, Halligan S, Williams A, et al. Effect of MRI on clinical outcome of recurrent fistula-in-ano. Lancet 2002;360:1661–2.

45. Van Assche G, Vanbeckevoort D, Bielen D, et al. Persistent fistula tracks in perianal Crohn's disease after long-term infliximab treatment: correlation with clinical out-come. Gastroenterology 2003;125:1025–31.

46. Bell SJ, Halligan S, Windsor AC, et al. Response of fistulating Crohn's disease to infliximab treatment assessed by magnetic resonance imaging. Aliment Pharmacol Ther 2003;17:387–93.

47. Ardizzone S, Maconi G, Colombo E, et al. Perianal fistulae following infliximab treatment: clinical and endosonographic outcome. Inflamm Bowel Dis 2004;10:91–6.

48. Karmiris K, Bielen D, Vanbeckevoort D, et al. Long-term monitoring of infliximab therapy for perianal fistulizing Crohn's disease by using magnetic resonance imaging. Clin Gastroenterol Hepatol 2011;9:130–6.

49. Savoye-Collet C, Savoye G, Koning E, et al. Fistulizing perianal Crohn's disease: contrast-enhanced magnetic resonance imaging assessment at 1 year on mainte-nance anti-TNF-alpha therapy. Inflamm Bowel Dis 2011;17:1751–8.

50. Sandborn WJ, Fazio VW, Feagan BG, et al. AGA technical review on perianal Crohn's disease. Gastroenterology 2003;125:1508–30.

51. Ardizzone S, Maconi G, Cassinotti A, et al. Imaging of perianal Crohn's disease. Dig Liver Dis 2007;39:970–8.

52. Ruffolo C, Citton M, Scarpa M, et al. Perianal Crohn's disease: is there something new? World J Gastroenterol 2011;17:1939–46.

53. Dudukgian H, Abcarian H. Why do we have so much trouble treating anal fistula? World J Gastroenterol 2011;17:3292–6.

54. Isbister WH, Kyle S. The management of anorectal abscess: An inexpensive and simple alternative technique to incision and "deroofing". Ann Saudi Med 1991;11: 385–90.

55. Sangwan YP, Schoetz DJ Jr, Murray JJ, et al. Perianal Crohn's disease. Results of local surgical treatment. Dis Colon Rectum 1996;39:529–35.

56. Lewis RT, Maron DJ. Anorectal Crohn's disease. Surg Clin North Am 2010;90:83–97.

57. Makowiec F, Jehle EC, Becker HD, et al. Perianal abscess in Crohn's disease. Dis Colon Rectum 1997;40:443–50.
58. Chung W, Ko D, Sun C, et al. Outcomes of anal fistula surgery in patients with inflammatory bowel disease. Am J Surg 2010;199:609–13.
59. Loungnarath R, Dietz DW, Mutch MG, et al. Fibrin glue treatment of complex anal fistulas has low success rate. Dis Colon Rectum 2004;47:432–6.
60. Vitton V, Gasmi M, Barthet M, et al. Long-term healing of Crohn's anal fistulas with fibrin glue injection. Aliment Pharmacol Ther 2005;21:1453–7.
61. Grimaud JC, Munoz-Bongrand N, Siproudhis L, et al. Fibrin glue is effective healing perianal fistulas in patients with Crohn's disease. Gastroenterology 2010; 138:2275–81.
62. Schwandner O, Fuerst A. Preliminary results on efficacy in closure of transsphincteric and rectovaginal fistulas associated with Crohn's disease using new biomaterials. Surg Innov 2009;16:162–8.
63. Schwandner O, Stadler F, Dietl O, et al. Initial experience on efficacy in closure of cryptoglandular and Crohn's transsphincteric fistulas by the use of the anal fistula plug. Int J Colorectal Dis 2008;23:319–24.
64. Ky AJ, Sylla P, Steinhagen R, et al. Collagen fistula plug for the treatment of anal fistulas. Dis Colon Rectum 2008;51:838–43.
65. Rojanasakul A, Pattanaarun J, Sahakitrungruang C, et al. Total anal sphincter saving technique for fistula-in-ano; the ligation of intersphincteric fistula tract. J Med Assoc Thai 2007;90:581–6.
66. Shanwani A, Nor AM, Amri N. Ligation of the intersphincteric fistula tract (LIFT): a sphincter-saving technique for fistula-in-ano. Dis Colon Rectum 2010;53:39–42.
67. Bleier JI, Moloo H, Goldberg SM. Ligation of the intersphincteric fistula tract: an effective new technique for complex fistulas. Dis Colon Rectum 2010;53:43–6.
68. Neal Ellis C. Outcomes with the use of bioprosthetic grafts to reinforce the ligation of the intersphincteric fistula tract (BioLIFT procedure) for the management of complex anal fistulas. Dis Colon Rectum 2010;53:1361–4.
69. Soltani A, Kaiser AM. Endorectal advancement flap for cryptoglandular or Crohn's fistula-in-ano. Dis Colon Rectum 2010;53:486–95.
70. Safar B, Sands D. Perianal Crohn's disease. Clin Colon Rectal Surg 2007;20:282–93.
71. Mueller MH, Geis M, Glatzle J, et al. Risk of fecal diversion in complicated perianal Crohn's disease. J Gastrointest Surg 2007;11:529–37.

Optimizing Immunomodulators and Anti-TNF Agents in the Therapy of Crohn Disease

Themistocles Dassopoulos, MD[a],*, Charles A. Sninsky, MD[b]

KEYWORDS

- Crohn disease • Azathioprine • 6-mercaptopurine
- Infliximab • Thiopurine methyltransferase
- 6 thioguanine nucleotides

Randomized controlled trials support the use of the thiopurines and anti-tumor necrosis factor α (anti-TNF) monoclonal antibodies (mAb's) in the treatment of Crohn disease (CD). Nonetheless, lack of response, loss of response, and toxicity pose significant clinical challenges. In this article, the authors review therapeutic approaches and laboratory assays that help optimize the use of these agents. The activity of the thiopurine methyltransferase (TPMT) enzyme should always be determined to avoid thiopurine use in individuals with absent TPMT. The role of metabolite-adjusted dosing in patients initiating thiopurine therapy is not settled. Metabolite concentrations help guide management in patients failing thiopurine therapy. Loss of response to anti-TNF mAb's is a common clinical scenario that is mitigated by scheduled maintenance therapy and by coadministration of immunomodulators. In the event of loss of response to infliximab, further management is guided by measuring the serum concentrations of infliximab and antibodies to infliximab. No commercial assays are presently available to guide therapy with adalimumab and certolizumab pegol. The effectiveness of the thiopurines and the anti-TNF mAb's is highest when these agents are (1) introduced earlier in the disease course, (2) continued indefinitely, and (3) combined as initial therapy.

Disclosures: Speaker for following: Janssen, UCB, Warner, Chilcott, Abbott and Prometheus.
[a] Gastroenterology Division, Washington University School of Medicine, 660 South Euclid Avenue, Box 8124, St Louis, MO 63110, USA
[b] Digestive Disease Associates, 6400 West Newberry Road Suite 302, Gainesville, FL 32605, USA
* Corresponding author.
E-mail address: themos@dom.wustl.edu

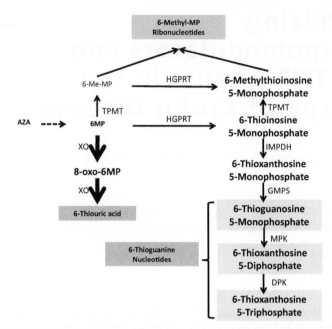

Fig. 1. Pathways for thiopurine metabolism. The majority of 6MP is catabolized by xanthine oxidase. The remaining substrate is anabolized to 6-MMPR and 6-TGN. DPK, diphosphate kinase; GMPS, guanine monophosphate synthetase; HGPRT, hypoxanthine guanine phosphoribosyl transferase; IMPDH, inosine monophosphate dehydrogenase; ITPase, inosine triphosphate pyrophosphatase; MPK, monophosphate kinase; XO, xanthine oxidase.

OPTIMIZING THIOPURINE THERAPY
Pharmacology and Metabolism

6-mercaptopurine (6MP) and its prodrug, (AZA), are purine analogs,[1] which are metabolized via three pathways. The majority of 6MP is catabolized by xanthine oxidase. Xanthine oxidase hydroxylates 6MP preferentially at the 8- position to form 8-oxo-6MP and then the 2- position to form 6-thiouric acid (**Fig. 1**). The remaining substrate is anabolized through two competing pathways: (1) TPMT converts 6MP to 6-methyl-mercaptopurine ribonucleotides (6-MMPR), which are inactive metabolites. (2) In a pathway involving several enzymatic steps, 6MP is converted to 6-thioguanine nucleotides (6-TGN; the sum of 6-thio- guanine monophosphate, -guanosine diphosphate and -guanosine triphosphate), which are believed to be the active metabolites.[2]

TPMT

The activity of TPMT is critically important in determining the balance between the production of 6-TGN and that of 6-MMPR. In 1980, Weinshilboum and Sladek[3] demonstrated that TPMT activity is determined by a genetic polymorphism. Alleles conferring normal (TPMT^N) or low/absent TPMT activity (TPMT^L) are inherited in codominant fashion. Approximately 90% of whites are homozygous for wild type alleles (TPMT^N/TPMT^N) and therefore exhibit normal or high enzymatic activity. The 10% of individuals who are heterozygotes (TPMT^N/TPMT^L) have intermediate enzyme activity. Finally, approximately 0.3% are homozygous for low activity alleles (TPMT^L/TPMT^L) and have low to absent TPMT activity.[3,4] TPMT^L/TPMT^L individuals generate very high 6-TGN concentrations and invariably develop profound leukopenia when treated with standard doses of AZA (2.5–3.0 mg/kg/day) or 6MP (1.0–1.5 mg/kg/day). Although such individuals have rarely been treated with miniscule thiopurine doses, treatment is best avoided. Conversely, individuals with normal or high TPMT activity achieve lower 6-TGN concentrations and lower rates of treatment response.[5–9] Individuals with TPMT heterozygosity/lower TPMT activity display the optimal AZA/ 6MP pharmacokinetics, achieving higher 6-TGN concentrations and response rates.[5–8] Nonetheless, other studies have not found a relation between TPMT activity and treatment outcome,[9–11] It must be kept in mind that although TPMT genotype generally correlates with enzymatic activity, some patients with two normal alleles have intermediate TPMT activity, whereas some heterozygotes actually have normal TPMT activity. The TPMT enzymatic assay is therefore more informative than TPMT genotyping.[12]

Whereas decreased TPMT activity is associated with early leukopenia, myelosuppression commonly occurs independently of a decreased TPMT enzymatic activity.[13,14] One study found that only 25% of leukopenic events were related to low-intermediate activity, whereas the remaining 75% were sporadic events unrelated to the TPMT activity.[13]

Standard dosing of thiopurines is based on weight (AZA 2.5–3.0 mg/kg/day and 6MP 1.0–1.5 mg/kg/day).[15] TPMT measurements may help to guide thiopurine dosing, in other words with standard dosage reserved for normal TPMT metabolizers but lower dosages used in intermediate metabolizers. A recent study suggested the utility of this approach.[10] Consecutive inflammatory bowel disease (IBD) patients starting AZA or 6MP were followed up for 9 months. The thiopurine dose was individualized using 6-TGN concentrations (range, 235–450 pmol/8 $\times$ 10^8 red blood cells [RBCs]) and clinical status. The mean initial dose (as AZA equivalents) was similar (approximately 1 mg/kg/d) for the two TPMT genotypes, but after 9 months the dose was 50% lower in the heterozygous group (0.9 vs 1.8 mg/kg/d, $P<.0001$). Despite lower doses, heterozygotes had two-fold higher median 6-TGN concentrations at the end of the follow-up period (505 vs 273 pmol/8 $\times$ 10^8 RBCs, $P = .02$). This difference was three-fold when the concentration was adjusted for dose (578 vs 183 pmol/8 $\times$ 10^8 per mg/kg/d, $P = .0007$). The results were similar if TPMT phenotype was used instead of genotype. The investigators concluded that initial AZA doses to attain therapeutic 6-TGN concentrations (>235 pmol/8 $\times$ 10^8 RBCs) in patients with IBD might be 1 and 3 mg/kg/d in intermediate and normal metabolizers, respectively.[10]

Although some current guidelines do not endorse pretreatment TPMT testing,[15,16] avoiding thiopurine therapy in patients with absent or very low TPMT activity should prevent life-threatening toxicities and associated costs of hospitalizations (**Table 1**). Indeed, two modeling studies found that TPMT testing is highly cost-effective[21] or even cost-saving[22] compared with a policy of no testing. The Food and Drug Administration recommends consideration of TPMT genotype or phenotype testing before initiating thiopurine therapy but also states that TPMT testing cannot substitute for blood count monitoring.[17] In regards to other enzymes in the thiopurine pathway, there are no confirmed pharmacogenetic variations predicting clinically relevant differences in effectiveness and toxicity.[23]

6-TGN

Studies addressing the correlation of 6-TGN concentrations with thiopurine effectiveness have yielded conflicting results. A metaanalysis found that patients with 6-TGN concentrations higher than 230 to 260 pmol/8 $\times$ 10^8 were more likely to be in

Table 1
Value of TPMT and metabolite testing in 2012

TPMT	• Avoiding thiopurines in patients with absent/low TPMT Comments: 1. TPMT testing may have a role in selecting the initial thiopurine dose (ie, AZA dose of 1.0 and 3.0 mg/kg/d in intermediate and normal metabolizers, respectively[10]). 2. Intermediate TPMT metabolizers may have higher success rates than normal metabolizers.[7,8] 3. TPMT testing cannot substitute for blood count monitoring.[17] 4. TPMT phenotype testing is preferred to genotype testing.[12]
6-TGN	• Characterizing thiopurine failures: ○ Underdosed patients ○ Noncompliant patients ○ Patients with active disease despite "therapeutic" 6-TGN concentrations, who should be switched to other agents ○ Preferential 6-MMPR metabolizers, in whom allopurinol shifts metabolism toward 6-TGN and probably improves outcome[18,19]
6-MMPR	• Monitoring compliance (in conjunction with 6-TGN measurements). Comments: 1. No role in predicting hepatotoxicity.[20] 2. Possible role (in conjunction with 6-MMPR measurements) in preferential 6-MMPR metabolizers, in whom allopurinol shifts metabolism toward 6-TGN.[18,19]

remission (62%) than those with concentrations below the threshold value (36%) (pooled odds ratio, 3.3; 95% confidence interval [CI], 1.7–6.3; $P<.001$).[24]

The potential value of 6-TGN (and 6-MMPR) measurements was bolstered by a study that assessed the effects of dose escalation on 6-TGN concentrations in 51 IBD patients for whom therapy failed.[18] Metabolite measurements were repeated at a median interval of 13 weeks after dose increase. All but 4 patients had "subtherapeutic" 6-TGN concentrations (<250 pmol/8×10^8 RBC) at baseline. The median starting 6MP dose was 0.87 mg/kg/day, with only 22 patients receiving more than the recommended daily dose of 1.0 mg/kg/day. Only 14 of 51 patients (27%) achieved remission (responders) with dose escalation. The change in dose (mg/kg/day) did not differ between responders and nonresponders (median [range]: 0.4 [−0.1 to +0.9] vs 0.56 [−0.15 to +1.2]; $P = .1$). Remission in responders coincided with significant increases in 6-TGN levels (183 [39–298] to 306 [168–853]; $P = .03$). There was a small increase in 6-TGN levels among nonresponders (136 [50–378] to 155 [90–707]; $P = .046$). 6-TGN levels were higher at baseline among the responders than the nonresponders ($P = .006$). The absolute change in 6-TGN levels from baseline to follow-up was significantly higher among the responders versus nonresponders (median: 122 [−2 to +627] vs 26 [−177 to +503]; $P = .0003$). Dose escalation had strikingly different effects on 6-MMPR levels in responders versus nonresponders. Median 6-MMPR levels rose insignificantly among responders from 498.5 (0–2000) to 2345 (264–11,591). Among nonresponders, median 6-MMPR levels increased from 2201 (0–14,412) at baseline to 9346 (0–45,095). The median changes of 6-MMPR were 1908 (+264 to +9591) versus 7986 (−201 to +35,134) ($P = .0057$). Thus, both at baseline and upon dose escalation, responders were characterized by 6-TGN production and nonresponders by 6-MMPR production. These differences were also reflected on the values of the metabolite ratio (6-MMPR÷6-TGN). Responders had lower ratios both at baseline (2.5 vs 18; P<.0007) and at follow-up (9.1 vs 66; P<.0001). Of note, dose escalation produced a similar 3.7-fold increase in the metabolite ratio of both responders and nonresponders. Surprisingly, the baseline TPMT activities did not differ between preferential 6-TGN producers (responders) and preferential 6-MMPR producers (nonresponders). The investigators concluded that metabolite testing identifies IBD patients who are resistant to 6MP/AZA therapy and are biochemically characterized by suboptimal 6-TGN and preferential 6-MMPR production upon dose escalation[18] These findings will require replication in prospective studies. In the future, it will also be important to assess the predictor value of the metabolite ratio by measuring it at shorter time intervals from any dosing changes.

Two clinical trials have compared individualized with standard, weight-based dosing.[25,26] An unblinded, randomized trial compared standard AZA dosing (2.5 mg/kg/d; n = 33) to 6-TGN–adjusted dosing (target 6-TGN 250-400 mol/8 × 10⁸ RBC; n = 25) in patients with active CD (Crohn disease activity index 150–450).[26] The primary end point of steroid-free remission at week 16 was achieved by 43.8% (14 of 32) patients in the standard group versus 44% (11 of 25) in the adjusted group (intent-to-treat analysis). Median 6-TGN concentrations in the adjusted arm were below the target range throughout the trial, and in fact were lower than those in the standard arm. The unblinded design, the selection of an initial dose without account for the baseline TPMT activity, and the nonattainment of target 6-TGN concentrations in the adjusted arm are significant limitations of the trial.

A multicenter double-blind, randomized controlled trial compared the efficacy and safety of weight-based AZA dosing (WD) to individualized AZA dosing (ID) in inducing and maintaining remission in adults and children with steroid-treated CD.[25] In the WD arm, the AZA dose was 2.5 mg/kg/d. In the ID group, the initial AZA dose was 1.0 mg/kg/d (if intermediate TPMT) or 2.5 mg/kg/d (if normal TPMT). Starting at week 5, the dose was adjusted to target 6-TGN concentrations of 250 to 400 pmol/8 × 10⁸ RBC, or up to a maximal dose of 4 mg/kg/d. The primary outcome was clinical remission (CR) at 16 weeks. The trial was stopped prematurely because of insufficient enrollment. In the intention-to-treat analysis, CR rates at week 16 were 40% (10 of 25) for the ID and 16% (4 of 25) WD groups (P = .11). In the per-protocol (PP) analysis (noncompliers excluded), week 16 CR rates were 60% (9 of 15) for the ID and 25% (3 of 12) WD groups respectively (P = .12). Median 6-TGN concentrations at week 16 among normal TPMT metabolizers in the ID arm (198 pmol/8 × 10⁸ RBCs) were below the target of 250 pmol/8 × 10⁸ RBCs, and not significantly higher than the corresponding concentrations of the normal TPMT metabolizers of the WD arm (150 pmol/8 × 10⁸ RBCs). It must be kept in mind that these (albeit nonsignificant) differences in 6-TGN concentrations reflected differences in the final doses at week 16 (median doses of 3.4 vs 2.3 mg/kg/day in the ID and WD arms respectively, P<.0001). As may have been predicted, intermediate TPMT metabolizers in the ID arm achieved higher 6-TGN concentrations than the normal TPMT metabolizers in the same arm (despite a much lower AZA dose: 1.5 vs 3.4 mg/kg/day): median 6-TGN concentrations 212 (88–413) versus 198 (81–246) pmol/8 × 10⁸ RBCs. At week 16, median (range) 6-TGN concentrations in PP remitters (n = 12) and nonremitters (n = 15) were 216 (127–413) and 154 (81–972) pmol/8 × 10⁸ RBCs respectively (P = .07). There were no differences in the frequencies of adverse events, including myelosuppression and hepatotoxicity. In summary, despite a trend in favor of ID over WD, there was no statistically significant difference in efficacy. In the PP analysis, remitters had higher 6-TGN concentrations than nonremitters, but this missed

Table 2
Interpretation of metabolite concentrations and suggested course of action in patients with active IBD in whom thiopurine therapy has failed

6TGN	6MMPR	Interpretation	Action
Low	Low	1. Underdosing 2. Non-compliance	1. Increase dose 2. Compliance
Low	Normal or high	Underdosed due to preferential 6MMPR production	Add allopurinol or switch therapy
Normal	Low, normal or high	Appropriately dosed	Switch therapy
High	Low, normal or high	Overdosed	Switch therapy

statistical significance ($P = .07$). The trial was limited by low statistical power and inability to achieve the target 6-TGN concentrations in the ID arm.[25]

6-MMPR

Elevated 6-MMPR concentrations have been associated with hepatotoxicity, prompting questions regarding the role of routine 6-MMPR monitoring. Dubinsky and colleagues[8] reported increased risk of hepatotoxicity with 6-MMPR concentrations greater than 5700 pmol/8 $\times$ 10^8 RBC, and Nygaard and colleagues[27] found that increasing 6-MMPR levels correlated with rises in alanine aminotransferase. However, elevated 6-MMPR concentrations are expected in many patients taking 6MP or AZA, and most of these patients will have normal liver biochemistries. Goldenberg and colleagues[20] found that 12% of patients on thiopurines had 6-MMPR levels greater than 5700, but none had liver chemistry abnormalities. Because measurement of 6-MMPR for purposes of hepatotoxicity monitoring has a low predictive value, patients are simply followed for symptoms and abnormal liver chemistries. Presently, the value of 6-MMPR metabolite measurements is limited to identifying noncompliers. As noted, 6-MMPR (and 6-TGN) testing may have a role in identifying patients with a 6-MMPR dominant metabolism who are likely to have failure of thiopurine dose escalation and may instead benefit from addition of allopurinol[18,19] (**Table 2**; also see **Table 1**).

Allopurinol Therapy

A pioneering study of the effects of allopurinol on metabolite concentrations and thiopurine effectiveness further supports the concept of a therapeutic window for 6-TGN concentrations.[19] Sparrow and colleagues[19] treated 20 thiopurine nonresponders who were 6-MMPR preferential metabolizers with combination allopurinol 100 mg orally daily and AZA or 6MP at 25% to 50% of the original dose. 6-TGN concentrations increased from 191 $\pm$ 17 to 400 $\pm$ 37 pmol/8 $\times$ 10^8 RBCs ($P<.001$), whereas 6-MMPR decreased from 10,605 $\pm$ 1278 to 2001 $\pm$ 437 pmol/8 $\times$ 10^8 RBCs ($P<.001$). In CD patients, the mean partial Harvey Bradshaw Index decreased from 4.9 $\pm$ 1.0 to 1.5 $\pm$ 0.3 ($P = .001$). In patients with ulcerative colitis, the mean Mayo Score decreased from 4.1 $\pm$ 0.7 to 2.9 $\pm$ 0.7 ($P = .13$). The addition of allopurinol also enabled a reduction in mean daily prednisone dosage from 17.6 $\pm$ 3.9 to 1.8 $\pm$ 0.7 mg ($P<.001$) and led to normalization of transaminases.[19] Allopurinol thus (a) shifted thiopurine metabolism toward production of 6-TGN in nonresponding, 6-MMPR preferential producers, (b) improved clinical responses, and (c) improved liver biochemistries. Subsequent, open-label studies have replicated these findings.[28–30]

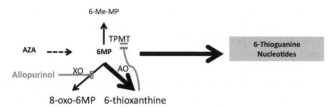

Fig. 2. Hypothesis for increased 6-TGN and decreased 6MMPR on thiopurine-allopurinol cotherapy. In the setting of xanthine oxidase inhibition by allopurinol, aldehyde oxidase hydroxylates 6MP at the 2 position to form 6-thio-xanthine, which is a potent inhibitor of TPMT. The formation of 6-Me-MP from 6MP is suppressed, and the synthesis of 6-TGN is enhanced. AO, aldehyde oxidase; XO, xanthine oxidase. (*From* Blaker PA, Monica Arenas A, Fairbanks L, et al. A Biochemical mechanism for the role of allopurinol in TPMT inhibition. Gastroenterology 2011;140:S–769.)

Randomized, placebo-controlled trials are needed to establish the effectiveness and safety of allopurinol in 6-MMPR preferential metabolizers. Allopurinol inhibits xanthine oxidase, but this activity would not be expected to produce simultaneous increases in 6-TGN concentrations and decreases in 6-MMPR concentrations. TPMT inhibition would intuitively seem the most likely mechanism. Investigators have recently postulated that, in the setting of xanthine oxidase inhibition by allopurinol, aldehyde oxidase hydroxylates 6MP at the 2 position to form 6-thio-xanthine, which is a potent inhibitor of TPMT[31] (**Fig. 2**).

TPMT Activity and Metabolite Concentrations in Clinical Practice

Testing of baseline TPMT enzyme activity is critical in avoiding thiopurines in patients with absent TPMT activity. TPMT testing may have a role in selecting the initial thiopurine dose, in other words 1.0 mg/kg/d in intermediate TPMT metabolizers versus 3.0 mg/kg/d normal TPMT metabolizers.[10] 6-TGN measurements are helpful in characterizing thiopurine failures. Patients for whom therapy fails fall into four groups: (1) noncompliers (absent-low 6-TGN and 6-MMPR concentrations); (2) underdosed patients (low but detectable 6-TGN and 6-MMPR concentrations) who will benefit from higher dosing; (3) patients with "therapeutic" 6-TGN concentrations, who should be given alternate therapies; and (4) patients with preferential 6-MMPR producers, for whom thiopurine dose escalation will likely fail and who should receive alternate therapies. Based on early data, another option in preferential 6-MMPR producers is combination thiopurine-allopurinol therapy (see **Tables 1** and **2**). A recent study demonstrated the clinical usefulness of metabolite monitoring in patients for whom thiopurines fail.[32] Based on weight-based criteria, 50% of 63 patients were underdosed. However, metabolite patterns showed that only 29% of patients were actually underdosed. Nine percent of patients were noncompliant, 53% had either appropriate (40%) or elevated (13%) 6-TGN concentrations, and 9% were preferential 6-MMPR producers. The clinical outcome improved in 40 of 46 (87%) of patients in whom the course of action taken followed the metabolite-directed algorithm, whereas 3 of 17 patients (18%) improved where discordant actions were taken ($P = .0001$; Fisher exact test). Fifteen patients (24%) avoided inappropriate escalation of therapy.[32]

OPTIMIZING ANTI-TNF THERAPY
Biology and Pharmacokinetics of the Anti-TNF Monoclonal Antibodies

The introduction of the anti-TNF mAb's (infliximab [IFX], adalimumab [ADA] and certolizumab pegol [CZP]) revolutionized the therapy of CD. Successive trials proved the efficacy of these agents in the induction and maintenance of remission of luminal and perianal CD. IFX and ADA consist of two TNF-binding domains linked to human immunoglobin G [IgG]1 Fc. ADA is humanized, whereas IFX is chimeric, containing a human Fc region and a murine variable region. CZP consists of a pegylated Fab fragment of a humanized IgG1 mAb. Lacking the Fc region, CZP cannot mediate antibody-dependent cell-mediated cytotoxicity and complement-dependent cytotoxicity. These mAb's interfere with the TNFα system through several mechanisms, including binding and neutralization of soluble as well as membrane-bound TNF (all three agents), apoptosis of T cells and monocytes (IFX and ADA), antibody-dependent cell-mediated cytotoxicity (IFX and ADA), complement-dependent cytotoxicity (IFX and ADA), reverse signaling via membrane TNF (IFX and ADA), and blockade of the CD40/CD40L pathway (IFX).[33–36] Suppression of mucosal inflammation is ultimately mediated by neutralization of soluble and membrane-bound TNF, death of activated immune cells by cytotoxicity and apoptosis, and downstream effects on inflammatory cytokines, adhesion molecules, and regulatory subpopulations of T cells and macrophages.[37–40]

A comprehensive discussion of the pharmacokinetics of the anti-TNF mAb's is beyond the scope of this review. In the context of anti-TNF mAb therapy for IBD, pharmacokinetic studies in this patient population, focused on IFX, have provided the following insights: (1) IFX pharmacokinetics conform to a two-compartment model with first-order distribution and elimination constants.[41] (2) IFX clearance is increased in the presence of antibodies to infliximab (ATI).[41–43] ATIs form complexes with IFX, which are likely cleared by the reticuloendothelial system.[44] Interestingly, one group reported that patients with higher serum albumin concentrations (SAC) maintained higher IFX concentrations, lower clearance, and longer half-life than patients with lower SAC.[45] These investigators postulated that alterations in the neonatal Fc receptor, which protects both albumin and IgG from intracellular degradation, may explain the observed SAC-IFX relationship.[45] (3) IFX clearance is decreased with coadministration of immunomodulators.[42,46]

There are no confirmed pharmacogenetic variations associated with response (or nonresponse) to the anti-TNF mAb's. (For a review, see Vermeire and colleagues.[47]) Ultimately, and despite a tendency to "lump" IFX, ADA, and CZP together, differences in the mechanisms of action and pharmacokinetics may translate into differences in short- and long-term response, as well as safety.

Immunogenicity of the Anti-TNF Monoclonal Antibodies

All three anti-TNF mAb's are immunogenic, irrespective of chimeric versus humanized structure.[48–54] Concerning IFX, the development of ATIs is mitigated by a policy of scheduled maintenance therapy[48,49,55,56] and by the concomitant administration of an immunomodulator, both among patients receiving IFX episodically, as well as among patients receiving scheduled maintenance therapy.[49,54,55,57] Similar to IFX, the frequency of anti-CZP antibodies is reduced by administering CZP regularly and by co-treating with immunomodulators. In PRECISE 2, the rates of antibody formation to CZP were lower in patients who received continuous therapy with CZP (18% among subjects who received induction CZP and maintenance placebo, vs 8% among subjects who received induction and maintenance CZP and maintenance placebo). Anti-CZP antibodies were also less frequent among subjects who received concomitant immunosuppressive agents: 24% versus 8% among subjects who only received induction CZP, and 12% versus 2% among subjects who received induction and maintenance CZP.[53] In PRECISE 3, anti-CZP antibodies were observed in 8.0% of patients in the continuous group versus 17.7% in the drug-interruption group.[51] In

PRECISE 1, the frequencies of CZP antibodies did not vary according to concomitant immunomodulatory therapy.[52] In an open label study of ADA, concomitant immunomodulator therapy at baseline did not did not influence the development of antibodies against ADA (AAA).[50] Because circulating IFX and ADA interfere with the ATI and AAA assays, these assays are indeterminate when the anti-TNF mAb is detected.

Optimizing Response to the Anti-TNF Monoclonal Antibodies

For the currently approved anti-TNF mAb's, response rates to induction therapy approximate 60% at 2 to 6 weeks,[48,52,53,58–60] with higher response rates seen in patients with shorter disease duration.[52,58,61] Despite the high rates of short response, 30% to 50% of the initial responders lose response over time while on scheduled maintenance therapy and require dose intensification.[48,50,52,62–65] Loss of response can occur through several mechanisms, including altered pharmacokinetics (for example, via increased clearance by antibodies to the anti-TNF mAb or a greater burden of inflammation), changes in the dominant mechanism of inflammation, or the development of other processes that decrease response, such as strictures, irritable bowel syndrome, or small bowel bacterial overgrowth.[66]

Maximizing initial response and mitigating loss of response to anti-TNF mAb's are therefore critically important. Clinical studies have revealed a number of approaches that improve outcomes. Higher rates of initial remission and response, and lower rates of loss of response are possible via a policy of high dose induction therapy, followed by scheduled (rather than episodic) maintenance therapy.[48,49,56,67]

Importantly, IFX trough concentrations correlate with IFX effectiveness in CD. Lower IFX trough concentrations are associated with a shorter duration of response while on episodic therapy[57] and with loss of response while on maintenance therapy.[55,68,69] Higher anti-TNF mAb trough concentrations are observed with concomitant immunomodulator therapy among patients treated episodically,[54,57] as well as in patients on scheduled maintenance therapy in the recent SONIC trial.[70] IFX trough concentrations are lower in patients with detectable ATIs.[48,54,57] Importantly, these data parallel those in rheumatoid arthritis (RA). In RA as in CD, low IFX concentrations correlate with treatment failure and ATIs are associated with lower IFX concentrations.[66,71–73] It must be emphasized that the rates of clinical remission in CD are significantly lower in patients with undetectable trough IFX, *whether or not ATIs are present.*[55] Therefore, trough IFX concentration is a primary determinant of efficacy/effectiveness *independent* of ATI formation. There are several corollaries to this observation: (1) in addition to ATIs, any processes that lead to suboptimal IFX concentrations, such as individual pharmacokinetic variability, will lead to lower IFX effectiveness[66,71]; (2) minimizing the development of ATIs should enhance efficacy; (3) theoretically, initial IFX response can be optimized and loss of IFX response can be restored by targeting trough concentrations above the threshold value. Only one commercial assay is available for measurement of IFX concentrations in the United States (Prometheus, San Diego, CA). Patients with IFX at or above 12 mcg/mL at 4 weeks after infusion, or a detectable IFX ($>$1.4 mcg/mL) at trough are considered to have therapeutic concentrations.[55,57]

In ADA-treated patients with rheumatoid arthritis, low ADA concentrations correlate with treatment failure and AAA.[74,75] Few data are available on the clinical relevance of ADA concentrations in CD. In an observational study,[50] ADA primary nonresponders and patients who lost response had lower trough serum concentration compared with those who maintained response. The presence of AAA was associated with lower ADA concentrations.[50] In a retrospective study, AAA was associated with lack of response.[76] ADA concentrations were not measured in that study. An analysis of

CLASSIC I found a dose-exposure-response relationship, but the overlap in serum ADA concentrations precluded the delineation of a predictive trough concentration.[77] Serum ADA concentrations did not correlate with clinical remission in CLASSIC II.[77] In CLASSIC I[59] and in one observational study,[50] concomitant AZA or 6MP therapy was not associated with any differences in ADA trough concentrations. Antibodies to CZP are associated with lower drug concentrations,[51] but there are no data correlating CZP concentrations with efficacy.

Whether concomitant immunomodulator therapy enhances anti-TNF efficacy was controversial until recently. One trial and two observational studies found higher response rates in patients treated with combination immunomodulator-IFX therapy.[64,65,78] However, post-hoc analyses of all but one of the pivotal IFX, ADA, and CZP trials did not demonstrate superior efficacy in subjects who also received an immunomodulator.[79] Observational studies also found no benefit to concomitant immunomodulator therapy compared with IFX alone[55] or ADA alone.[50]

The SONIC trial has settled the question of combination AZA-IFX therapy in one group of patients, namely those who have active CD and are naïve to both AZA and IFX.[70] The trial randomized 508 immunomodulator- and biologic-naïve patients with active CD (40% on prednisone or budesonide) to three arms: AZA (2.5 mg/kg/d) monotherapy, IFX monotherapy, or combination therapy for 26 weeks. The primary end point of clinical remission at week 26 was observed in 30.0%, 44.4%, and 56.8% of the AZA, IFX, and combination groups, respectively (AZA vs IFX, $P = .006$; IFX vs combination, $P = .02$; and AZA vs combination, $P<.001$). Mucosal healing rates at week 26 were 16.5%, 30.1%, and 43.9% (AZA vs IFX, $P = .02$; IFX vs combination, $P = .06$; and AZA vs combination, $P<.001$). Patients were followed to week 30 and given the option of continuing in the extended phase of the trial through week 50, which 280 patients did. Patients who did not enter the study extension were assumed to have had treatment failure at week 50. In this analysis of the entire 508-patient study population, steroid-free remission rates at 50 weeks were 46.2% in the combination group, 34.9% in the IFX group, and 24.1% in the AZA group (combination vs AZA, $P<.001$; IFX vs AZA, $P = .03$; combination vs IFX, $P = .04$). For the subgroup of 280 patients in the extension phase, 72.2% of those in the combination group, 60.8% of those in the IFX group, and 54.7% of those in the AZA group maintained steroid-free remission at week 50 (combination vs AZA, $P = .010$; IFX vs AZA, $P = .32$; combination vs IFX therapy, $P = .07$). The fraction of patients with infusion reactions and the fraction with antibodies to IFX at week 30 were significantly lower in the combination arm compared with IFX monotherapy (infusion reactions: 5.0% versus 16.6%; $P<.001$ and ATIs 0.9% vs 14.6%). Conversely, median trough IFX concentrations were significantly higher in the combination arm compared with the IFX arm both at week 30 (3.5 vs 1.6 μg/mL; $P<.001$) and at week 46 (3.8 vs 1.0 μg/mL; $P<.001$). Finally, infections and serious infections did not differ among the groups.[70]

It must be noted that the SONIC trial likely underestimated the efficacy of AZA therapy for several reasons. Intermediate TPMT metabolizers, who represent 10% of the population and probably achieve higher response rates compared with normal TPMT metabolizers, were excluded. Moreover, more than 60% of subjects in the AZA arm were not receiving steroids; in other words, were not on any inductive therapy. Finally, evaluating mucosal healing at 26 weeks is probably too soon for a slow-acting drug, like AZA. Unfortunately, the SONIC investigators did not perform a multivariate analysis to identify the relative contribution of AZA cotherapy and higher IFX concentrations toward treatment success. This is an important question because the thiopurines probably enhance IFX efficacy by suppressing inflammation directly, as well as by augmenting IFX concentrations. Combination therapy was also found superior to IFX monotherapy in a recent trial in ulcerative colitis.[80]

In summary, the following conclusions can be drawn regarding means of optimizing anti-TNF therapy: (1) With all three anti-TNF mAb's, higher rates of short- and long-term response are possible via high dose induction therapy, followed by scheduled maintenance therapy. (2) Trough concentrations of IFX correlate with effectiveness. (3) AZA-IFX combination therapy is superior to IFX monotherapy in patients with active CD naïve to immunomodulators and biologics. (4) AZA-IFX combination therapy leads to higher IFX concentrations than IFX monotherapy in patients with active CD naïve to immunomodulators and biologics. It is not known whether concomitant immunomodulator therapy enhances the efficacy of ADA and CZP.

Managing Loss of Response to Anti-TNF mAb's

As reviewed, low IFX trough concentrations are associated with loss of response. There are conflicting data on the value of ADA concentrations, and there are no data on CZP concentrations. In addition, there are no commercially available assays for the measurement of ADA and CZP. The following discussion thus focuses on managing patients with loss of response to IFX.

Loss of response to IFX should never be equated with bowel inflammation that has become refractory to IFX therapy. After intercurrent infection, particularly with *Clostridium difficile*, is considered, disease activity should be assessed with standard tests, such as colonoscopy, imaging studies, and serum and fecal inflammatory markers. If there is no active disease, or if the symptoms are out of proportion to the objectively assessed disease activity, then the clinician must consider other processes, such as a flare of irritable bowel syndrome, bile acid diarrhea, or the development of stricture(s) or small bowel bacterial overgrowth. Intuitively, individuals with active disease and low IFX concentrations, or undetectable circulating IFX *and* no detectable ATIs, would benefit from dose escalation. Conversely, individuals with IFX within the therapeutic window (IFX ≥12 mcg/mL at 4 weeks after infusion, or detectable trough IFX[55,57]) would benefit from non-IFX-based therapy. Although switching to ADA or CZP may be effective, non-anti-TNF therapy may be preferable in these patients who may have developed inflammation resistant to TNF suppression. The management of individuals with undetectable trough IFX *and* detectable ATIs may involve increasing the IFX dose to circumvent the effects of the ATIs, or switching to another therapy.

The clinical utility of IFX and ATI concentrations was addressed in a retrospective study of 155 patients.[81] The management of individuals with detectable ATIs (increasing the IFX dose vs switching to another therapy) was also assessed. The main indications for testing were loss of response to IFX (49%), partial response after initiation of IFX (22%), and possible autoimmune/delayed hypersensitivity reaction (10%). ATIs were identified in 35 patients (23%) and therapeutic IFX concentrations in 51 (33%). Of 177 tests assessed, the results impacted treatment decisions in 73%. In ATI-positive patients, change to another anti-TNF mAb was associated with a complete or partial response in 92%, whereas dose escalation produced a response in only 17%. In patients with subtherapeutic IFX concentrations, dose escalation was associated with complete or partial clinical response in 86%, whereas changing to another anti-TNF mAb yielded a response in 33% of patients. The investigators concluded that (1) increasing the IFX dose in ATI-positive patients is ineffective, and (2) in patients with subtherapeutic IFX concentrations, dose escalation is a good alternative to changing to another anti-TNF mAb.[81] The investigators did not address

Table 3
Interpretation of IFX and ATI concentrations and suggested course of action in patients with active CD and loss of response to IFX

IFX	ATI	Interpretation	Action
Undetectable	Undetectable	Suboptimal dosing	Increase dose or frequency
Low	[a]	Suboptimal dosing	Increase dose or frequency
Therapeutic	[a]	IFX therapy failing	Switch to non-anti-TNF therapy
Undetectable	Detectable	Increased clearance of IFX by ATIs	Switch to another anti-TNF mAb

[a] The ATI assay is indeterminate if there is circulating IFX.

the predictive value of the actual ATI titer or the time-point of ATI detection. A high ATI titer at 4 weeks precludes continued IFX therapy, whereas a low ATI titer at 8 weeks may not obviate continued IFX therapy. In contrast, Baert and colleagues[57] found that it was the *titer*, not the mere presence of ATIs that mattered. The median duration of response among patients with ATI concentrations less than 8.0 μg/mL was 71 days (95% CI, 57–88), as compared with 35 days (95% CI, 28–42) among those with ATI concentrations at or above 8.0 μg/mL ($P<.001$). Duration of response was the same in patients with undetectable ATI (<1.7 μg/mL) and patients with ATI concentrations between 1.7 and 7.9 μg/mL. Further data are needed on patients with detectable ATI at trough. **Table 3** summarizes the interpretation of IFX and ATI concentrations and suggested course of action in patients with active CD and loss of response to IFX.

In the absence of commercial assays for ADA and CZP, loss of response to these agents is guided by the clinician's impression of the most likely underlying mechanism. Shorter and/or abrogated response suggests altered pharmacokinetics leading to lower drug concentrations, and should be managed by dosage or frequency increases. Absolute lack of response implies the development of either anti-TNF refractoriness or antibodies to the agents, and is most prudently managed by switching to non-anti-TNF therapy.

THE THIOPURINES VIS-À-VIS THE ANTI-TNF MAB'S

The "rise" of the anti-TNF agents has by no means relegated the thiopurines to the back stage. Indeed, we have developed a more sophisticated understanding of the relative positioning of the thiopurines and the anti-TNF mAb's in the management of CD. Whereas AZA and 6MP produce lower short-term remission rates than the anti-TNF mAb's, remission rates are greater than 30% at 1 year.[70,82] In contrast to the high rates of loss of response seen with anti-TNF monotherapy, thiopurine-induced remission is durable.[83,84] AZA, and probably 6MP as well, augment the efficacy of IFX via targeting other inflammatory pathways and improving IFX pharmacokinetics. Given the ten-fold greater expense of biologics, upfront anti-TNF therapy may not be cost-effective compared with initial thiopurine therapy. Mathematical models and long-term outcome data from patient registries and population studies will help assess the relative cost-effectiveness of different treatment approaches.

Several questions remain: (1) Is AZA-IFX combination therapy superior to IFX monotherapy in patients for whom AZA fails? (2) Do immunomodulators enhance the efficacy of ADA or CZP in immunomodulator-naïve and immunomodulator-experienced patients? (3) Do trough ADA and CZP concentrations correlate with efficacy? (4) How does a strategy of initial combination therapy compare with a strategy of initiating a thiopurine, and then adding an anti-TNF agent for thiopurine failure? Future investigations will also pursue molecular biomarkers to inform other decisions, such as selecting patients suited to thiopurine versus anti-TNF therapy, identifying nonresponders early (without waiting to see clinical nonresponse), and selecting patients in whom anti-TNF induction can serve as bridge therapy to thiopurine maintenance, or patients who can be converted from combination therapy to monotherapy.

REFERENCES

1. Sahasranaman S, Howard D, Roy S. Clinical pharmacology and pharmacogenetics of thiopurines. Eur J Clin Pharmacol 2008;64:753.
2. Lennard L. The clinical pharmacology of 6-mercaptopurine. Eur J Clin Pharmacol 1992;43:329.
3. Weinshilboum RM, Sladek SL. Mercaptopurine pharmacogenetics: monogenic inheritance of erythrocyte thiopurine methyltransferase activity. Am J Hum Genet 1980;32:651.
4. Lennard L. Thiopurine methyltransferase in the treatment of Crohn's disease with azathioprine. Gut 2002;51:143.
5. Ansari A, Arenas M, Greenfield SM, et al. Prospective evaluation of the pharmacogenetics of azathioprine in the treatment of inflammatory bowel disease. Aliment Pharmacol Ther 2008;28:973.
6. Ansari A, Hassan C, Duley J, et al. Thiopurine methyltransferase activity and the use of azathioprine in inflammatory bowel disease. Aliment Pharmacol Ther 2002;16:1743.
7. Cuffari C, Dassopoulos T, Turnbough L, et al. Thiopurine methyltransferase activity influences clinical response to azathioprine in inflammatory bowel disease. Clin Gastroenterol Hepatol 2004;2:410.
8. Dubinsky MC, Lamothe S, Yang HY, et al. Pharmacogenomics and metabolite measurement for 6-mercaptopurine therapy in inflammatory bowel disease. Gastroenterology 2000;118:705.
9. Lowry PW, Franklin CL, Weaver AL, et al. Measurement of thiopurine methyltransferase activity and azathioprine metabolites in patients with inflammatory bowel disease. Gut 2001;49:665.
10. Gardiner SJ, Gearry RB, Begg EJ, et al. Thiopurine dose in intermediate and normal metabolizers of thiopurine methyltransferase may differ three-fold. Clin Gastroenterol Hepatol 2008;6:654.
11. Gonzalez-Lama Y, Bermejo F, Lopez-Sanroman A, et al. Thiopurine methyl-transferase activity and azathioprine metabolite concentrations do not predict clinical outcome in thiopurine-treated inflammatory bowel disease patients. Aliment Pharmacol Ther 2011;34:544.
12. Winter JW, Gaffney D, Shapiro D, et al. Assessment of thiopurine methyltransferase enzyme activity is superior to genotype in predicting myelosuppression following azathioprine therapy in patients with inflammatory bowel disease. Aliment Pharmacol Ther 2007;25:1069.
13. Colombel JF, Ferrari N, Debuysere H, et al. Genotypic analysis of thiopurine S-methyltransferase in patients with Crohn's disease and severe myelosuppression during azathioprine therapy. Gastroenterology 118:1025, 2000.
14. Gisbert JP, Luna M, Mate J, et al. Choice of azathioprine or 6-mercaptopurine dose based on thiopurine methyltransferase (TPMT) activity to avoid myelosuppression. A prospective study. Hepatogastroenterology 2006;53:399.
15. Lichtenstein GR, Abreu MT, Cohen R, et al. American Gastroenterological Association Institute technical review on corticosteroids, immunomodulators, and infliximab in inflammatory bowel disease. Gastroenterology 2006;130:940.

16. Travis SP, Stange EF, Lemann M, et al. European evidence based consensus on the diagnosis and management of Crohn's disease: current management. Gut 2006; 55(Suppl 1):i16.

17. Imuran (azathioprine) [package insert]. San Diego (CA): Prometheus Laboratories I; 2009.

18. Dubinsky MC, Yang H, Hassard PV, et al. 6-MP metabolite profiles provide a biochemical explanation for 6-MP resistance in patients with inflammatory bowel disease. Gastroenterology 2002;122:904.

19. Sparrow MP, Hande SA, Friedman S, et al. Effect of allopurinol on clinical outcomes in inflammatory bowel disease nonresponders to azathioprine or 6-mercaptopurine. Clin Gastroenterol Hepatol 2007;5:209.

20. Goldenberg BA, Rawsthorne P, Bernstein CN. The utility of 6-thioguanine metabolite levels in managing patients with inflammatory bowel disease. Am J Gastroenterol 2004;99:1744.

21. Winter J, Walker A, Shapiro D, et al. Cost-effectiveness of thiopurine methyltrans- ferase genotype screening in patients about to commence azathioprine therapy for treatment of inflammatory bowel disease. Aliment Pharmacol Ther 2004;20:593.

22. Priest VL, Begg EJ, Gardiner SJ, et al. Pharmacoeconomic analyses of azathioprine, methotrexate and prospective pharmacogenetic testing for the management of inflammatory bowel disease. Pharmacoeconomics 2006;24:767.

23. Smith MA, Marinaki AM, Sanderson JD. Pharmacogenomics in the treatment of inflammatory bowel disease. Pharmacogenomics 2010;11:421.

24. Osterman MT, Kundu R, Lichtenstein GR, et al. Association of 6-thioguanine nucle- otide levels and inflammatory bowel disease activity: a meta-analysis. Gastroenterol- ogy 2006;130:1047.

25. Dassopoulos T, Martin CF, Galanko J, et al. A Randomized trial of metabolite-adjusted versus weight-based dosing of azathioprine (AZA) in Crohn's disease (CD). Gastro- enterology 2009;136:A–519.

26. Reinshagen M, Schutz E, Armstrong VW, et al. 6-thioguanine nucleotide-adapted azathioprine therapy does not lead to higher remission rates than standard therapy in chronic active crohn disease: results from a randomized, controlled, open trial. Clin Chem 2007;53:1306.

27. Nygaard U, Toft N, Schmiegelow K. Methylated metabolites of 6-MP are associated with hepatotoxicity. Clin Pharmacol Ther 2004;75:274.

28. Ansari A, Elliott T, Baburajan B, et al. Long-term outcome of using allopurinol co-therapy as a strategy for overcoming thiopurine hepatotoxicity in treating inflam- matory bowel disease. Aliment Pharmacol Ther 2008;28:734.

29. Govani SM, Higgins PD. Combination of thiopurines and allopurinol: adverse events and clinical benefit in IBD. J Crohns Colitis 2010;4:444.

30. Rahhal RM, Bishop WP. Initial clinical experience with allopurinol-thiopurine combi- nation therapy in pediatric inflammatory bowel disease. Inflamm Bowel Dis 2008;14: 1678.

31. Blaker PA, Monica Arenas A, Fairbanks L, et al. A Biochemical mechanism for the role of allopurinol in TPMT inhibition. Gastroenterology 2011;140:S–769.

32. Haines ML, Ajlouni Y, Irving PM, et al. Clinical usefulness of therapeutic drug moni- toring of thiopurines in patients with inadequately controlled inflammatory bowel disease. Inflamm Bowel Dis 2011;17:1301.

33. Danese S, Sans M, Scaldaferri F, et al. TNF-alpha blockade down-regulates the CD40/CD40L pathway in the mucosal microcirculation: a novel anti-inflammatory mechanism of infliximab in Crohn's disease. J Immunol 2006;176:2617.

34. Horiuchi T, Mitoma H, Harashima S, et al. Transmembrane TNF-alpha: structure, function and interaction with anti-TNF agents. Rheumatology (Oxford) 2010;49:1215.

35. Nesbitt A, Fossati G, Bergin M, et al. Mechanism of action of certolizumab pegol (CDP870): in vitro comparison with other anti-tumor necrosis factor alpha agents. Inflamm Bowel Dis 2007;13:1323.

36. Van den Brande JM, Braat H, van den Brink GR, et al. Infliximab but not etanercept induces apoptosis in lamina propria T-lymphocytes from patients with Crohn's disease. Gastroenterology 2003;124:1774.

37. Arijs I, De Hertogh G, Machiels K, et al. Mucosal gene expression of cell adhesion molecules, chemokines, and chemokine receptors in patients with inflammatory bowel disease before and after infliximab treatment. Am J Gastroenterol 2011;106: 748.

38. Li Z, Arijs I, De Hertogh G, et al. Reciprocal changes of Foxp3 expression in blood and intestinal mucosa in IBD patients responding to infliximab. Inflamm Bowel Dis 2010; 16:1299–310.

39. Veltkamp C, Anstaett M, Wahl K, et al. Apoptosis of regulatory T lymphocytes is increased in chronic inflammatory bowel disease and reversed by anti-TNFalpha treatment. Gut 2011;60:1345.

40. Vos AC, Wildenberg ME, Duijvestein M, et al. Anti-tumor necrosis factor-alpha antibodies induce regulatory macrophages in an Fc region-dependent manner. Gastroenterology 2011;140:221.

41. Ternant D, Aubourg A, Magdelaine-Beuzelin C, et al. Infliximab pharmacokinetics in inflammatory bowel disease patients. Ther Drug Monit 2008;30:523.

42. Fasanmade AA, Adedokun OJ, Blank M, et al. Pharmacokinetic properties of infliximab in children and adults with Crohn's disease: a retrospective analysis of data from 2 phase III clinical trials. Clin Ther 2011;33:946.

43. Fasanmade AA, Adedokun OJ, Ford J, et al. Population pharmacokinetic analysis of infliximab in patients with ulcerative colitis. Eur J Clin Pharmacol 2009;65:1211.

44. van der Laken CJ, Voskuyl AE, Roos JC, et al. Imaging and serum analysis of immune complex formation of radiolabelled infliximab and anti-infliximab in responders and non-responders to therapy for rheumatoid arthritis. Ann Rheum Dis 2007;66:253.

45. Fasanmade AA, Adedokun OJ, Olson A, et al. Serum albumin concentration: a predictive factor of infliximab pharmacokinetics and clinical response in patients with ulcerative colitis. Int J Clin Pharmacol Ther 2010;48:297.

46. Klotz U, Teml A, Schwab M. Clinical pharmacokinetics and use of infliximab. Clin Pharmacokinet 2007;46:645.

47. Vermeire S, Van Assche G, Rutgeerts P. Role of genetics in prediction of disease course and response to therapy. World J Gastroenterol 2010;16:2609.

48. Hanauer SB, Feagan BG, Lichtenstein GR, et al. Maintenance infliximab for Crohn's disease: the ACCENT I randomised trial. Lancet 2002;359:1541.

49. Hanauer SB, Wagner CL, Bala M, et al. Incidence and importance of antibody responses to infliximab after maintenance or episodic treatment in Crohn's disease. Clin Gastroenterol Hepatol 2004;2:542.

50. Karmiris K, Paintaud G, Noman M, et al. Influence of trough serum levels and immunogenicity on long-term outcome of adalimumab therapy in Crohn's disease. Gastroenterology 2009;137:1628.

51. Lichtenstein GR, Thomsen OO, Schreiber S, et al. Continuous therapy with certolizumab pegol maintains remission of patients with Crohn's disease for up to 18 months. Clin Gastroenterol Hepatol 2010;8:600.

52. Sandborn WJ, Feagan BG, Stoinov S, et al. Certolizumab pegol for the treatment of Crohn's disease. N Engl J Med 2007;357:228.

53. Schreiber S, Khaliq-Kareemi M, Lawrance IC, et al. Maintenance therapy with certolizumab pegol for Crohn's disease. N Engl J Med 2007;357:239.
54. Vermeire S, Noman M, Van Assche G, et al. Effectiveness of concomitant immunosuppressive therapy in suppressing the formation of antibodies to infliximab in Crohn's disease. Gut 2007;56:1226.
55. Maser EA, Villela R, Silverberg MS, et al. Association of trough serum infliximab to clinical outcome after scheduled maintenance treatment for Crohn's disease. Clin Gastroenterol Hepatol 2006;4:1248.
56. Rutgeerts P, Feagan BG, Lichtenstein GR, et al. Comparison of scheduled and episodic treatment strategies of infliximab in Crohn's disease. Gastroenterology 2004;126:402.
57. Baert F, Noman M, Vermeire S, et al. Influence of immunogenicity on the long-term efficacy of infliximab in Crohn's Disease. N Engl J Med 2003;348:601.
58. Colombel JF, Sandborn WJ, Rutgeerts P, et al. Adalimumab for maintenance of clinical response and remission in patients with Crohn's disease: the CHARM trial. Gastroenterology 2007;132:52.
59. Hanauer SB, Sandborn WJ, Rutgeerts P, et al. Human anti-tumor necrosis factor monoclonal antibody (adalimumab) in Crohn's disease: the CLASSIC-I trial. Gastroenterology 2006;130:323.
60. Targan SR, Hanauer SB, van Deventer SJ, et al.A short-term study of chimeric monoclonal antibody cA2 to tumor necrosis factor alpha for Crohn's disease. Crohn's Disease cA2 Study Group. N Engl J Med 1997;337:1029.
61. Schreiber S, Colombel JF, Bloomfield R, et al. Increased response and remission rates in short-duration Crohn's disease with subcutaneous certolizumab pegol: an analysis of PRECiSE 2 randomized maintenance trial data. Am J Gastroenterol 2010;105:1574.
62. Billioud V, Sandborn WJ, Peyrin-Biroulet L. Loss of response and need for adalimumab dose intensification in Crohn's disease: a systematic review. Am J Gastroenterol 2011;106:674.
63. Chaparro M, Panes J, Garcia V, et al. Long-term durability of infliximab treatment in Crohn's disease and efficacy of dose "escalation" in patients losing response. J Clin Gastroenterol 2011;45:113.
64. Rudolph SJ, Weinberg DI, McCabe RP. Long-term durability of Crohn's disease treatment with infliximab. Dig Dis Sci 2008;53:1033.
65. Rutgeerts P, D'Haens G, Targan S, et al. Efficacy and safety of retreatment with anti-tumor necrosis factor antibody (infliximab) to maintain remission in Crohn's disease. Gastroenterology 1999;117:761.
66. Yanai H, Hanauer SB. Assessing response and loss of response to biological therapies in IBD. Am J Gastroenterol 2011;106:685.
67. Loftus EV, Pan X, Zurawski P, et al. Adalimumab real-world dosage pattern and predictors of weekly dosing: Patients with Crohn's disease in the United States. J Crohns Colitis 2011;5:550–4.
68. Ainsworth MA, Bendtzen K, Brynskov J. Tumor necrosis factor-alpha binding capacity and anti-infliximab antibodies measured by fluid-phase radioimmunoassays as predictors of clinical efficacy of infliximab in Crohn's disease. Am J Gastroenterol 2008;103:944.
69. Steenholdt C, Bendtzen K, Brynskov J, et al. Cut-off levels and diagnostic accuracy of infliximab trough levels and anti-infliximab antibodies in Crohn's disease. Scand J Gastroenterol 2011;46:310.
70. Colombel JF, Sandborn WJ, Reinisch W, et al. Infliximab, azathioprine, or combination therapy for Crohn's disease. N Engl J Med 2010;362:1383.

71. Bendtzen K, Geborek P, Svenson M, et al. Individualized monitoring of drug bioavailability and immunogenicity in rheumatoid arthritis patients treated with the tumor necrosis factor alpha inhibitor infliximab. Arthritis Rheum 2006;54:3782.

72. Mulleman D, Chu Miow Lin D, Ducourau E, et al. Trough infliximab concentrations predict efficacy and sustained control of disease activity in rheumatoid arthritis. Ther Drug Monit 2010;32:232.

73. St Clair EW, Wagner CL, Fasanmade AA, et al. The relationship of serum infliximab concentrations to clinical improvement in rheumatoid arthritis: results from ATTRACT, a multicenter, randomized, double-blind, placebo-controlled trial. Arthritis Rheum 2002;46:1451.

74. Bartelds GM, Wijbrandts CA, Nurmohamed MT, et al. Clinical response to adalimumab: relationship to anti-adalimumab antibodies and serum adalimumab concentrations in rheumatoid arthritis. Ann Rheum Dis 2007;66:921.

75. Radstake TR, Svenson M, Eijsbouts AM, et al. Formation of antibodies against infliximab and adalimumab strongly correlates with functional drug levels and clinical responses in rheumatoid arthritis. Ann Rheum Dis 2009;68:1739.

76. West RL, Zelinkova Z, Wolbink GJ, et al. Immunogenicity negatively influences the outcome of adalimumab treatment in Crohn's disease. Aliment Pharmacol Ther 2008;28:1122.

77. Li JL, Paulson SK, Chiu YL, et al. Evaluation of potential correlations between serum adalimumab concentration and remission in patients with Crohn's disease in classic I and II. Gastroenterology 2010;138 S–101.

78. Parsi MA, Achkar JP, Richardson S, et al. Predictors of response to infliximab in patients with Crohn's disease. Gastroenterology 2002;123:707.

79. D'Haens GR, Panaccione R, Higgins PD, et al. The London Position Statement of the World Congress of Gastroenterology on Biological Therapy for IBD with the European Crohn's and Colitis Organization: when to start, when to stop, which drug to choose, and how to predict response? Am J Gastroenterol 2011;106:199.

80. Panaccione R, Ghosh G, Middleton M, et al. Infliximab, azathioprine, or infliximab + azathioprine for treatment of moderate to severe ulcerative colitis: the UC Success Trial. Gastroenterology 2011;140:S.

81. Afif W, Loftus EV Jr, Faubion WA, et al. Clinical utility of measuring infliximab and human anti-chimeric antibody concentrations in patients with inflammatory bowel disease. Am J Gastroenterol 2010;105:1133.

82. Lemann M, Mary JY, Duclos B, et al. Infliximab plus azathioprine for steroid-dependent Crohn's disease patients: a randomized placebo-controlled trial. Gastroenterology 2006;130:1054.

83. Lemann M, Mary JY, Colombel JF, et al. A randomized, double-blind, controlled withdrawal trial in Crohn's disease patients in long-term remission on azathioprine. Gastroenterology 2005;128:1812.

84. Treton X, Bouhnik Y, Mary JY, et al. Azathioprine withdrawal in patients with Crohn's disease maintained on prolonged remission: a high risk of relapse. Clin Gastroenterol Hepatol 2009;7:80.

Patient-Specific Approach to Combination Versus Monotherapy with the Use of Antitumor Necrosis Factor α Agents for Inflammatory Bowel Disease

Shane M. Devlin, MD, FRCPC[a],*, Adam S. Cheifetz, MD[b], Corey A. Siegel, MD, MS[c], on behalf of the BRIDGe group

KEYWORDS

- Antitumor necrosis factor α • Thiopurines • Methotrexate
- Crohn disease • Inflammatory bowel disease • Infliximab
- Adalimumab • Certolizumab-pegol • Infection • Lymphoma

There is little debate that monoclonal antibodies directed against tumor necrosis factor-α (anti-TNFα) represent important tools in our armamentarium in the management of inflammatory bowel disease (IBD). However, the beneficial effects

The BRIDGe (Building Research in IBD Globally) group is comprised of Leonard Baidoo, University of Pittsburgh, Pittsburgh, Pennsylvania; Brian Bressler, University of British Columbia, Vancouver, British Columbia, Canada; Adam S Cheifetz, Beth Israel Deaconess Medical Center, Harvard Medical School, Boston, Massachusetts; Shane M. Devlin, The University of Calgary, Calgary, Alberta, Canada; Laura E. Raffals, Mayo Clinic, Rochester, Minnesota; Peter M. Irving, Guy's and St. Thomas' Hospitals London, United Kingdom; Jennifer Jones, University of Saskatchewan, Saskatoon, Saskatchewan, Canada; Gilaad G. Kaplan, The University of Calgary, Calgary, Alberta, Canada; Patricia L. Kozuch, Jefferson University, Philadelphia, Pennsylvania; Gil Y. Melmed, Cedars-Sinai Medical Center, Los Angeles, California; Corey A. Siegel, Dartmouth-Hitchock Medical Center, Lebanon, New Hampshire; Miles P. Sparrow, Department of Gastroenterology, The Alfred Hospital, Melbourne, Australia; Fernando S. Velayos, University of California San Francisco, San Francisco, California.

[a] Division of Gastroenterology and Hepatology, The University of Calgary, 3280 Hospital Drive NW, Calgary, Alberta T2N4N1, Canada
[b] Center for Inflammatory Bowel Disease, Beth Israel Deaconess Medical Center, Harvard Medical School, Boston, MA, USA
[c] Dartmouth Medical School and The Dartmouth Institute for Health Policy and Clinical Practice, Dartmouth-Hitchock Medical Center, Lebanon, NH, USA
* Corresponding author.
E-mail address: devlins@ucalgary.ca

Gastroenterol Clin N Am 41 (2012) 411–428
doi:10.1016/j.gtc.2012.01.012
0889-8553/12/$ – see front matter © 2012 Elsevier Inc. All rights reserved.

of systemic therapy for IBD, including immunosuppressive (IS) agents such as azathioprine/6-mercaptopurine (AZA/6-MP), methotrexate (MTX), corticosteroids, and anti-TNFα therapy must be countered against established risks. Because of the wealth of data now supporting the use of anti-TNFα–based therapy, the debate has switched from whether or not to use such treatments to how to optimize their use in individual patients. The debate over the use of concomitant anti-TNFα and IS therapy (combination therapy) versus anti-TNFα monotherapy is central to this question and represents a point of significant consternation for clinicians. This review provides an overview and historical perspective on this question and also discusses a clinically useful approach for individualizing treatment decisions.

THE HISTORY OF THE COMBINATION THERAPY VERSUS MONOTHERAPY DEBATE (HOW DID WE GET HERE ANYWAY?)

With the advent of anti-TNFα therapy in the 1990s with infliximab (IFX), practitioners had at their disposal a rapidly acting and highly efficacious therapy for both luminal and perianal Crohn disease (CD).[1–4] However, because of the significant cost of these therapies and a less clear understanding of the benefits of scheduled maintenance therapy, episodic use of IFX was common both in clinical practice and in clinical trials.[2,4–7] It soon became apparent that the episodic use of IFX was associated with increased immunogenicity as measured by higher levels of antibodies to IFX (ATI) (**Table 1**).[8,9] Rates of ATI were as high as 75% in one study.[6] In a study by Maser and colleagues,[7] episodic use of IFX was associated with ATI in 39% of patients versus only 16% in those treated with scheduled maintenance therapy with IFX. These data are highly relevant when considering the debate regarding combination versus monotherapy, because it was clear that administration of a concomitant IS reduced

Table 1
Incidence of antibodies to IFX stratified by concomitant use of immunosuppressants and by IFX treatment strategy

Study	CON-IS/ATI Pos (%)	No CON-IS/ATI Pos (%)	P Value
Episodic Therapy			
Baert[6]	43	75	<.01
Farrell[8]	24	63	.007[a]
Hanauer[9]	16	38	.003
Maser[7]	0	60	.018
Vermeire[10]	46	73	<.001
Scheduled Maintenance Therapy			
Hanauer[9] (5mg/kg)	7	11	.42
Hanauer[9] (10mg/kg)	4	8	.42
Maser[7]	13	15	.9
Van Assche[11]	5	12.5	.43
Colombel (SONIC)[12]	0.9	14.6	NR
Feagan (COMMIT)[13]	4	20.4	.01

Abbreviations: ATI: antibodies to IFX; CON-IS, concomitant immunosuppressant used; No CON-IS, no concomitant immunosuppressant used; NR, not reported; Pos, positive.
   [a] In observational cohort.

Table 2
IFX levels stratified by concomitant use of immunosuppressants and by IFX treatment strategy

Study	IFX Level/CON-IS	IFX Level/No CON-IS	P Value
Episodic Therapy			
Baert[6a]	RR 1.93 for IFX >12 μg/mL[b]	Reference	<.001
Vermeire[10a]	6.45 μg/mL (3–11.6)	2.42 (1–10.8)	.065
Scheduled Maintenance Therapy			
Maser[7c]	Reported as similar but no data provided		NA
Van Assche[11c]	2.87 μg/mL (1.35–4.72)	1.65 μg/mL (0.54–3.68)	<.0001
Colombel (SONIC)[12c]	3.5 μg/mL	1.6 μg/mL	<.001
Feagan (COMMIT)[13c]	6.35 μg/mL	3.75 μg/mL	P = NS

Abbreviations: CON-IS: concomitant immunosuppressant used; NA, not applicable; No CON-IS, no concomitant immunosuppressant used; NS, nonsignificant; RR, relative risk.
[a] IFX levels were drawn 4 weeks after an infusion.
[b] 12 μg/mL represents the median IFX level 4 weeks postinfusion for the total cohort.
[c] Represents trough IFX levels.

the development of ATI and was associated with higher IFX drug levels in patients receiving episodic IFX (**Table 2**; also see **Table 1**).[6,10]

The optimal approach regarding concomitant IS therapy is more uncertain with scheduled maintenance anti-TNFα therapy, not only with IFX but also later with adalimumab and certolizumab pegol. The results of several large randomized controlled trials (RCTs) were undertaken for all three anti-TNFα agents, with approximately 40% of patients entering these respective studies on concomitant immunosuppressive therapy (primarily AZA/6-MP). Retrospective analyses were performed to determine if there was a clinical difference, based on the Crohn Disease activity index (CDAI), between those on combination therapy versus anti-TNFα monotherapy.[2,4,14–16] Lichtenstein and colleagues[18] combined the clinical efficacy rates, infection and serious infection rates, as well as drug pharmacokinetics for all patients in the Accent I and Accent II trials for CD as well as those patients enrolled in the ACT 1 and ACT 2 trials[17] for moderate to severe ulcerative colitis (UC). They found that concomitant administration of IS did not result in any difference in efficacy or exert any change in drug pharmacokinetics.[18] Similarly, retrospective subgroup analyses of the CHARM trial for adalimumab and the Precise-2 trial for certolizumab pegol failed to demonstrate a difference in CDAI-defined response when patients were stratified by baseline use of a concomitant IS agent.[15,19] However, these studies represent retrospective, post hoc analyses for which the studies under question were not powered. Moreover, they lack the more robust determination of objective end points such as mucosal healing. With respect to pharmacokinetic data for adalimumab and certolizumab pegol, there are less data with respect to the effect of concomitant IS therapy. In the CLASSIC-II study of adalimumab in CD, 3.8% of patients developed antibodies to adalimumab (AAA) with monotherapy versus no patients on combination therapy; however, this result must be interpreted with caution because only 7 of 269 patients developed AAA, making the clinical relevance uncertain.[20] In the Precise-2 trial of certolizumab pegol for CD, there was a numerically higher rate of antidrug antibodies in patients on monotherapy versus those on combination therapy (12% vs 2%, respectively).[16]

To address the question from a different angle, Van Assche and colleagues[11] studied whether patients on combination therapy could safely discontinue the IS agent. They conducted an RCT in which patients in remission on IFX in combination with an IS were randomized to continue their IS agent in combination with IFX or to discontinue IS therapy and continue with IFX monotherapy. There was no statistical difference in the predefined clinical end point (dose change of IFX) at 104 weeks, nor a difference in rates of mucosal healing. However, there was a statistically higher C-reactive protein (CRP) and lower trough IFX levels in those on monotherapy, leading many to speculate that the potential deleterious effects of IS withdrawal may be a problem in a time frame longer than the duration of this study.

At this point in time the data seemed to indicate an apparent lack of benefit from the addition of an IS agent in CD (and UC when considering the ACT data). Then, data emerged that implied that there were higher rates of opportunistic infections with combination therapy,[21] and there was a general acceptance that the use of thiopurines was associated with an increased rate of non-Hodgkin lymphoma (NHL) (statistically significant in younger male patients).[22,23] In addition, great concern arose around case reports of hepatosplenic T cell lymphoma (HSTCL) in young male patients treated with thiopurines and anti-TNFα therapy.[24] Therefore, there seemed to be a paradigm shift away from combination therapy, particularly among pediatric gastroenterologists. There was a need for further data to clarify these issues in order to determine whether there truly was a benefit with combination therapy and to better ascertain the true significance of HSTCL. The importance of this question was compounded by the fact that, with the exception of natalizumab, at that time practitioners had no other biologic agents at their disposal for the treatment of CD and UC; thus, optimization of therapy was paramount.

No discussion about the issue of combination versus monotherapy can be complete without acknowledging the importance of serum drug levels of anti-TNFα agents. Increasingly, it has become apparent that the absolute serum level of IFX is an important factor in determining response to this therapy.[7,25] Although less clear from available data, the same is probably true of adalimumab.[26] As discussed later, this factor may be the explanation for the increased efficacy of combination therapy (see **Table 2**).

WHAT ARE THE INFECTIOUS RISKS ASSOCIATED WITH COMBINATION THERAPY?

With respect to the risk of infection, it is generally agreed that the use of IS therapy is associated with risk, but quantifying that risk is challenging because there are less controlled data available for IS use than for anti-TNFα therapy. Controlled data come from large RCTs for anti-TNFα agents, in which consistently approximately 40% of patients entered on an IS agent. A recent metaanalysis of all anti-TNFα trials in CD evaluated safety and efficacy.[27] The safety analysis of this study found that anti-TNFα therapy was not associated with an increased risk of infectious complications when compared with CD patients not treated with anti-TNFα. Because there was general consistency in the trials with respect to the proportion of patients on IS in both treatment arms, one could infer that combination therapy is not associated with increased risk. However, none of the individual trials were powered or stratified for such an analysis, and the length of most trials was 1 year or less, thus providing a more limited opportunity to address this question. Similarly, in two recent RCTs designed to explicitly explore the benefit of combination therapy with IFX with an IS (see later discussion), there was no difference in infectious adverse events in patients on combination therapy compared with monotherapy.[12,13] This finding is in contrast to data from a case-control study from the Mayo

Clinic in which the use of combination therapy was associated with a significantly increased risks of opportunistic infection (OI).[21] However, on close inspection of this study, the majority of risk came from the combination of IS and corticosteroids and not the combination of IS and anti-TNFα.

Perhaps the best way to estimate the risk of infection with IS monotherapy versus combination therapy is to look at real-life patients. A study by Marehbian and colleagues[28] provides a good example of this approach, in which they examined claims data from over 22,000 patients in the United States between 2002 and 2005. They calculated the relative rates of adverse events related to having CD, and to medications for CD by comparing with referent patients on no therapy for CD and to over 100,000 control patients without IBD.[28] In this study, two groups of CD patients were studied: (1) prevalent CD patients representing patients with existing CD and (2) a longitudinal cohort representing patients with CD diagnosed within 1 year in an effort to model an inception cohort. Compared with the general population, patients in the prevalent cohort treated with IS agents alone had rate ratios for OI, herpes zoster, and sepsis of 3.63, 2.54, and 1.28, respectively, but these ratios were not statistically significant. When an IS was used in combination with anti-TNFα, the rate ratios were 6.18, 4.15, and 1.75, respectively, and still not statistically significant. The use of combination therapy in the prevalent cohort was, therefore, associated with numerically higher (but not statistically significant) rates of infectious adverse events. It is worth noting, however, that adding corticosteroids was associated with even higher rates when used in combination with other therapies, a phenomenon consistent with other databases.[29] For longitudinal patients treated with an IS and an anti-TNFα agent in combination, only sepsis was significantly elevated with a hazard ratio of 1.73 (confidence interval [CI] 1.17–2.54). Again, when corticosteroids were added to combination therapy, the absolute rates increased and the hazard ratios became significant for candidiasis and sepsis. Taken as a whole, this real-life data representing a very large cohort of patients supports the fact that combination therapy with an IS and an anti-TNFα agent leads to a slightly increased, but not statistically significant, risk of infectious adverse events. Corticosteroids seem to confer the greatest risk, which is perhaps the most important and consistent message practitioners should consider.

IS THERE AN INCREASED RISK OF NHL WITH COMBINATION THERAPY, AND HOW SHOULD WE APPROACH THE RISK OF HSTCL?

Before addressing the issue of NHL related to therapy, one must first address whether or not CD itself is associated with an increased risk of NHL. A number of studies have found no association between CD and NHL. One study by Bernstein and colleagues[30] found a statistically significant association in younger male patients, independent of treatment, but this finding has not been replicated by others.[30–32] There are now clear and relatively consistent data that the use of AZA/6-MP is associated with an increased risk of NHL. A metaanalysis of six studies by Kandiel and colleagues[22] found a pooled relative risk of 4.18 (95% CI 2.07–7.51; 11 observed cases, 2.63 expected). However, this result included patients with both CD and UC, and both NHL and Hodgkin lymphoma. When more closely evaluating these data, there were 4 cases of NHL in 11,012 patient-years of exposure in patients with CD. This result calculates to an absolute risk of 3.6 NHL per 10,000 patient-years. A more recent French cohort study (CESAME cohort) evaluated over 19,000 patients with IBD (approximately 60% CD, 40% UC/IBD unspecified) among whom 23 new cases of lymphoproliferative disease were diagnosed (22 of 23 NHL, 1 of 23 Hodgkin disease).[33] The multivariate-adjusted hazard ratio of lymphoproliferative disease in patients treated with AZA/6-MP was 5.28 (2.01–13.9). There is a paucity of data to draw on with respect to determining if MTX is associated with any increased risk of NHL, but a case-control study in patients with rheumatoid arthritis (RA) failed to demonstrate any increased risk.[34] However, this association represents an area where data are lacking in IBD.

Determining if there is an increased risk of NHL in the context of anti-TNFα therapy is challenging by virtue of the rarity of the event. Ascertaining whether combination therapy is associated with even greater risk of NHL than with IS alone is confounded by the fact that, historically, the majority of patients treated with anti-TNFα therapy had been previously exposed to IS therapy. One of the most comprehensive attempts at addressing this issue came in the form of a metaanalysis of several study types evaluating the risks of NHL in CD patients treated with anti-TNFα therapy.[23] A total of 26 studies met entry criteria, representing almost 9000 patients and more than 20,000 patient-years of anti-TNFα exposure. The crude rate was 6.1 per 10,000 patient-years compared with the expected rate from the SEER (Surveillance Epidemiology and End Results) database, which was 3.23. When stratified by age and gender, the standardized incident ratio (SIR) was significant only in men aged 20 to 54 (SIR 5.4, 95% CI 1.3–18.1). Of the 13 patients with NHL identified in this metaanalysis, 11 had been exposed to IS therapy, thus making a determination of the risk of anti-TNFα alone impossible.

To examine real-life, the study by Marehbian and colleagues[28] provides some insight from a large US sample of CD patients treated with a variety of therapies. In the prevalent CD population, IS monotherapy was associated with a rate ratio of lymphoma (when compared with the general population) of 1.66 (95% CI 0.95–2.88). For anti-TNFα monotherapy, the corresponding rate ratio in this cohort was 2.10 (95% CI 0.82–5.40) and for combination therapy the rate ratio was 0.63 (95% CI 0.08–4.64). None of these comparisons were statistically significant.

Taken cumulatively, it seems that AZA/6-MP is associated with a slightly increased risk of NHL. Whether monotherapy with anti-TNFα is independently associated with an increased risk is uncertain. If combination therapy itself increases the risk of NHL further, the magnitude of the effect is small.

A separate discussion is warranted with respect to HSTCL. This rare but aggressive and almost universally fatal form of NHL was first described in 1990 and is the result of clonal expansion of $\gamma\delta$ or $\alpha\beta$ T cells.[35] The flurry of case reports beginning in 2006 in the context of patients treated with IFX and azathioprine led to a Food and Drug Administration (FDA) black box warning being added to the IFX package insert later that year.[24]. A recent review of all reports of HSTCL submitted to the FDA found a total of 25 cases, of which 88% were in patients with IBD.[36] Although the majority were younger male patients taking combination therapy, a number of cases on IS monotherapy have been reported, and 16% of cases were in women. Furthermore, 16% of patients were older than 65 years of age, implying that the risk is not isolated to any single age or gender group. It is not possible to calculate an accurate rate of occurrence because the denominator of exposed patients in the highest risk group (young men) is not currently available. However, the absolute rarity of the event can still provide us with some reassurance.

WHAT IS THE BENEFIT OF COMBINATION THERAPY?

As with many issues relevant to the use of anti-TNFα therapy for IBD, the use of the same therapies in rheumatologic disorders such as RA can offer some insight. The question of the benefit of combination therapy in the context of RA is questioned to a significantly lesser degree because it has been repeatedly demonstrated that the concomitant administration of MTX is associated with improved clinical response, but also a reduction in immunogenicity and higher IFX blood levels.[37–41]

A recent French study evaluated 121 consecutive IBD patients (23 UC, 98 CD) being treated with IFX (for at least 12 months) and evaluated important clinical end points in those receiving concomitant IS therapy with either AZA or MTX (for at least 6 months) versus those on IFX monotherapy.[42] The investigators divided the patient follow-up into semesters, with a semester being a 6-month block of time. They then evaluated exacerbations of IBD, perianal complications, dose escalation, and switch to adalimumab by semesters with and without IS therapy. Overall, semesters with combination therapy were associated with fewer disease exacerbations, perianal complications, and a switch to adalimumab than those with monotherapy (19.3% vs 32% $P = .003$, 4.1% vs 11.8% $P = .03$, 1.1% vs 5.3%, $P = .006$).

The best way to properly address the question surrounding the benefit of combination versus monotherapy in IBD is through prospective RCTs designed specifically to address this issue. Fortunately, we now have four such trials from which we can draw some conclusions.[11–13,43]

The first trial to examine this question evaluated whether an IS could safely be withdrawn when a patient was already on and responding well to combination therapy with IFX.[11] As noted previously, there was no clinical difference at 2 years in terms of a need for a change in IFX dosing or in mucosal healing, but there was a difference in CRP and IFX pharmacokinetics that favored combination therapy.

The largest and most definitive attempt at examining this question of combination versus monotherapy is the Study of Biologic and Immunomodulator Naïve Patients in Crohn Disease (SONIC).[12] The SONIC trial randomized 508 patients with active, moderate to severe CD who were naïve to IS and biologic therapy to either AZA alone (n = 170) at a dose of 2.5 mg/kg, IFX induction and maintenance alone (n = 169), or combination therapy with AZA and IFX together (n = 169). The primary end point was corticosteroid-free remission at 26 weeks, but important secondary end points included mucosal healing at 26 weeks (among patients with ulceration noted at baseline), corticosteroid-free remission at week 50, as well as IFX pharmacokinetics and determination of ATI. The primary end point was achieved in the AZA alone group in 30%, with IFX monotherapy in 44% and in 57% of patients on combination therapy (both IFX groups were statistically significantly superior to AZA alone ($P = .006$ IFX vs AZA, $P<.001$ IFX/AZA vs AZA). Strikingly, mucosal healing was noted in only 16.5% of patients with AZA alone, versus 30% and 43.9% of patients treated with IFX monotherapy and combination therapy, respectively ($P = .02$ IFX vs AZA, $P<.001$ IFX/AZA vs AZA). ATI were noted in 14.6% of patients treated with IFX monotherapy versus 0.9% of patients treated with combination therapy. Moreover, median trough IFX levels in patients treated with monotherapy were 1.6 μg/mL versus 3.5 μg/mL in patients in the combination therapy group, and rates of corticosteroid-free remission were higher in patients with higher trough IFX levels.

The SONIC trial provides the most resounding evidence that combination therapy (in this case with a thiopurine) is superior to monotherapy with IFX alone, and certainly superior to AZA monotherapy. The rate of infections was nearly equivalent across the three groups, and fortunately, there were no cases of lymphoma. However, SONIC was still too small to understand how rare adverse events might impact the benefit-risk tradeoff with combination therapy. To address this issue, a recent decision analysis studied how often rare adverse events (such as sepsis or lymphoma) would have to occur with combination therapy to change the overall benefit in favor of IFX monotherapy. At baseline, using SONIC as a model, over a 1-year period, AZA/IFX combination therapy is the favored treatment strategy. For the model results to change (ie, the risks of combination therapy to outweigh the benefits), the rate of serious infections on combination therapy would have to be 20% and the rate of NHL 3.9%. These rates are 5 and 65 times higher than what has been seen in the literature and seem higher than what is clinically realistic. Therefore, the conclusions were that in most cases, even when considering rare adverse events, the benefits of combination therapy outweigh its risks.[44]

However, it is important to recognize a few important caveats in terms of the generalizability of SONIC. First and foremost, all patients were naïve to IS and anti-TNFα. Additionally, patients had a shorter disease duration (<3 years) than most patients having entered prior RCTs for anti-TNFα agents. Therefore, these data may or may not apply equally to a patient with a longer disease duration who starts an anti-TNFα agent after failure of AZA/6-MP (a typical example of a patient entering prior anti-TNFα trial).

The third trial to evaluate the issue of combination therapy is a multicenter RCT evaluating IFX induction and maintenance with or without subcutaneous MTX for patients with moderate to severely active CD (COMMIT trial).[13] In this Canadian study, patients with moderate to severely active CD were treated with a per-protocol corticosteroid induction and taper in conjunction with either IFX induction and maintenance (n = 63) or IFX in combination with 25 mg MTX subcutaneously weekly (n = 63). The primary end point was time to treatment failure, defined as failure to achieve corticosteroid-free remission at week 14 or maintain corticosteroid-free remission out to week 50. At week 50, 30.6% of patients in the MTX/IFX group had failure of treatment versus 29.8% of those on IFX alone (P = .63). Pharmacokinetic data from COMMIT demonstrated that 4% of patients on combination therapy developed ATI versus 20.4% of patients on IFX monotherapy (P = .01).[45] In patients treated with MTX, the median trough IFX level was 6.35 verus 3.75 in those on monotherapy, and patients with detectable trough IFX were numerically more likely to be a treatment success (72%) than those with no detectable trough IFX (52%). None of the pharmacokinetic comparisons were statistically significant.

There are important similarities and differences between the SONIC and COMMIT trials that are relevant to combination versus monotherapy debate. On the surface, the results seem discordant and could potentially leave the practitioner with more questions than answers. However, the study populations and the study designs warrant further discussion. As noted previously, the SONIC population represents patients with a shorter disease duration, many of whom were requiring some amount of corticosteroids, but there was no per-protocol corticosteroid induction and taper. In COMMIT, all patients received a full corticosteroid induction, so this trial is really a comparison of triple induction and dual maintenance versus double induction and single-therapy maintenance. It is important to reflect on the very high rates of corticosteroid-free remission in both treatment arms in COMMIT, rates that are far in excess of those reported in adult anti-TNFα trials previously. This result has led many to conclude that corticosteroid induction may further optimize response and that perhaps this response could serve as an explanation as to why no clinical difference was noted between the two groups (eg, a "ceiling effect"). Another key difference is the absence of mucosal healing data in the COMMIT trial, so one can only speculate as to whether there would have been a difference in this end point. Perhaps the most important similarity to SONIC that proponents of combination therapy will point out is the similarity in the immunogenicity and pharmacokinetic data between the two trials, both favoring combination therapy. Whether AZA is a superior combination therapy agent to MTX cannot be concluded from these trials because of the important differences noted previously. As seen in SONIC, there was no increase in the rate of infections in patients treated with combination as compared with IFX monotherapy.

The fourth and most recent trial to evaluate this question was a multicenter RCT evaluating different treatment strategies in 231 patients with mild to moderately active UC for whom corticosteroids were failing (UC-SUCCESS).[43] Patients had to be naïve to AZA (or had stopped AZA ≥3 months prior to entry) and anti-TNFα. Patients were randomized to AZA, IFX induction and maintenance, or the combination of both. The primary end point was corticosteroid-free remission at week 16 with secondary end points including response and mucosal healing. The primary end point was met in 22% of patients in the AZA treatment group, 24% in the IFX group, and 40% in the combination therapy group ($P<.05$ compared with IFX and AZA groups). There was a stepwise increase in mucosal healing rates at week 16 in the three groups at 37% with AZA monotherapy, 55% with IFX monotherapy, and 63% with combination therapy ($P<.05$ for both IFX groups compared with AZA). No pharmacokinetic data are available currently from this study. Despite the discordantly low rate of clinical remission with IFX monotherapy at 16 weeks in this study, the findings as a whole seem to favor combination therapy.

WHAT DOES COMBINATION THERAPY MEAN: AZA? MTX? EITHER?

The term *combination therapy* can mean different things when one considers that the concomitant immunosuppressive medication used may not always be AZA/6-MP. Combination therapy with weekly MTX, either subcutaneously or orally, is not uncommon and is likely more prevalent in Canada and Europe than the United States. The use of subcutaneously administered MTX has been found to be an effective induction and maintenance agent in patients with CD.[46,47] The use of oral MTX has been studied in a more limited fashion in CD and UC, and small studies have demonstrated good bioavailability in patients with IBD.[48–50] However, as cited previously, there are no data with respect to whether MTX is associated with an increased risk of NHL in IBD with only limited data in RA suggesting that it is not. With respect to whether or not MTX is associated with similar benefits to AZA/6-MP in terms of reduction of immunogenicity, improved pharmacokinetics, and improved efficacy, one can draw on a few data sources. In the COMMIT trial there was a favorable pharmacokinetic profile associated with MTX use that was similar to that seen in the SONIC trial. A study by Vermeire and colleagues[10] evaluated the use of concomitant IS therapy in episodically administered IFX and demonstrated that both MTX and AZA were equally effective in reducing the formation of ATI, but in this study MTX was given parentally (see **Table 1**).[10] In the previously noted French study, combination therapy with AZA was associated with statistically lower rates of IBD exacerbations, perianal complications, dose escalation, and a lower mean CRP when compared with combination therapy with oral or parentally administered MTX.[42] One can borrow data from RA, in which case the administration of low dose oral MTX weekly was associated with improved IFX pharmacokinetcs.[41] There are no data supporting the use of this approach in IBD. Despite this lack, the use of 7.5 to 12.5 mg of weekly oral MTX as a combination IS agent is fairly common practice in IBD, especially in view of concerns surrounding NHL and

HSTCL with AZA/6-MP. This approach represents an important and as yet unanswered research question in IBD.

ONE SIZE DOES NOT FIT ALL: A SYSTEMATIC APPROACH TO DEVELOP AN ALGORITHM FOR WHEN TO USE COMBINATION THERAPY

When contemplating a patient's potential risk of disease progression, there is significant heterogeneity in the possible outcomes. Whether predicted by clinical, endoscopic, serologic, or genetic markers, some patients are destined for a more complicated disease course in both CD and UC.[51-54] However, all practitioners will appreciate that there are patients whose disease course is more indolent and for whom rapid progression of disease does not occur. Obviously, the manner of treatment can reasonably be quite distinct in the two circumstances. Similarly, risk associated with therapy may well be heterogeneous. Therefore, the application of a standard algorithmic approach to the management of IBD is difficult. When considering the question of monotherapy versus combination therapy, individual patient characteristics need to be considered.

To address this clinically important question, the Building Research in IBD Globally (BRIDGe) group sought to apply an established RAND/University of California Los Angeles (UCLA) panel consensus methodology to explore the risks and benefits of combination therapy across a variety of permutations of clinical patient characteristics. This methodology is an established technique using a modified Delphi panel approach, which can be used to combine available literature and its interpretation by expert opinion to determine the appropriateness of certain health care interventions. In this case the discussion focused on the appropriateness of using a concomitant IS when the decision has already been made to initiate anti-TNFα therapy.[55,56]

Because the debate centered around efficacy balanced against risk, as a prelude to the RAND/UCLA panel, members of the BRIDGe group undertook a comprehensive literature review of the following topics: (1) analysis of the results of the SONIC and COMMIT trials,[12,13] (2) available data on pharmacokinetics of anti-TNFα in the context of IS therapy, (3) predictors of response to anti-TNFα therapy, (4) efficacy and safety of combination therapy in the rheumatology literature, and (5) lymphoma risk with combination therapy in IBD. Some of the data referred to in this review were not available at the time of the RAND/UCLA panel.

In an effort to make the findings of the RAND/UCLA panel relevant and interpretable, the authors reflected on the fact that a practitioner might approach a patient with short duration of complicated CD with poor prognostic factors who was naïve to IS and anti-TNFα therapy differently than someone with long-established, perhaps more indolent disease. Therefore, the authors created different scenarios in which a practitioner would contemplate the issue of combination therapy versus anti-TNFα monotherapy. To organize these seemingly complex and diverse concepts, the authors organized patient scenarios into five chapters, and within each chapter they modified the scenario based on clinical characteristics. The five chapters they evaluated included (1) steroid and immunomodulator-naïve, starting anti-TNFα (ie similar to SONIC trial); (2) steroid-induced, starting anti-TNFα concurrently for maintenance (ie similar to COMMIT); (3) failure of immunomodulators and starting anti-TNFα (ie similar to many patients enrolled in clinical trials and similar to usual clinical practice); (4) attenuation to anti-TNFα monotherapy, switching to a second anti-TNFα agent; and (5) In remission for 6 months or longer on anti-TNFα with combination therapy (ie a question of *withdrawal vs continuation* of concomitant IS therapy, similar to the study population presented by Van Assche and colleagues.[11] Superimposed on scenarios within each chapter, the authors modified the clinical characteristics around the following variables: sex, age, disease duration, disease extent, presence or absence of perianal involvement, and surgical history. By modifying the clinical variables across the five chapters, a total of 134 unique patient scenarios were presented to each member of the BRIDGe group.

For each of the 134 scenarios, each member independently rated the use of combination therapy on a scale of 1 to 9 (1–3, inappropriate, 4–6, uncertain, and 7–9 appropriate). (Note that for chapter 5, the same scale was used but the rater was evaluating withdrawal of, rather than addition of, an IS agent). For the purpose of the study, "appropriate" was defined as benefit of combination therapy exceeding any additional risk imposed by IS therapy (reverse in chapter 5 as noted). In addition to the unique clinical scenarios, members were also asked whether their response was influenced by smoking status, which anti-TNFα agent was being used, and whether gender or age influenced their decision.

After independently rating each scenario, the BRIDGe group convened in January 2009, at which point each scenario was discussed and clarified when necessary. Members then confidentially rerated each scenario, and median scores were calculated and an accepted RAND/UCLA disagreement index was applied to determine areas of agreement and disagreement. Overall, in 63 of 134 scenarios, the use of combination therapy was believed to be appropriate, in 60 of 134 it was uncertain, and in only 11 scenarios was an inappropriate rating applied (**Tables 3** and **4** list sample scenarios and their rating and the 11 scenarios deemed inappropriate). However, in five of 11 inappropriate ratings, it was believed to be inappropriate to *withdraw* IS therapy in the context of clinical remission on combination therapy (ie a recommendation *favoring* combination therapy). Disagreement was noted statistically in only six of 134 scenarios. The results of the ratings of the 134 scenarios were used to construct an online tool that practitioners can use to gauge the cumulative rating of the BRIDGe group. This tool, available at www.BRIDGeIBD.com, allows a practitioner to input the clinical variables of a given patient and then output a rating of appropriate, inappropriate, or uncertain with respect to the use of combination therapy for that specific patient. To date, over 3000 visitors have accessed this site from over 60 different countries.

As an important example of how clinical variables can influence decision-making, in no scenario involving extensive or complicated CD (regardless of gender or age) was combination therapy believed to be inappropriate, and in the majority of scenarios it was believed to be appropriate. The scenarios in which combination therapy was believed to be inappropriate (see **Table 4**) were predominantly in either younger male patients with more limited disease or older patients with more limited disease, both in the context of failure of IS monotherapy. Presumably, this rating was driven by the concern for HSTCL or NHL in younger male patients and the increased risk of infection in older patients.

With respect to the influence of other factors such as which anti-TNFα agent was prescribed, smoking status, gender, and age, some interesting findings were noted. Respondents were more likely to use combination therapy in patients who were actively smoking. In patients over age 25, gender did not influence their decision, but generally there was reluctance to prescribe combination therapy in those over 60 years of age. Respondents believed it was more appropriate to use combination therapy with IFX than with adalimumab or certolizumab pegol. Whether more recent data highlighting the importance of immunogenicity with adalimumab (not available at the time of the RAND panel) would influence this sentiment is unknown but worth exploring.[57]

Table 3
Selection of scenario ratings within each of five chapters

Chapter	Disease Extent/Behavior	Patient Characteristics	Recommendation
Chapter 1: Medication-naïve (ie SONIC population)	Limited disease/no perianal involvement	Male <26, disease duration >2 y	Inappropriate[a]
	Extensive/complicated disease	Male <26 years, disease duration ≤2 y	Appropriate[a]
Chapter 2: Steroid-induced (ie, COMMIT population)	Limited disease/no perianal involvement	Male or female, any age, 1 or more resection	Appropriate
	Limited disease/no perianal involvement	Male or female, any age, no resections	Uncertain
Chapter 3: Failure of immunomodulator	Limited disease/perianal involvement	Male <26, no resections	Inappropriate
	Extensive/complicated disease	Male or female, any age, extensive resection(s)	Appropriate
Chapter 4: Attenuated response while on anti-TNFα monotherapy, now switching anti-TNFα	Limited disease/no perianal involvement	Male or female, any age, no resection	Uncertain
	Limited disease/no perianal involvement	Male, <26, extensive resection(s)	Appropriate
Chapter 5: Appropriateness of immunomodulator *withdrawal* in patients in clinical remission on combination therapy for 6 months	Limited disease/no perianal involvement	Male or female, any age, no resection	Appropriate
	Extensive/complicated disease	Male or female, any age, extensive resection(s)	Inappropriate[b]

For complete ratings of all 134 scenarios, see Supplementary Table 2 in Melmed et al ref[56] or go to www.BRIDGeIBD.com.

[a] Denotes disagreement defined by statistically measurable variability in panelist ratings.

[b] Denotes that *withdrawal* of immunomodulator is inappropriate (ie, combination therapy is more appropriate).

Table 4
Scenarios with a rating of inappropriate

Chapter	Disease Extent/Behavior	Patient Characteristics	Recommendation
Chapter 1: Medication-naïve (ie SONIC population)	No scenario was deemed inappropriate		NA
Chapter 2: Steroid induced (ie, COMMIT population)	No scenario was deemed inappropriate		NA
Chapter 3: Failure of immunomodulator	Limited disease, perianal involvement	Male <26, no resection(s)	Inappropriate
		Older, no resection(s)	Inappropriate
	Limited disease, no perianal involvement	Male <26, no resection(s)	Inappropriate
		Male <26, 1 resection	Inappropriate
		Older, no resection(s)	Inappropriate
		Female <26, no resection(s)	Inappropriate
Chapter 4: Attenuated response while on anti-TNFα monotherapy, now switching anti-TNFα	No scenario was deemed inappropriate		NA
Chapter 5: Appropriateness of immunomodulator withdrawal in patients in clinical remission on combination therapy for 6 months	Limited disease, perianal involvement	Female <26, extensive resection(s)	Inappropriate[a]
	Extensive/complicated	Male <26, extensive resection(s)	Inappropriate[a]
		Female <26, extensive resection(s)	Inappropriate[a]
		Older 1 resection	Inappropriate[a]
		Older, extensive resection(s)	Inappropriate[a]
			Inappropriate[a]

Abbreviation: NA, not applicable.

[a] In these scenarios it was deemed inappropriate to *withdraw* immunosuppressive agent (ie *combination therapy was deemed more appropriate*).

CAN WE WITHDRAW THE ANTI-TNFα AGENT WHEN A PATIENT ON COMBINATION THERAPY IS DOING WELL?

A prospective study evaluating the question of withdrawal of the anti-TNFα agent in patients in remission on combination therapy gives us important information.[58] In this study, patients in clinical remission on combination therapy with AZA for more than 6 months were followed prospectively after IFX withdrawal. All patients had a baseline mucosal assessment and determination of laboratory parameters. Approximately 50% of patients had a relapse of Crohn symptoms after withdrawing IFX. Two important findings emerged from those who relapsed. First, there were predictors for recurrence of symptoms (such as presence of endoscopic lesions, elevated CRP), which could guide decisions for when it may be safe to withdraw IFX. Second, nearly 90% of those who relapsed after withdrawal of IFX (but still on AZA) regained response after reinitiating IFX without any signs of infusion or delayed hypersensitivity reactions. Replication and longer term follow-up is required before incorporating this plan into routine practice, but this work certainly raises interest in the idea of anti-TNFα withdrawal.

WHAT ARE THE QUESTIONS WE NEED ANSWERED?

It is apparent when considering the myriad clinical scenarios that a clinician can encounter that we lack data to address the question of combination versus monotherapy in all patients. There are a number of scenarios in which we completely lack data. This list includes but is not limited to the following: (A) Can we use low dose oral MTX as combination therapy and expect to see benefit both pharmacokinetically and clinically? (B) Does adding an IS agent after initiation of anti-TNFα make sense and will it confer any benefit? (C) Is combination therapy beneficial for all anti-TNFα agents? Clear answers to these questions would allow for a more well-defined algorithmic approach than we are capable of devising currently.

SUMMARY

It is likely that the debate surrounding combination versus monotherapy will continue for the foreseeable future, because there will always be a risk-benefit ratio that must be taken into account with IBD therapy. However, because more studies now include a thoughtful approach with respect to concomitant IS therapy with inclusion of objective end points such as mucosal healing and drug pharmacokinetics, it is anticipated that this issue will become clearer over time, which will benefit patients and practitioners. The BRIDGe approach described in this review is a useful tool but must be taken in the context of the subjectivity of much of the analyzed data and the individual perspectives that influenced the results. It cannot in any way be interpreted as a clinical practice guideline or standard of care, but rather a tool that seeks to interpret and incorporate the available literature and, it is hoped, aid clinicians in making sense of the conflicting data in this area. The decision regarding the risks and benefits of combination therapy must be carefully weighed in each individual patient.

REFERENCES

1. Targan SR, Hanauer SB, van Deventer SJ, et al. A short-term study of chimeric monoclonal antibody cA2 to tumor necrosis factor alpha for Crohn's disease. Crohn's Disease cA2 Study Group. N Engl J Med 1997;337:1029–35.
2. Hanauer SB, Feagan BG, Lichtenstein GR, et al. Maintenance infliximab for Crohn's disease: the ACCENT I randomised trial. Lancet 2002;359:1541–9.

3. Present DH, Rutgeerts P, Targan S, et al. Infliximab for the treatment of fistulas in patients with Crohn's disease. N Engl J Med 1999;340:1398–405.
4. Sands BE, Anderson FH, Bernstein CN, et al. Infliximab maintenance therapy for fistulizing Crohn's disease. N Engl J Med 2004;350:876–85.
5. Rutgeerts P, Feagan BG, Lichtenstein GR, et al. Comparison of scheduled and episodic treatment strategies of infliximab in Crohn's disease. Gastroenterology 2004;126:402–13.
6. Baert F, Noman M, Vermeire S, et al. Influence of immunogenicity on the long-term efficacy of infliximab in Crohn's disease. N Engl J Med 2003;348:601–8.
7. Maser EA, Villela R, Silverberg MS, et al. Association of trough serum infliximab to clinical outcome after scheduled maintenance treatment for Crohn's disease. Clin Gastroenterol Hepatol 2006;4:1248–54.
8. Farrell RJ, Alsahli M, Jeen YT, et al. Intravenous hydrocortisone premedication reduces antibodies to infliximab in Crohn's disease: a randomized controlled trial. Gastroenterology 2003;124:917–24.
9. Hanauer SB, Wagner CL, Bala M, et al. Incidence and importance of antibody responses to infliximab after maintenance or episodic treatment in Crohn's disease. Clin Gastroenterol Hepatol 2004;2:542–53.
10. Vermeire S, Noman M, Van Assche G, et al. Effectiveness of concomitant immuno-suppressive therapy in suppressing the formation of antibodies to infliximab in Crohn's disease. Gut 2007;56:1226–31.
11. Van Assche G, Magdelaine-Beuzelin C, D'Haens G, et al. Withdrawal of immunosup-pression in Crohn's disease treated with scheduled infliximab maintenance: a randomized trial. Gastroenterology 2008;134:1861–8.
12. Colombel JF, Sandborn WJ, Reinisch W,et al. Infliximab, azathioprine, or combination therapy for Crohn's disease. N Engl J Med;362:1383–95.
13. Feagan B, McDonald JW, Panaccione R, et al. A randomized trial of methotrexate in combination with infliximab for the treatment of Crohn's disease. Gastroenterology 2008;135:294.
14. Hanauer SB, Sandborn WJ, Rutgeerts P, et al. Human anti-tumor necrosis factor monoclonal antibody (adalimumab) in Crohn's disease: the CLASSIC-I trial. Gastro-enterology 2006;130:323–33 [quiz: 591].
15. Colombel JF, Sandborn WJ, Rutgeerts P, et al. Adalimumab for maintenance of clinical response and remission in patients with Crohn's disease: the CHARM trial. Gastroenterology 2007;132:52–65.
16. Schreiber S, Khaliq-Kareemi M, Lawrance IC, et al. Maintenance therapy with certoli-zumab pegol for Crohn's disease. N Engl J Med 2007;357:239–50.
17. Rutgeerts P, Sandborn WJ, Feagan BG, et al. Infliximab for induction and mainte-nance therapy for ulcerative colitis. N Engl J Med 2005;353:2462–76.
18. Lichtenstein GR, Diamond RH, Wagner CL, et al. Clinical trial: benefits and risks of immunomodulators and maintenance infliximab for IBD-subgroup analyses across four randomized trials. Aliment Pharmacol Ther 2009;30:210–26.
19. Thomsen OO, Schreiber S, Khaliq-Kareemi M, et al. Rapid onset of response and remission to subcutaneous certolizumab pegol and lack of influence of concomitant baseline medications in active Crohn's Disease: results from the open-label induction phase of the Precise 2 Study. Gastroenterology 2007;132:A–505.
20. Sandborn WJ, Hanauer SB, Rutgeerts P, et al. Adalimumab for maintenance treat-ment of Crohn's disease: results of the CLASSIC II trial. Gut 2007;56:1232–9.
21. Toruner M, Loftus EV Jr, Harmsen WS, et al. Risk factors for opportunistic infections in patients with inflammatory bowel disease. Gastroenterology 2008;134:929–36.

22. Kandiel A, Fraser AG, Korelitz BI, et al. Increased risk of lymphoma among inflammatory bowel disease patients treated with azathioprine and 6-mercaptopurine. Gut 2005;54:1121–5.

23. Siegel CA, Marden SM, Persing SM, et al. Risk of lymphoma associated with combination anti-tumor necrosis factor and immunomodulator therapy for the treatment of Crohn's disease: a meta-analysis. Clin Gastroenterol Hepatol 2009; 7:874–81.

24. Rosh JR, Gross T, Mamula P, et al. Hepatosplenic T-cell lymphoma in adolescents and young adults with Crohn's disease: a cautionary tale? Inflamm Bowel Dis 2007;13:1024–30.

25. Seow CH, Newman A, Irwin SP, et al. Trough serum infliximab: a predictive factor of clinical outcome for infliximab treatment in acute ulcerative colitis. Gut;59:49–54.

26. Karmiris K, Paintaud G, Noman M, et al. Influence of trough serum levels and immunogenicity on long-term outcome of adalimumab therapy in Crohn's disease. Gastroenterology 2009;137:1628–40.

27. Peyrin-Biroulet L, Deltenre P, de Suray N, et al. Efficacy and safety of tumor necrosis factor antagonists in Crohn's disease: meta-analysis of placebo-controlled trials. Clin Gastroenterol Hepatol 2008;6:644–53.

28. Marehbian J, Arrighi HM, Hass S, et al. Adverse events associated with common therapy regimens for moderate-to-severe Crohn's disease. Am J Gastroenterol 2009;104:2524–33.

29. Lichtenstein GR, Feagan BG, Cohen RD, et al. Serious infections and mortality in association with therapies for Crohn's disease: TREAT registry. Clin Gastroenterol Hepatol 2006;4:621–30.

30. Bernstein CN, Blanchard JF, Kliewer E, et al. Cancer risk in patients with inflammatory bowel disease: a population-based study. Cancer 2001;91:854–62.

31. Lewis JD, Bilker WB, Brensinger C, et al. Inflammatory bowel disease is not associated with an increased risk of lymphoma. Gastroenterology 2001;121:1080–7.

32. Loftus EV Jr, Tremaine WJ, Habermann TM, et al. Risk of lymphoma in inflammatory bowel disease. Am J Gastroenterol 2000;95:2308–12.

33. Beaugerie L, Brousse N, Bouvier AM, et al. Lymphoproliferative disorders in patients receiving thiopurines for inflammatory bowel disease: a prospective observational cohort study. Lancet 2009;374:1617–25.

34. Baecklund E, Iliadou A, Askling J, et al. Association of chronic inflammation, not its treatment, with increased lymphoma risk in rheumatoid arthritis. Arthritis Rheum 2006;54:692–701.

35. Farcet JP, Gaulard P, Marolleau JP, et al. Hepatosplenic T-cell lymphoma: sinusal/sinusoidal localization of malignant cells expressing the T-cell receptor gamma delta. Blood 1990;75:2213–9.

36. Parakkal D, Sifuentes H, Semer R, et al. Hepatosplenic T-cell lymphoma in patients receiving TNF-alpha inhibitor therapy: expanding the groups at risk. Eur J Gastroenterol Hepatol 2011;23:1150–6.

37. Maini R, St Clair EW, Breedveld F, et al. Infliximab (chimeric anti-tumour necrosis factor alpha monoclonal antibody) versus placebo in rheumatoid arthritis patients receiving concomitant methotrexate: a randomised phase III trial. ATTRACT Study Group. Lancet 1999;354:1932–9.

38. Smolen JS, Han C, Bala M, et al. Evidence of radiographic benefit of treatment with infliximab plus methotrexate in rheumatoid arthritis patients who had no clinical improvement: a detailed subanalysis of data from the anti-tumor necrosis factor trial in rheumatoid arthritis with concomitant therapy study. Arthritis Rheum 2005;52:1020–30.

39. Lipsky PE, van der Heijde DM, St Clair EW, et al. Infliximab and methotrexate in the treatment of rheumatoid arthritis. Anti-Tumor Necrosis Factor Trial in Rheumatoid Arthritis with Concomitant Therapy Study Group. N Engl J Med 2000;343:1594–602.
40. St Clair EW, van der Heijde DM, Smolen JS, et al. Combination of infliximab and methotrexate therapy for early rheumatoid arthritis: a randomized, controlled trial. Arthritis Rheum 2004;50:3432–43.
41. Maini RN, Breedveld FC, Kalden JR, et al. Therapeutic efficacy of multiple intravenous infusions of anti-tumor necrosis factor alpha monoclonal antibody combined with low-dose weekly methotrexate in rheumatoid arthritis. Arthritis Rheum 1998;41: 1552–63.
42. Sokol H, Seksik P, Carrat F, et al. Usefulness of co-treatment with immunomodulators in patients with inflammatory bowel disease treated with scheduled infliximab maintenance therapy. Gut;59:1363–8.
43. Panaccione R, Ghosh S, Middleton S, et al. Infliximab, azathioprine, or infliximab + azathioprine for treatment of moderate to severe ulcerative colitis: The UC Success Trial. Gastroenterology 2011;140:A–202.
44. Siegel CA, Finlayson SR, Sands BE, et al. Adverse events do not outweigh benefits of combination therapy for Crohn's disease in a decision analytic model. Clin Gastroenterol Hepatol 2012;10:46–51.
45. Feagan BG, McDonald JW, Panaccione R, et al. Methotrexate for the Prevention of antibodies to infliximab in patients with Crohn's disease. Gastroenterology 2010;138: S–167.
46. Feagan BG, Rochon J, Fedorak RN, et al. Methotrexate for the treatment of Crohn's disease. The North American Crohn's Study Group Investigators. N Engl J Med 1995;332:292–7.
47. Feagan BG, Fedorak RN, Irvine EJ, et al. A comparison of methotrexate with placebo for the maintenance of remission in Crohn's disease. North American Crohn's Study Group Investigators. N Engl J Med 2000;342:1627–32.
48. Oren R, Arber N, Odes S, et al. Methotrexate in chronic active ulcerative colitis: a double-blind, randomized, Israeli multicenter trial. Gastroenterology 1996;110: 1416–21.
49. Oren R, Moshkowitz M, Odes S, et al. Methotrexate in chronic active Crohn's disease: a double-blind, randomized, Israeli multicenter trial. Am J Gastroenterol 1997;92: 2203–9.
50. Moshkowitz M, Oren R, Tishler M, et al. The absorption of low-dose methotrexate in patients with inflammatory bowel disease. Aliment Pharmacol Ther 1997;11:569–73.
51. Beaugerie L, Seksik P, Nion-Larmurier I, et al. Predictors of Crohn's disease. Gastroenterology 2006;130:650–6.
52. Allez M, Lemann M, Bonnet J, et al. Long term outcome of patients with active Crohn's disease exhibiting extensive and deep ulcerations at colonoscopy. Am J Gastroenterol 2002;97:947–53.
53. Dubinsky MC, Lin YC, Dutridge D, et al. Serum immune responses predict rapid disease progression among children with Crohn's disease: immune responses predict disease progression. Am J Gastroenterol 2006;101:360–7.
54. Siegel CA, Siegel LS, Hyams JS, et al. Real-time tool to display the predicted disease course and treatment response for children with Crohn's disease. Inflamm Bowel Dis;17:30–8.
55. Brook RH. The RAND/UCLA appropriateness method. Clinical practice guideline development: methodology perspectives. Rockville (MD): Public Health Service, AHCR; 1994.

56. Melmed GY, Spiegel BM, Bressler B, et al. The appropriateness of concomitant immunomodulators with anti-tumor necrosis factor agents for Crohn's disease: one size does not fit all. Clin Gastroenterol Hepatol;8:655–9.

57. Bartelds GM, Krieckaert CL, Nurmohamed MT, et al. Development of antidrug antibodies against adalimumab and association with disease activity and treatment failure during long-term follow-up. JAMA;305:1460–8.

58. Louis E, Vernier-Massouille G, Grimaud JC, et al. Infliximab discontinuation in Crohn's disease patients in stable remission on combined therapy with immunosuppressors: a prospective ongoing cohort study. Gastroenterology 2009;136:146.

Disability in Inflammatory Bowel Disease

Bincy P. Abraham, MD, MS*, Joseph H. Sellin, MD

KEYWORDS

- Disability • Unemployment • Crohn disease
- Ulcerative colitis
- Inflammatory bowel disease

It is surprising how little is known about disability in patients with inflammatory bowel disease (IBD). There are sparse data on IBD-related disability compared with other chronic inflammatory diseases such as multiple sclerosis.[1] Even advocacy organizations such as the Crohn and Colitis Foundation of America (CCFA) have little information on the extent of disability of its membership.[2] Perhaps the reason for this shortage relates to the lack of a standardized instrument to evaluate disability as well as multiple challenges in defining disability in these patients. Although defining disability may be important in research that provides a better understanding of the impact of disease and treatment on those with IBD, the definition has real-world implications for those individuals in terms of their financial security, access to medical care, and the ability to work and function in society.

DEFINING DISABILITY

There are major differences in how disability is defined. Disability generally implies chronic limitations that preclude the ability to resume normal daily activities. In this sense, individuals with acute and relatively short-term flares of ulcerative colitis (UC) or Crohn disease (CD) may not be considered disabled. Several large population-based studies suggest that disease activity may be greatest in the first 2 years after diagnosis of IBD and then plateau for many patients.[3–5] Delineating the differences between sick leave and disability may be an important component of the process. Another corollary includes the duration of disability and the expectation that an individual with IBD will shed a disabled status. Thus, setting an appropriate time frame is a necessary component of defining IBD disability.

Most disability studies have traditionally focused on work and employment. There are aspects of work force disability, which can be defined as unemployment versus employment, which can be divided further into full-time versus part-time or even

Section of Gastroenterology and Hepatology, Baylor College of Medicine, 1709 Dryden Street, Suite 800, Houston, TX 77030, USA
* Corresponding author.
E-mail address: bincya@bcm.edu

Gastroenterol Clin N Am 41 (2012) 429–441
doi:10.1016/j.gtc.2012.02.001
0889-8553/12/$ – see front matter © 2012 Elsevier Inc. All rights reserved.

occupation-specific disability. For example, almost all physicians in the United States carry occupation-specific disability, which provides benefits when they are unable to perform adequately in their own specialty or subspecialty. This system contrasts with other disability insurance systems, which may be focused on whether the individual can perform any job. Disability benefits from a private insurer may have different criteria compared with a governmental organization. Besides work disability, specific physical and psychosocial factors of disability can exist as well.

There are no generally accepted measures of disability for IBD patients. Development of such an index would be useful for evaluation of several aspects of IBD care. A major effort to create an index has been undertaken by a World Health Organization initiative, based on the International Classification of Functioning, Disability, and Health (ICF) Core Sets.[6] Its development was based on information from several preparatory studies (a systematic literature review, a qualitative study, an expert survey, and a cross-sectional study) and an international consensus conference of 20 experts in the field of IBD from 17 countries.

The advantages include the establishment of an international standard and the ability to compare results between various institutions and different countries, potentially identify environmental factors that impact disability, implement and evaluate medical interventions in a more patient-oriented way, and establish a common language between the different health care professionals, patients, and policy makers and thereby disburden the life of the patients and improve their health and functioning.[1] The ICF approach includes components of community support and governmental rules/regulations in defining disability. Including factors of activities and participation from a social setting to employment and education as well as attitudes of the patient creates some overlap with the Inflammatory Bowel Disease Questionnaire (IBDQ). This broad approach in evaluation of disability increases the potential of the ICF to become a valuable research tool but makes it more difficult to be applied to making "insurance" decisions about one individual's disability in Peoria.

Although the bulk of disability research has focused on what patients with IBD cannot do, there is a flip side: can medical or surgical intervention significantly reduce the burden of the disease. Bernstein[7] points out several benefits in utilizing this newly standardized tool to evaluate disability outcomes in IBD patients: Showing reduced disability in prescription drug users could help the pharmaceutical industry convince those who pay for health care of the long-term benefits of treatments, especially the expensive biologic therapies. Knowing potential short-term and long-term disability after surgery could help clinicians and patients decide on the potential benefit of surgery. If research shows no difference in disability for IBD patients with quiescent disease compared with the general population, this information may increase access to affordable health insurance. Although not a focus of this article, the question of health care insurability after a diagnosis of IBD is a major concern of patients, at least in the United States. A better understanding of the frequency and degree of IBD-related disability may have an effect on insurability, which, in either subtle or not-so-subtle ways, may alter the balance between working and disability.

In Spain, Vergara and colleagues[8] have validated a questionnaire to assess disability in CD patients. In this CD perceived work disability questionnaire (CPWDQ), individuals with CD estimate the impact on their ability to function. It showed good correlations ($r = 0.59$, $P<.01$) to clinical activity and overall work impairment, $r = 0.66$ ($P<.01$). The investigators found that CPWDQ scores were higher in patients with active disease versus those with inactive disease ($P<.001$), prior sick leave versus none ($P<.01$), and in those requiring hospitalization versus none ($P<.01$).

Physical Disability

Previous studies that evaluated physical disability looked at the physical component summary (PCS) of the short form (SF-36) scale. In Lichtenstein and colleagues'[9] study, patients in CD activity index (CDAI) remission at week 54 had a mean PCS score 46.6, which is close to the general US population and higher than the mean score for patients who are not in CDAI remission (37.4) (P<.0001).[9]

Interestingly, Walker and colleagues[10] found IBS patients had significantly higher medically unexplained physical symptoms and disability ratings than patients with IBD. Feagan and colleagues[11] found significant differences in those with SF-36 PCS scores who were unemployed, employed part-time, or employed full-time ranging from lower to higher scores, respectively (P<.0001).[11]

Psychosocial Disability

Our current best estimates for psychosocial disability are through quality of life measurements. A study of CD patients in CDAI remission had mean mental component summary (MCS) score of 49.8, essentially the same as the general US population. But those patients not in CDAI remission at week 54 had an MCS score 41.3, much lower than that of the general US population (P<.0001).[9]

In Feagan and colleagues'[11] study, the IBDQ total score and the emotional, social, and systemic dimensions of the IBDQ, along with SF-36 MCS scores, were each significantly different (P<.05), with the lowest scores in patients unemployed, higher scores in patients employed part-time, and the highest scores in patients employed full-time.[11] The total score and the social dimension score were most significantly affected and had the greatest difference (P<.0001).

Work/Financial Disability

Most disability studies have traditionally focused on work and employment. Employment status may be affected by disease severity and/or activity, but a host of other factors may come into play. The Americans with Disability Act addresses this issue by attempting to minimize those logistics that may preclude an individual with some disabilities from continuing to work. Individuals may consider themselves disabled, in other words self-reported disability, but may not qualify for disability insurance. Also, disability status for most insurance programs is a binary calculation: either disabled or not disabled. There is no partial disability status.

There is a considerable range of estimates of the incidence of work disability in IBD. Using data from the National Health Interview Survey, an estimated 31.5% of individuals with IBD were out of the labor force, which was twice as high as the non-IBD population.[12] Another study found that at 10 years following IBD diagnosis, over 70% of patients were fully capable of work capacity, where less than 10% were partially capable and about 20% were incapable.[13] Lichtenstein and colleagues'[9] study showed 49% of patients were employed full time, 12% part time, and 39% unemployed.

Several small case-control studies on work status in IBD reported almost similar employment rates in patients and controls.[5,11,12] Comparable employment rates in Crohn patients relative to control subjects were found in the Netherlands.[14]

Other studies did find increased work disability in IBD patients: A fourfold increased risk of chronic work disability in Crohn disease compared with controls was found in a study in England and Wales (odds ratio [OR]: 4.0; 95% confidence interval [CI]: 2.2–7.3).[15] Another case-control study showed that patients with CD had significantly more long-term unemployment compared with controls, and up to 30% of the patients actively concealed their illness from their employers.[16] A study of 106 patients reported significantly more patients (80%) than controls (24%) had experienced periods of unemployment and missed more work days than those without CD.[17] Compared with the general population, patients with IBD were twice as likely to be unemployed, however, had a low rate of reporting themselves as disabled (1.3%).[18] In a postal questionnaire conducted in the Netherlands where 69% of IBD patients and 48% of controls responded, employment was 6.5% lower compared with controls (95% CI: 4.0–9.0), and chronic work disability was 17.1% higher than expected (95% CI: 15.1–19.1). For those who were employed, 62% of patients versus 53% of controls had one or more episodes of sick leave during the past year ($P = .002$).[19]

Baseline data from the ACCENT I trial showed that 48% of CD patients were employed full time, 13% employed part time, and 39% were unemployed.[9] Based on the TREAT registry report of September 2000, 16% of patients were not working due to CD. Full-time workers missed an average of 3.3 workdays per month compared with 2.4 workdays missed by part-time workers, and an overall disability rate of 25%.[11] Given that this was an international study, it is interesting to note that there was a large variation in disability rates depending on the country, ranging from a low of 20% in the United States to a high of 34% in Europe.

There are several factors that may explain this considerable variability among studies. Patient selection may be a major determinant. The more community-based patient population will have a lower rate of disease severity and disability than a tertiary referral center. The ACCENT 1 data and the TREAT registry may have selected for a large proportion of patients with more severe disease. However, the geographic variations within TREAT probably reflect socioeconomic factors and government regulations that affect the ability to obtain disability in one country versus another. Thus, similar disease severity may entitle an individual to disability in one country but not another.

Another estimate from a health insurance claims database stated that 15% to 25% of patients with CD require hospitalization in a given year.[20,21] Rogala and colleagues[22] showed that despite similar employment rates in IBD and non-IBD populations, there was a three times increased short-term disability in IBD population reported as reduced activity at work/home, having been confined to bed, and requiring extra effort due to illness, than those in the community sample.[22]

Disability as a Function of Governmental Policy/Economics

In the United States individuals may purchase private disability insurance or rely on Social Security Disability Insurance (SSDI). There are significantly different standards for defining what qualifies as disability between the two (see later discussion). In the United States, at least, the most widely applicable definition of IBD disability is that embodied in the SSDI regulations. The Americans with Disabilities Act forbids disability discrimination in the workplace, with a goal to keep disabled individuals working.

In studies, considerable variety in rates of disability were found. Procaccini and Bickston[23] reported that 20.4% of individuals were disabled but that approximately one-third of these (7%) had been denied disability. Anathakrishnan and colleagues[24] found that 5.3% of CD patients at a university referral center were receiving SSDI. In a Norwegian cohort, the average disability pension in 1995 to 1999 in IBD patients was 8.8%, identical to the general population.[25] An earlier study in Germany found that 3% of all German employees with IBD were granted a disability pension.[26]

PREDICTORS OF DISABILITY

Certain factors can predict an increased risk of disability.

CD Versus UC

In general, CD seemed to affect employment more than UC.[27] The OR of chronic work disability in CD was 5.4 (95% CI: 3.7–7.8) compared with 2.6 (95% CI: 1.8–3.6) in UC.[19] CD patients reported somewhat more frequent sick leave than UC patients ($P = .04$), and days absent at work were higher in CD compared with UC patients ($P = .04$).[19] The sick leave numbers for those with CD were twice as high, whereas UC patients were only slightly higher than the background Norwegian population.[25] In Sweden, patients with CD received an early pension threefold more frequently than patients with UC.[28]

Disease Characteristics

Interestingly, shorter disease duration predicted a higher likelihood of unemployment.[11] No studies have evaluated medications specifically as a marker of disability. Certain clinical courses suggest a greater risk, including more than two operations, more than two medical hospitalizations, and a lower quality of life.[11,24] Prior bowel resection predicted a higher likelihood of unemployment and of receiving disability compensation.[11]

Not surprisingly, patients in remission are more likely to be working than those with active disease.[9,27] Thirty-one percent of the IBD population who experienced symptoms in the past 12 months were not in the labor force. This rate was greater than for the IBD group without symptoms (18.5%) and the non-IBD group (14.8%).[12] Other variables of disease severity such as number of visits to the specialist, taking IBD-related drugs, hospitalization, or surgery in the past year were also significantly associated with sick leave ($P<.001$).[19] Within IBD patients, the risk of sick leave was associated with self-reported disease severity during the past year (OR for no episode of bowel symptoms compared with continuous disease 0.07 (95% CI: 0.02–0.22), OR for one episode of disease compared with continuous disease 0.17 (95% CI: 0.05–0.55), and OR for several episodes of disease activity compared with continuous disease activity 0.3 (95% CI: 0.1–0.7).[19]

This statement is somewhat self-evident: more severe disease leads to a greater chance of disability. However, some studies have not found a strong correlation between disease activity indices and disability. This result raises the possibility that there may be cumulative morbidity associated with disease that leads to disability. In the ACCENT I trial data, a higher number of patients went from unemployed status to employed status (31%) if they were in remission at week 54 of the study, compared with only 16% if they were not in remission at that time.[9] Patients' mean work hours lost decreased the longer the patients were in remission per CDAI criteria.

Quality of Life

IBD-related sick leave turned out to be the variable with the strongest association to the patient's health-related quality of life (HRQOL) as measured by the SF-36 and Norwegian-IBDQ.[25] Both disability pension and sick leave were significantly associated with the patients' HRQOL. Quality of life (IBDQ SF-36) scores were significantly higher in employed patients.[11]

Family-related factors may also play a role. The mother's positive affect was significantly inversely correlated with adolescent depression and functional disability described by the 15-item Functional Disability Index[15] and frequency of bowel movements.[29]

Extra-Intestinal Manifestations

Self-reported joint complaints were associated with sick leave (OR: 3.19; 95% CI: 1.15–8.86; $P<.03$).[19] Although no significant differences in HRQOL scores were found between those with PSC-IBD and non-PSC IBD in Anathakrishnan and colleagues'[24] small retrospective study, permanent work disability defined by receipt of Social Security disability payments was found in 7.7% of PSC-IBD patients compared with 0% of non-PSC-IBD patients ($P = .013$).[24]

Employment Type

Sonnenberg[26] reported that of all German employees, work-disabled IBD patients were more likely to have a white-collar job than all the other work-disabled subjects. However, the investigator states that this result may simply reflect the higher prevalence of IBD among white-collar workers.

Age

There are conflicting data for age as a risk factor for disability. Some studies find that younger patients are more likely to be disabled, others not.[11,30] Whether this result reflects greater disease activity early in the disease, development of coping mechanisms over time, or national differences in societal benefit plans remains unclear. If younger age is a true risk, it would argue against the importance of cumulative morbidity.

A Norwegian study found that the patients receiving disability pension or unemployed patients had higher mean age (7% unemployed under 30 vs 43% unemployed in 60–67 years of age range) than those not receiving disability or employed.[25] In contrast, patients reporting sick leave or IBD-related sick leave had lower mean age than those not reporting any sick leave ($P<.001$).[25] Relative to controls, the risk of chronic work disability was more increased in younger ($P = .02$) and higher educated ($P = .02$) patients compared with controls in Boonen and colleagues'[19] study as well. The IBD group with symptoms was a younger group (32.6% were aged 30–39 years) than the IBD group without symptoms (46.5% were aged 50–64 years).[12] Younger age predicted a higher likelihood of unemployment, as well as part-time employment.[11] Sonnenberg's[30] study from Germany found that in Crohn patients, the largest fraction of disability pensions was given to patients younger than 40 years, with a small peak at age 60 to 64 years. UC patients had similar distributions as well.[30]

Gender

There has been conflicting information on gender as an influence on disability. Although some studies showed no differences,[19] others found a female predominance.[11] In Germany, female patients with IBD had an increased risk for disability than their male counterparts.[30] Specifically, disability in CD was twice as common in women than men ($P<.001$), whereas disability in UC was equal.[30] In a Norwegian cohort, women with CD had a three to four times higher disability rate (22.5%) than men with CD and women and men with UC.[25] Although no specific findings within their study explained this difference, the investigators suggested that differing coping mechanisms between genders may account for the difference.[31–33]

Marital status and domestic arrangements may also be a determinant in employment status.[12] However, marital status did not change the results of chronic work disability significantly.[19] Smoking habits were not associated with increased disability.

Lower Educational Levels

Procaccini and Bickston[23] found that, in the United States, the chance of maintaining employment was a function of level of education, with 91% of those with postgraduate education and 72% of those with a college degree continuing to work, whereas only 42% of high school graduates were still in the work force.

Longobardi and colleagues[12] also concluded that a higher level of education, in the United States, was one of the most important factors in determining work status in patients with IBD. However, a study from the Netherlands found the opposite, that those with low education had an almost four times higher association of work disability than those with high education (OR 3.8; 95% CI: 2.4–6.2).[19] However, the risk to be chronically work-disabled was higher among higher educated patients in this study. Thus, there may be important factors beyond the disease itself that impact disability status.

A PRIMER ON DISABILITY BENEFITS

Physicians have an integral role in the disability process. However, most physicians have limited knowledge of the complexities of how the system works. Patients may ask physicians to fill out forms with what seem like bewildering and sometimes bizarre questions like, "Can the patient stand for two hours?" Nevertheless, a clear understanding of the details of the disability process allows the physician to be both an advisor and an advocate for the IBD patient.

Competing agendas have led to a convoluted, confusing, and opaque disability system in the United States that attempts to balance providing for those in need, minimizing cost, and eliminating fraud. Individual, societal, and governmental cost of this system can be staggering. Because there are significant differences in qualifications for sick leave and disability from country to country, the authors focus their comments exclusively on the disability systems in the United States. Data on how many individuals receive disability support from private insurers and private employers are not readily available. Therefore it is difficult to obtain a comprehensive and accurate picture of disability in the United States. It is probable, however, that the majority of claims are handled through the principal government insurance programs, Social Security Income (SSI) and Social Security Disability Insurance (SSDI). SSI is a needs-based income support program that is financed by general tax dollars, not by Social Security. SSDI is based on prior work history, not necessarily financial need. However, disability qualifications for both are the same and administered by Social Security. The authors focus on the most common program, SSDI.

SSDI was designed to help workers who are permanently and totally disabled. With waxing and waning symptoms, an individual with IBD may be unable to work at some point in time but not be "permanently disabled." That variation may make the bureaucratic distinction between prolonged sick leave and disability problematic.

For SSDI, once granted disability benefits, the individual will continue to collect indefinitely because the benefits have no expiration date. Of almost 600,000 medical reviews conducted on beneficiaries in 2009, Social Security expects less than 1% to leave because of improved health. There has been a concerted effort to allow individuals with disability to transition back to the workforce while maintaining some benefits. However, this effort has met with limited success; only 13,656 beneficiaries out of 12.5 million disabled returned to work over the last 2 years. And not even one-third earned enough to drop benefits. SSDI costs have been increasing rapidly. In the United States, 8.2 million people collected disability benefits totaling $115 billion; this number is approximately a 60% increase over the last 10 years (**Fig. 1**).

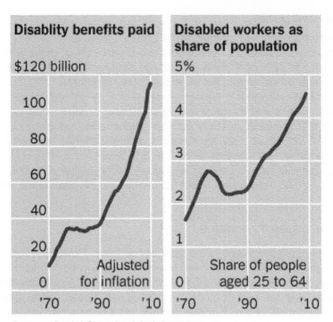

Fig. 1. Change over time of disability benefits paid and percentage of disabled workers as share of the population. (*From* Rich M. Disabled, but Looking for Work. New York Times, April 7, 2011; with permission.)

Although there may be many reasons for increasing disability claims, for example aging population, the difficult job market may be an important contributory factor. For the last 5 years, Social Security has spent more in benefits to disabled workers than taken in by payroll taxes. The Disability Trust Fund is projected to run out of money by 2018. However, despite these macroeconomic considerations, for an individual, the benefits are modest; average monthly payment is less than $1000.

It is clear that disability insurance is fraught with potential for abuse. The General Accounting Office estimated that 20% of disability recipients were not entitled to benefits. A recent investigation revealed that employees of the Long Island Railroad qualified for disability at the startling rate of greater than 90% in the year prior to retirement. Private insurers may have financial incentives to deny/delay payment to improve their own bottom line.[34–36] Thus, depending on one's perspective, the system may be much too lax or hard-hearted.

The application process is cumbersome and swamped with an increasing number of applications. The initial step is a review by state agencies, where two-thirds of the applicants are turned down. Most do not pursue further claims. But there is an appeal system before federal administrative law judges. The average wait for resolution of an application has nearly doubled over the last few years.[37] Lawyers specializing in disability law are subject to federal regulations with fees set by SSI. They may be a valuable asset to navigate the currents and eddies of the disability system for the IBD patient.

Patients with IBD have more initial denials and less overall success in gaining benefits (33%) than the general population (39%).[38] The greater rate of denial may reflect the challenges of establishing disability criteria for individuals with IBD

Table 1
Factors that influence obtaining disability

Increases Chance of Obtaining Disability	Does Not Increase Chance of Obtaining Disability

• Significant Intestinal Obstruction
• At least two of the following, at least 60 days apart:
  –Anemia
  –Hypoalbuminemia
  –Tender abdominal mass unresponsive to narcotics
  –Draining abscess/fistula with pain
  –Involuntary weight loss (10% of baseline)
  –PEG/parenteral nutrition
	• Diarrhea
	• Incontinence
	• Pain
	• Fatigue
	• Enteral/parenteral feeding alone
	• Ostomies

Abbreviation: PEG, percutaneous endoscopic gastrostomy.

compared with other chronic illnesses. There is understandably an emphasis on objective findings for each disease-specific disability.

For IBD, new regulations were published in October 2007 without consultation from CCFA or other interested parties. The updated criteria include significant intestinal obstruction or at least two of the following documented 60 days apart: anemia, hypoalbuminemia, tender abdominal mass not responding to narcotic analgesics, draining abscess or fistulae with pain, involuntary weight loss of greater than 10%, and a requirement for either enteral or parenteral nutrition (**Table 1**).[39] Essentially, objective findings count such as labs, imaging, operative reports, but subjective findings do not.

It is noteworthy that what is not on the list is what many would consider some of the most "disabling" aspects of IBD including diarrhea, incontinence, pain, and fatigue. If none of the specific criteria are present, then benefits may still be granted because of a limited functional reserve capacity. This capacity is the criterion that relies on questions of how long one can stand or whether one can lift 5 pounds. There are also certain questions that must be answered (**Box 1**).

From the medical perspective of a patient with IBD, where the lack of insurance benefits may jeopardize care, the most important aspect of SSDI is the linkage to Medicare. Obtaining SSDI benefits is not the same as acquiring Medicare or other medical insurance. When Medicare benefits were initially extended to the disabled in the 1970s, a 2-year waiting period was established as a cost-containment measure. There are now 2.5 million individuals in that 2-year gap. Because eliminating the gap would cost somewhere between $5 and $9 billion, it is unlikely to occur in the

Box 1
Steps to qualify for social security disability benefits

1. Is the claimant employed? (If so, disability denied)
2. Does the claimant have a severe impairment, ie, inability to perform basic work-related functions?
3. Does the claimant have one of the disease-specific predefined criteria?
4. Can the claimant perform his previous occupation or do any other possible work?
5. Is there any functional residual capacity?

foreseeable future. There is an added trap: in some states SSDI benefits make individuals too rich to qualify for Medicaid. When the recent health care reforms go into effect, they may eliminate many of these considerations. There are indirect costs of IBD disability as well including work/school absenteeism, unpaid/underpaid employment, lower quality of life, and even early retirement.

SPECIAL ISSUES IN DISABILITY
Pediatric Disability

Pediatric patients with IBD face many unique challenges in medical management, physical development, psychosocial adaptation, and education. Therefore, understanding and measuring disability in the child or adolescent with IBD may differ significantly from the adult IBD population. Work and employment considerations do not apply to this younger group of patients. Education may be considered the equivalent of employment/work in the pediatric IBD patient.

Bernstein and colleagues[27] found fewer patients with IBD achieved postsecondary education than the general population. Marri and Buchman,[40] on the other hand, showed that a similar level of education was attained by IBD patients as that of the general population. It was acknowledged, however, that students did face difficulties based on quality of life measurements from patients and teachers on missed school time and physical inconveniences.

Psychosocial issues, especially depression and anxiety disorders, may play a role, especially in future outcomes for these patients in regard to obtaining and keeping employment, learning social skills, and future risk of disability as an adult. No validated instrument currently evaluates disability specifically for the pediatric IBD population. A real need exists to develop the appropriate instruments to define and evaluate disability in children and adolescents with IBD.

Family Medical Leave Act for Parents

Parents and caregivers of children with IBD can also be directly affected because of sick leave taken for their child. In order to help maintain employment security, the Family Medical Leave Act (FMLA) for parents applies to employees working under the same employer for at least 12 months. Employers are required to give the parents up to 12 weeks of unpaid leave during a year to care for an immediate family member. Children with (active and in some cases inactive) IBD are covered as a serious health condition under the FMLA.

Social Security Disability in Children

Medically impaired children up to the age of 18 may be eligible for SSI and may receive benefits including Medicaid if the income and resources of the parents and child are within allowed limits. As in adults, the rules for meeting the SSI criteria for disability are stringent. Jaff and colleagues[41] have outlined detailed information on obtaining SSI in children: To become eligible, parents must have worked enough to be insured under the Social Security system and the child must not be doing any substantial work and must have a medically proven condition that causes marked and severe functional limitations that are expected to last at least 12 months.[41] They advocate that the health care team should write a letter in support of an application for SSI that tracks the listing of impairments as closely as possible and attach the evidence including diagnostic tests relevant to the patient's case. A full list of disability criteria for children and adults can be found online at http://www.ssa.gov/disability/professionals/bluebook/.

SUMMARY

Disability can include different aspects of patient's quality of life from physical to psychosocial to employment. Disability in IBD patients contributes to loss of workplace personnel, increased sick leave, and other indirect costs to society. Considerations for more expensive treatment regimens should include their potential to reduce indirect costs to the individual patients and to society in general. The recently developed tool could help establish specific criteria in a set of these diseases that have varied effects and severity.

REFERENCES

1. Peyrin-Biroulet L, Cieza A, Sandborn WJ, et al. Disability in inflammatory bowel diseases: developing ICF core sets for patients with inflammatory bowel diseases based on the International Classification of Functioning, Disability, and Health. Inflamm Bowel Dis 2010;16:15–22.
2. Sellin J. Disability in IBD: the devil is in the details. Inflamm Bowel Dis 2010;16:23–6.
3. Langholz E, Munkholm P, Davidsen M, et al. Course of ulcerative colitis: analysis of change in disease activity over years. Gastroenterology 1994;107:3–11.
4. Munkholm P, Langholz E, Davidsen M, et al. Disease activity courses in a regional cohort of Crohn's disease patients. Scand J Gastroenterol 1995;30:699–706.
5. Timmer A. How often and for how long are IBD patients expected to be sick, off work or in hospital each year? Inflamm Bowel Dis 2008;14:S48.
6. Peyrin-Biroulet L, Cieza A, Sandborn WJ, et al. Development of the first disability index for inflammatory bowel disease based on the international classification of functioning, disability and health. Gut 2011;61:241–7.
7. Bernstein CN. Trying to optimize a tool to measure disability in IBD. Nat Rev Gastroenterol Hepatol 2011;8:478–80.
8. Vergara M, Montserrat A, Casellas F, et al. Development and validation of the Crohn's disease perceived work disability questionnaire. Inflamm Bowel Dis 2011;17:2350–7.
9. Lichtenstein GR, Yan S, Bala M, et al. Remission in patients with Crohn's disease is associated with improvement in employment and quality of life and a decrease in hospitalizations and surgeries. Am J Gastroenterol 2004;99:91–6.
10. Walker EA, Gelfand AN, Gelfand MD, et al. Psychiatric diagnoses, sexual and physical victimization, and disability in patients with irritable bowel syndrome or inflammatory bowel disease. Psychol Med 1995;25(6):1259–67.
11. Feagan BG, Bala M, Yan S, et al. Unemployment and disability in patients with moderately to severely active Crohn's disease. J Clin Gastroenterol 2005;39:390–5.
12. Longobardi T, Jacobs P, Bernstein CN. Work losses related to inflammatory bowel disease in the United States: results from the National Health Interview Survey. Am J Gastroenterol 2003;98:1064–72.
13. Binder V, Hendriksen C, Kreiner S. Prognosis in Crohn's disease–based on results from a regional patient group from the county of Copenhagen. Gut 1985;26:146–50.
14. Russel MG, Dorant E, Volovics A, et al. High incidence of inflammatory bowel disease in The Netherlands: results of a prospective study. The South Limburg IBD Study Group. Dis Colon Rectum 1998;41:33–40.
15. Thompson NP, Fleming DM, Charlton J, et al. Patients consulting with Crohn's disease in primary care in England and Wales. Eur J Gastroenterol Hepatol 1998;10:1007–12.
16. Mayberry MK, Probert C, Srivastava E, et al. Perceived discrimination in education and employment by people with Crohn's disease: a case-control study of educational achievement and employment. Gut 1992;33:312–4.

17. Sorensen VZ, Olsen BG, Binder V. Life prospects and quality of life in patients with Crohn's disease. Gut 1987;28:382–5.
18. Bernstein CN, Kraut A, Blanchard JF, et al. The relationship between inflammatory bowel disease and socioeconomic variables. Am J Gastroenterol 2001;96:2117–25.
19. Boonen A, Dagnell PC, Feleus A, et al. The impact of inflammatory bowel disease on labor force participation. Inflamm Bowel Dis 2002;8:382–9.
20. Feagan BG, Vreeland MG, Larson LR, et al. Annual cost of care for Crohn's disease: A payor perspective. Am J Gastroenterol 2000;95:1955–60.
21. Decision Resources, Inc. Crohn's Disease [annual report]. Waltham (MA): Decision Resources, Inc., 2002.
22. Rogala L, Miller N, Graff LA, et al. Population-based controlled study of social support, self-perceived stress, activity and work issues, and access to health care in inflammatory bowel disease. Inflamm Bowel Dis 2008;14(4):526–35.
23. Procaccini NJ, Bickston SJ. Disability in the inflammatory bowel diseases: impact of awareness of the Americans with Disabilities Act. Pract Gastroenterol 2007;31: 16–23.
24. Anathakrishnan AN, Weber L, Knox JF, et al. Permanent work disability in Crohn's disease. Am J Gastroenterol. 2008;103:154–61.
25. Bernklev T, Jahnsen J, Henriksen M, et al. Relationship between sick leave, unemployment, disability, and health-related quality of life in patients with inflammatory bowel disease. Inflamm Bowel Dis 2006;12:402–12.
26. Sonnenberg A. Disability and need for rehabilitation among patients with inflammatory bowel disease. Digestion 1992;51(3):168–78.
27. Bernstein CN, Kraut A, Blanchard JF, et al. The relationship between inflammatory bowel disease and socioeconomic variables. Am J Gastroenterol 2001;96:2117–25.
28. Blomqvist P, Ekbom A. Inflammatory bowel diseases: health care and costs in Sweden in 1994. Scand J Gastroenterol 1997;32 (11):1134–9.
29. Tojek TM, Lumley MA, Corlis M, et al. Maternal correlates of health status in adolescents with inflammatory bowel disease. J Psychosom Res 2002;52:173–9.
30. Sonnenberg A. Disability from inflammatory bowel disease among employees in West Germany. Gut 1989;30:367–70.
31. Gafvels C, Wandell PE. Coping strategies in men and women with type 2 diabetes in Swedish primary care. Diabetes Res Clin Pract 2006;71:280–9.
32. Kristofferzon ML, Lofmark R, Carlsson M. Coping, social support and quality of life over time after myocardial infarction. J Adv Nurs 2005;52:113–24.
33. van Wijk CM, Kolk AM. Sex differences in physical symptoms: the contribution of symptom perception theory. Soc Sci Med 1997;45:231–46.
34. Walsh MW. Insurers Faulted as Overloading Social Security. New York Times. April 1, 2008; section A1. Available at: http://www.nytimes.com/2008/04/01/business/01disabled.html?scp=1&sq=April%201,%202008%20disability&st=cse. Accessed February 16, 2012.
35. Walsh MW. Senate Asks 9 Insurers to Furnish Information. New York Times. July 25, 2008. Available at: http://www.nytimes.com/2008/07/25/business/25insure.html?scp=3&sq=July%2025,%202008%20disability&st=cse. Accessed February 16, 2012.
36. Walsh MW. Disability Insurer Found Guilty of Social Security Fraud. New York Times. October 24, 2008; section B2.
37. Eckholm E. Disability Cases Last Longer as Backlog Rises. New York Times. December 10, 2007; section A1. Available at: http://www.nytimes.com/2007/12/10/us/10disability.html?pagewanted=all. Accessed February 16, 2012.

38. Government Accountability Office. SSA Actions Could Enhance Assistance to Claimants with Inflammatory Bowel Disease and Other Impairments. In: Social Security Disability Insurance. Report to Congressional Committees. United States Government Accountability Office; 2005. Available at: www.gao.gov/cgi-bin/getrpt? GAO-04-495. Accessed February 16, 2012.
39. Social Security Administration 20 CFR Parts 404,416.
40. Marri SR, Buchman AL. The education and employment status of patients with inflammatory bowel diseases. Inflamm Bowel Dis 2005;11:171–7.
41. Jaff JC, Arnold J, Bousvaros A. Effective advocacy for patients with inflammatory bowel disease: communication with insurance companies, school administrators, employers, and other health care overseers. Inflamm Bowel Dis 2006;12:814–23.

Clinical Predictors of Aggressive/Disabling Disease: Ulcerative Colitis and Crohn Disease

Wojciech Blonski, MD, PhD[a,b], Anna M. Buchner, MD, PhD[a],
Gary R. Lichtenstein, MD[a],*

KEYWORDS
- Clinical predictors • Ulcerative colitis • Crohn disease
- Inflammatory bowel disease • Aggressive disease

Inflammatory bowel disease (IBD) is classically characterized by periods of remission and clinical relapse. In some patients disease may take an aggressive course that involves frequent relapses, continued active disease, intensified medical treatment, or even a surgical approach. It is important to determine clinical factors that predict the aggressive course of disease to implement appropriate therapy to prevent patients from developing complications and to improve their quality of life. This review discusses clinical factors that have been suggested to predict an aggressive course of disease in patients with ulcerative colitis (UC) and Crohn disease (CD).

ULCERATIVE COLITIS
Introduction

UC is a chronic inflammatory disorder involving the colon.[1] The cause of UC remains unknown; however, it has been suggested that genetic, immunologic, and environmental factors may play a role.[2] Patients with UC may present with varied clinical

Gary R. Lichtenstein, MD, POTENTIAL CONFLICT OF INTEREST DECLARATION: Abbott Corporation, Consultant; Alaven, Consultant; Bristol-Myers Squibb, Research; Centocor Orthobiotech, Consultant, Research; Elan, Consultant; Ferring, Consultant, Research; Millenium Pharmaceuticals, Consultant; Proctor and Gamble, Consultant, Research; Prometheus Laboratories, Inc, Consultant, Research; Salix Pharmaceuticals, Consultant, Research; Schering-Plough Corporation, Consultant; Shire Pharmaceuticals, Consultant, Research; UCB, Consultant, Research; Warner Chilcotte, Consultant, Research; Wyeth, Consultant.
a Division of Gastroenterology, Perelman School of Medicine of the University of Pennsylvania, 9 Penn Tower, 1 Convention Avenue, Philadelphia, PA 19104–4283, USA
b Department of Gastroenterology, Medical University, 213 Borowska Street, 50–556 Wroclaw, Poland
* Corresponding author. Division of Gastroenterology, Perelman School of Medicine of the University of Pennsylvania, 9 Penn Tower, 1 Convention Avenue, Philadelphia, PA 19104–4283.
E-mail address: grl@uphs.upenn.edu

Gastroenterol Clin N Am 41 (2012) 443–462
doi:10.1016/j.gtc.2012.01.008
0889-8553/12/$ – see front matter © 2012 Elsevier Inc. All rights reserved.

gastro.theclinics.com

presentations and extraintestinal manifestations.[2] It has been estimated that there are 1 million people afflicted with IBD in the United States, with approximately half attributable to UC, and similar numbers in Europe.

Over 50% of patients using corticosteroids[3] and 15% using immunomodulators[4] and infliximab[5] may experience adverse events. It is thus appropriate for physicians and other health care providers who treat them to recognize which patients have a high propensity for having disease that will be active and aggressive in the near future. In such patients, other therapeutic interventions may modify disease activity. The term *disabling* or *aggressive* UC has not been specifically defined in the literature. For this review the authors have defined aggressive or disabling UC as disease with frequent clinical relapses that require intensification in medical treatment or surgical approach.

Thus, a pressing question that remains largely unanswered is which specific variables predict the presence of UC with an aggressive course. The most commonly cited variables predictive of relapse have been severity of disease at time of initial presentation,[6] younger patient age,[7] female sex,[8] time from recent relapse,[7] lack of primary sclerosing cholangitis (PSC) diagnosis,[9] therapy with mesalamine or systemic corticosteroids,[8] nonadherence to mesalamine,[10] and having had a recent colonoscopy.[11] However, there are several limitations to these studies. There has not been one single study that has conclusively demonstrated which variables accurately predict patient clinical relapse.

Natural history

The disease course is characterized typically by periods of active and inactive disease, a pattern reported to occur in 80% to 90% of UC patients.[2,12] Data from a large, long-duration population-based cohort study has demonstrated that 9% of patients have severe, 71% of patients moderate, and 20% of patients mild disease activity of UC at the time of presentation.[13] An intermittent course of the disease after the first flare was observed in 40% to 65% of patients, whereas a continuous course was present in 5% to 10% of patients.[14,15] Among 1161 patients with UC evaluated in years 3 to 7 after initial diagnosis, 25% were in remission, 18% had continuously active disease every year, and 57% had intermittent relapses.[12] After 25 years of follow-up, an intermittent course was observed in 90% of patients (**Fig. 1**).[12]

Population-based studies have also observed that approximately 50% of patients were symptom-free at any time during follow-up.[12,14] Disease activity in the preceding years and the duration of activity were predictive of the subsequent clinical course in the following years (**Fig. 2**).[12] There was a significant correlation observed between the activity of UC in the first 2 years after initial diagnosis with an increased chance of 5 consecutive years with active disease ($P<.00001$).[12] There was a 30% probability of a 1-year remission-free course in patients after the relapse.[12] On the other hand, an annual risk of relapse for patients in remission for 1 year was estimated at 20%.[12] Patients who experienced relapse had a 10% to 20% risk of yearly relapse 10 years after the first relapse.[12]

Predictors of colectomy

According to the most recent guidelines by the American College of Gastroenterology, absolute indications for surgery in UC include presence of exsanguinating hemorrhage, perforation of the colon, and documented or strongly suspected colon cancer (high grade dysplasia, low grade dysplasia in flat mucosa).[16] Colectomy is also recommended in patients with severe UC with or without toxic megacolon who do not respond to conventional medical therapy, or in those with

Per cent of patients

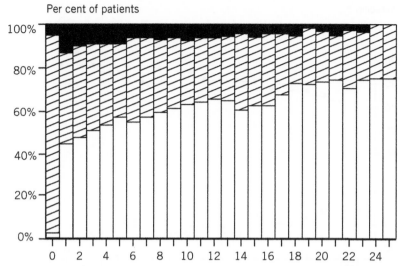

Fig. 1. Percentage of patients in remission (□), with continuous disease activity within the year (■), and with intermittent disease activity within the year (▨) in all years after diagnosis. The calculation is based on all study patients in the actual year of observation except for patients undergoing colectomy. (*From* Langholz E, Munkholm P, Davidsen M, et al. Course of ulcerative colitis: analysis of changes in disease activity over years. Gastroenterology 1994; 107:3–11; with permission.)

a less severe form of UC but with symptoms that are medically intractable or with intolerable medication side effects.[16] The rates of colectomy differ among studies, in part because of different proportions of patients with extensive and limited disease.[2] A population-based cohort study from Denmark observed that the rate of colectomy decreased with every year of disease, with the highest rate of 10% during the first year after diagnosis, 3% in the second year after diagnosis, and a constant 1% rate per year after 4 years of disease duration.[14] Another population-based study reported a 10-year cumulative rate of colectomy of 24%, 15-year rate of 30%, and a 25-year rate of 30%.[17]

Several studies attempted to determine factors predictive of colectomy in patients with UC and suggested that increased number of stools (>8 per day) or 3 to 8 stools along with increased serum C-reactive protein (CRP >45 mg/L) on the third day of hospitalization, the endoscopic appearance of rectal mucosa (deep ulcerations) upon hospital admission,[18] and disease extent (pancolitis) at diagnosis were predictors of colectomy.[17,19] A multivariate regression model of the data from the population-based study after stratification according to the initial extent of UC determined that patients at initial presentation of UC with mucopus in the stool (relative hazard coefficient 2.53, 95% confidence interval [CI] 1.16–5.53), fever (relative hazard coefficient 2.87, 95% CI 1.44–5.69) or poor general condition (relative hazard coefficient 2.54, 95% CI 1.22–1.66) were at an increased risk of colectomy.[20] Another model from a multicenter prospective inception cohort study of 617 UC patients determined that extensive colitis increased the risk of colectomy fourfold (hazard ratio [HR] = 4.1, 95% CI, 2.0–8.4).[21] Data from population-based inception IBD cohort from southeastern Norway (the IBSEN cohort) determined that extensive colitis and increased erythrocyte sedimentation rate (ESR ≥30 mm/h) at the time of diagnosis were independent

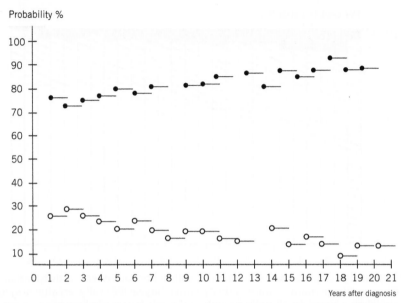

Fig. 2. One-year probabilities of staying in remission (●) and for having relapse (○) for patients in remission the previous year. The point and the adherent line indicates the probability level within a year. The lines are not coherent, indicating that the analysis only deals with 2 consecutive years and does not allow longitudinal comparison for a period longer than 2 years. (*From* Langholz E, Munkholm P, Davidsen M, et al. Course of ulcerative colitis: analysis of changes in disease activity over years. Gastroenterology 1994;107:3–11; with permission.)

factors that increased the risk of requiring a future colectomy threefold (HR = 2.98, 95% CI 1.25–7.08 and HR = 2.94, 95% CI 1.58–5.46, respectively).[22] It should be noted that this result is before the era of anti-tumor necrosis factor α (anti-TNF) therapy. It is uncertain what effect treatment with anti-TNF therapy would have on this patient population.

A retrospective case-control study of 246 patients with UC done in the era of anti-TNF therapy for UC found that the requirement to hospitalize a patient to control disease (odds ratio [OR] = 5.37, 95% CI 2.00–14.46) and the use of infliximab (OR = 3.12, 95% CI 1.21–8.07) were independent predictors of future colectomy.[23]

Mortality

The risk of death from UC decreased significantly after introduction of glucocortico-steroids.[2] Published in 2007, a metaanalysis of 10 population-based inception cohort studies highlighted that patients with UC had a risk of death that is similar to people in the general population, noting a standardized mortality ratio (SMR) of 1.1 (95% CI, 0.9–1.2, $P = .42$).[24] Overall, among all deaths in patients with UC, the disease itself only accounted for 17%.[24] The most common causes of UC-related morality were colorectal cancer (37%) and complications during or after surgery (44%).[24] Recent data from IBSEN study with 10-year follow-up also did not observe a significant increased risk of death in patients with UC, with an overall SMR of 1.24 (95% CI 0.93–1.62).[22]

Clinical Predictors of Aggressive/Disabling Disease

Clinical predictors of extent of progression of disease

Disease extent (as measured endoscopically) may progress over the 10-year time period after initial diagnosis in 10% to 30% of patients experiencing proctitis or proctosigmoiditis at the first recurrence of previously diagnosed disease.[25–27] According to the population-based study, the cumulative probability of progression of proctosigmoiditis was 53% after 25 years of disease. Disease progression was seen in 9% within the first year of disease, with a constant intensity of 5% per year during subsequent 10 years, and then with subsequent decrease to a stable rate of 2.5% per year.

The severity of UC is roughly proportionate to the amount of colon that is involved with macroscopically visible inflammation as determined endoscopically.[28] In four studies it was observed that anywhere from 14% to 37% of patients with UC have pancolitis, 36% to 41% have disease extending beyond the rectum, and about 44% to 49% have disease confined to the rectum at the time of disease diagnosis.[6,12,14,20]

An analysis of data from a cohort of 470 patients who were seen at the Cleveland Clinic in a referral-based center presenting with either proctitis or left-sided colitis at initial diagnosis determined that 53.8% of patients had an extension of their disease over time.[6] Patients were followed for at least 5 years with a mean duration of 12.7 years.[6] Clinical factors present at the time of diagnosis that were associated with an increased risk of disease extension included younger age (20–30 years) (OR 0.886, 95% CI 0.78–1.0), presence of toxic, fulminant, or severe colitis (OR = 14.8, 95% CI 3.5–63.1), left-sided colitis (OR = 2.5, 95% CI 1.6–3.9) and presence of joint symptoms (OR = 3.7, 95% CI 1.6–8.6).[6] Patients with pancolitis ($P<.001$) and left-sided ($P<.002$) UC had significantly greater frequencies of observed complications: toxic, fulminant, or severe colitis (24% and12.6% vs 3.7%), toxic dilatation (21.1% and 9.5% vs 2.9%), bleeding (25.2% and 17.9% vs 9.5%), and undergoing surgery (60.7% and 51.6% vs 14.2%) compared with those with proctitis.[6] Data from multivariable logistic regression analysis from a Scandinavian population-based cohort study indicated that abdominal pain (relative hazard coefficient of 3.59, 95% CI 1.76–7.35) and diarrhea (relative hazard coefficient of 5.54, 95% CI 2.25–13.64) when present at diagnosis were two independent predictors of progression of disease extent.[20]

Primary sclerosing cholangitis

Several studies observed that patients with UC who had concurrent PSC had a milder clinical course of UC than those with UC but without PSC.[9,29] Patients with UC only had received treatment with systemic and local corticosteroids significantly more often and were hospitalized more frequently because of disease activity than UC patients with PSC.[9,29] Another study evaluating 30 patients with PSC who underwent orthotopic liver transplantation and survived more than 12 months observed that among 16 patients who had concomitant UC, the activity of UC worsened in 50% of cases in the posttransplant period when compared with the pretransplant UC course; on the other hand, de novo UC developed after liver transplantation in 25% of patients without pretransplant IBD and follows a mild course.[30] However, studies have suggested that patients with UC and PSC are at increased risk of colon cancer when compared with those with UC only.[31,32] Patients with both UC and PSC had 48.1% cumulative incidence of colorectal cancer and dysplasia after 28 years.[31,32] A case-control study of 40 patients with extensive UC and PSC matched 1:2 to patients with extensive UC alone and determined that there is a significantly increased absolute cumulative risk of developing colorectal dysplasia/carcinoma in the former when compared with the latter group of patients after 10 (9% vs 2%), 20 (31% vs 5%), and 25 (50% vs 10%) (P<.001 for all comparisons) years from diagnosis.[32]

Medications

Corticosteroids. A population-based study from Olmsted County, Minnesota, described the natural history of treatment with corticosteroids in patients with UC.[33] It was observed that among patients treated with corticosteroids, 54% achieved complete remission, 30% partial response, and 16% no response over first 30 days.[33] An analysis of the course of disease over 1 year showed that 49% of patients achieved prolonged response, 22% became corticosteroid-dependent, and 29% required colectomy.[33] Because of the frequent occurrence of corticosteroid dependence and need of surgery, treatment with corticosteroids has been considered a marker of poor prognosis.[33]

Patients with a severe flare of UC are usually treated initially with intravenous glucocorticosteroids. Retrospective analysis of data from four hospital centers in Scandinavia obtained from 97 patients with severe UC who received corticosteroids intravenously determined that increased CRP level (≥25 mg/L) (P = .012) and the presence of increased bowel movement frequency (>4 per day) (P<.001) on the third day of treatment with high dose corticosteroids were independent predictors of corticosteroids resistance and colectomy within 30 days after admission to the hospital.[34] Multivariable logistic regression analysis of clinical, biological, or endoscopic factors gathered from 53 patients with UC and 1 patient with CD identified that the presence of an increased number of bowel movements (>7 per day) on the third day of hospitalization (adjusted OR 21.0, 95% CI 3.6–124.3) and male sex (adjusted OR 8.2, 95% CI 1.2–55.5), were independent factors predictive of corticosteroid failure in patients with severe IBD colitis.[35]

Azathioprine. Azathioprine is recommended in patients with UC as a maintenance treatment in those with inadequately sustained remission on 5-aminosalicylic acid agents or in corticosteroid-dependent patients allowing for corticosteroid sparing.[16] Data from a multicenter retrospective study of 127 patients with UC illustrated that withdrawal of azathioprine in patients with UC in remission is associated with an increased risk of relapse.[36] Multivariable logistic regression analysis determined clinical predictors of disease relapse after discontinuation of azathioprine.[36] Lack of remission during treatment with azathioprine (HR = 2.4, 95% CI 1.4–3.9), extensive disease beyond splenic flexure versus left-sided colitis (HR = 1.8, 95% CI 1.1–3.0) or versus distal colitis (HR = 2.0, 95% CI 1.1–3.7), and short duration (3–6 months) of treatment with azathioprine (HR = 2.8, 95% CI 1.3–6.1) increased the risk of UC relapse by a factor of two- to threefold.[36]

Nonsteroidal antiinflammatory drugs. Several studies assessed an association between the use of nonsteroidal antiinflammatory drugs (NSAIDs) and the course of IBD. A prospective case-control analysis determined that current (within 45 days) and recent (within 45 and 180 days) use of NSAIDs was associated with a significantly increased risk of emergency admissions to the hospital because of exacerbation of UC with a respective unadjusted odds ratios of 2.54 (95% CI 1.09–5.91) and 2.45 (95% CI 1.19–5.03).[37] Another prospective case-control study observed 20-fold increased odds of exacerbation or new onset of disease among IBD patients when compared with controls with irritable bowel syndrome (IBS) who were taking NSAIDs less than 1 month before onset of symptoms with confirmed association between

NSAID use and disease activity (OR = 20.3, 95% CI 2.6–159.7).[38] The relationship between the use of NSAIDs and disease activity was found in 31% and 2% of IBD and IBS patients, respectively.[38] Data from retrospective analyses determined a significant association between IBD relapse and use of NSAIDs (adjusted OR = 6.31, 95% CI, 1.16–34.38, P = .03).[39] Early clinical relapse of IBD within 9 days of NSAIDs ingestion was observed in 17% to 28% of users of nonselective NSAIDs (23% of UC patients and 20% of CD patients, $P>.6$).[40] A randomized double blind placebo controlled trial with celecoxib showed no risk of UC flare after 2 weeks of use when compared with placebo with similar respective relapse rates of 3% and 4% (P = .719).[41]

Nonadherence to mesalamine. Nonadherence to mesalamine has been found to increase the risk of UC recurrence fivefold (HR 5.5, 95% CI 2.3–13) based on data from a prospective cohort study of 99 patients.[42] A systematic review of the literature determined that nonadherence to mesalamine was associated with increased morbidity and greater risk of symptomatic relapse, reduced quality of life, and possible increased risk of colorectal cancer.[43]

Nonsmoking status

Recent metaanalysis of 12 case-control studies and 1 prospective cohort study that examined the relationship between UC and smoking when compared with non-IBD controls indicated that current smoking had a protective effect on the development of UC (OR = 0.58, 95% CI 0,45–0.75) by reducing the risk of UC by 42%.[44] Patients who quit smoking were found to be at an increased risk of UC compared with current smokers (OR 1.79, 95% CI 1.37–2.34).[44] Small studies and case reports observed that intermittent smokers may experience symptomatic improvement during smoking[45–47] and that nonsmokers with UC who start smoking may achieve remission.[45] An analysis of the effect of smoking habits on the course of UC performed in 209 patients showed that current smoking status after disease onset was associated with a decreased risk of hospitalization when compared with nonsmoking status (less than 100 cigarettes in the lifetime) (adjusted relative risk [RR] = 0.5, 95% CI 0.3–0.8).[48] On the contrary, the adjusted risk of colectomy was similar between current smokers and nonsmokers (RR = 1.1, 95% CI 0.4–2.8).[48] Those who stopped smoking before the disease onset were 1.5-fold more likely to be hospitalized because of disease activity than nonsmokers (adjusted RR = 1.5, 95% CI 1.0–2.2), and the odds were particularly increased in those who smoked at least 21 pack-years (adjusted RR = 2.4, 95% CI 1.3–4.6).[48] A nonsignificantly increased risk of colectomy was found in patients who stopped smoking after UC diagnosis when compared with nonsmokers (adjusted RR = 2.2, 95% CI 0.8–6.3).[48] However those who smoked at least 41 pack-years had significant and nearly 18-fold higher risk of colectomy than nonsmokers (adjusted RR = 17.9, 95% CI 2.4–131.7).[48] A group of French researchers observed significantly increased rates of duration of time with active UC (54 vs 35 per 100 person-years, $P<.01$), years with hospital admissions (9 vs 4 per 100 person-years, $P<.05$), and years with medical therapy with oral (13 vs 3 per 100 person-years, $P<.01$) or intravenous (4 vs 0 per 100 person-years, $P<.01$) corticosteroids and azathioprine (5 vs 0 per 100 person-years, $P<.01$) after cessation of smoking when compared with these parameters measured before discontinuation of smoking in 32 patients.[49]

Colonoscopy

A significant association between performing colonoscopy and developing a subsequent increase in UC disease activity as measured by the UC Simple Clinical Colitis

Activity Index (SCCAI) was recently suggested based on a multivariate mixed modeling performed in 51 patients with UC in remission.[11] It was observed that shorter time from colonoscopy preparation (week 1 vs week 4, $P = .0127$), higher baseline SCCAI ($P<.0001$) and the use of prednisone ($P = .0120$) were factors predictive of increased disease activity after colonoscopy.[11] However, the use of thiopurines ($P = .0045$) was protective against an increase in disease activity following colonoscopy.[11] It should be noted that 6 of 51 patients (12%) experienced relapse within a week after colonoscopy with only 1 of them continuing to relapse 4 weeks after the colonoscopy.[11]

Clinical factors predictive of relapse in patients with UC determined by multivariate logistic regression analyses

Several prospective studies have identified multiple clinical factors affecting the probability of UC relapse using multivariable logistic regression analysis during follow-up ranging from 6 months to 10 years (**Table 1**).[7,8,50–52]

The identified clinical factors that were considered independent predictors of disease relapse included younger age (20–30 years old) (HR = 0.4, 95% CI 0.2–0.7), history of multiple relapses in women (HR = 1.6, 95% CI 1.2–1.9), plasmacytosis on rectal biopsy specimens (HR = 4.5, 95% CI 1.7–11.9),[7] use of mesalamine (HR = 1.9, 95% CI, 1.6–2.2), use of glucocorticosteroids (HR = 5.6, 95% CI, 4.5–6.9), female sex (HR = 1.2, 95% CI, 1.1–1.3), cessation of smoking during the study period (HR = 1.3, 95% CI, 1.1–1.6),[8] presence of pit patterns in rectal mucosa (RR = 2.06, 95% CI 1.34–3.17),[50] or absence of minute defects of colonic epithelium (HR = 0.24, 95% CI 0.072–0.801) on magnifying colonoscopy[51] or regular magnifying colonoscopy findings (OR = 0.03, 95% CI 0.01–0.24.[52] A recent prospective population-based study of 354 patients with UC who were evaluated after 1 year and 5 years of follow-up periods determined based on multivariable logistic regression analysis that factors predictive of mucosal healing after 1 year of follow-up included duration of education greater than 12 years (OR = 2.08, 95% CI 1.27–3.43) and extensive disease at the time of initial diagnosis (OR = 2.56, 95% CI 1.38–4.75).[53] It was also determined that the presence of mucosal healing at 1 year was associated with decreased risk of future colectomy at 5 years (RR = 0.22, 95% CI 0.06–0.79).[53]

Summary

Controlled data focusing on factors that predict an aggressive course of UC are limited. In the medical literature there is a lack of consistent definition of aggressive and disabling UC. Most patients with UC have an intermittent, relapsing-remitting course, with a minority of patients having continuous disease activity. Therapy with rectal mesalamine and systemic immunomodulators has greatly reduced the relapse rate and has lowered the necessity of using systemic corticosteroids, agents which may actually increase the relapse rate.

Patients with PSC and patients who are taking azathioprine tended to have a lower relapse rate, whereas those patients who were ex-smokers, female, or of younger age have been shown to have an elevated risk of relapse. Additionally, patients who have basal plasmacytosis on rectal biopsy or abnormal endoscopic findings on magnifying colonoscopy also tended to have increased risk of relapse. There are still not enough data to conclusively judge which factors are responsible for greater relapse rates, however. Significant limitations exist because of shortcomings of the studies that have been published. Therefore, a large multicenter prospective study, as well as additional other studies, are required to conclusively assess such factors.

Table 1
Clinical factors predictive of clinical relapse of ulcerative colitis as determined by multivariable logistic regression analyses

Author and Year Study Design	Design	Patients (n)	Risk Factors	Hazard Ratio (95% CI)	Comment
Hoie et al 2007[8]	Population-based inception cohort	771	Female sex	1.2 (1.0–1.5)	Factors predictive of first clinical relapse within 10-year follow-up
			High level of education	1.4 (1.1–1.8)	
			Mesalamine rx during follow-up	2.1 (1.7–2.7)	
			Corticosteroids rx during follow-up	7.1 (5.1–9.7)	
			Female sex	1.2 (1.1–1.3)	Factors predictive of all clinical relapses within 10-year follow-up
			Smoking cessation during study vs never smoking	1.3 (1.1–1.6)	
			Mesalamine rx during follow-up	1.9 (1.6–2.2)	Clinical relapse: increase in disease symptoms causing changes in medical treatment or necessitating surgery
			Corticosteroids rx during follow-up	5.6 (4.5–6.9)	
Bitton et al 2001[7]	Prospective longitudinal	74	Younger age (20–30 y) (per decade)	0.4 (0.2–0.7)	Factors predictive of shorter time to clinical relapse: worsening of bowel function and rectal bleeding within 12-month follow-up
			Basal plasmacytosis on rectal biopsy	4.5 (1.7–11.9)	
			Greater number of prior relapses in women (per prior relapse)	1.6 (1.2–1.9)	
Nishio et al 2006[50]	Prospective cohort	113	Pit patterns in rectal mucosa on magnifying colonoscopy	2.06 (1.53–3.17)	Factors predictive of clinical relapse within 12-month follow-up Remission: Disease Activity Index ≤3
Fujiya et al 2002[51]	Prospective cohort	18	Absence of minute defects of colonic epithelium on magnifying colonoscopy	0.24 (0.072–0.801)	Factors predictive of clinical relapse within 6-month follow-up Relapse: Rachmilewitz score ≥5
Watanabe et al 2009[52]	Prospective longitudinal	57	Regular findings on magnifying colonoscopy	0.03 (0.01–0.24)	Factors predictive of clinical relapse within 12-month follow-up Relapse: presence of diarrhea, bloody stool, abdominal pain

Abbreviation: rx, treatment.

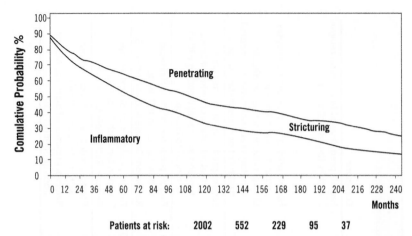

Fig. 3. Kaplan-Meier estimates of remaining free of penetrating complication (upper curve) and free of stricturing and/or penetrating complication (lower curve) in 2002 patients with Crohn disease since onset (diagnosis) of the disease. The number of patients at risk referred to the number of patients at risk for any complication. (*From* Cosnes J, Cattan S, Blain A, et al. Long-term evolution of disease behavior of Crohn's disease. Inflamm Bowel Dis 2002;8:244–50. *With permission from* John Wiley and Sons (2002).)

CROHN DISEASE
Introduction

CD is a disease of unknown cause; however, it has been suggested that genetic, bacterial, immunologic, and environmental factors may play role in the pathogenesis of disease.[54] The Vienna classification of CD separated the clinical behavior of disease into three distinct categories: inflammatory (nonstricturing nonpenetrating) (B1), stricturing (B2), and penetrating (B3).[55] A retrospective analysis of disease behavior on a group of 297 CD patients from a referral center showed that 80% of patients had inflammatory type, 10% had stricturing, and 10% had penetrating disease behavior at the time of diagnosis.[56] Long-term retrospective assessment (20-year period) of the disease course among 2002 CD patients from a referral center determined that the disease progressed over time from inflammatory to more aggressive stricturing and/or penetrating disease.[57] After 5 and 20 years of having CD, 48% and 12% of patients, respectively, had inflammatory disease; 12% and 18% of patients, respectively, had stricturing; and 40% and 70% of patients, respectively, had penetrating behavior (**Fig. 3**).[57] The tendency to develop complicated behavior (B2 or B3) was related to disease location with 94% and 78% of patients with disease of terminal ileum and colon, respectively, having complications at 20 years, (**Fig. 4**).[57]

The term *disabling CD* has been somewhat arbitrarily defined by Beaugerie and colleagues[58] in 2006. The investigators proposed to label patients as having disabling CD as those patients presenting with CD and at least one of the following criteria: having received more than 2 courses of corticosteroids and/or corticosteroid dependence, hospitalization because of disease relapse, development of CD complications, the presence of disabling symptoms for more than 12 months during a 5-year follow-up period (including the following symptoms: diarrhea with nocturnal stools and/or fecal urgency, intense abdominal pain caused by intestinal obstruction, fever, fatigue, joint pain, painful uveitis or pyoderma gangrenosum), requirement of therapy

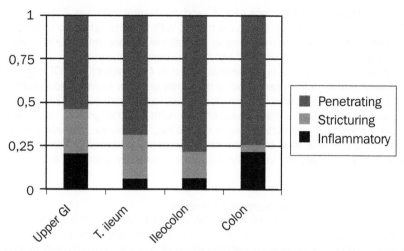

Fig. 4. Kaplan-Meier 20-year cumulative incidence of stricturing and penetrating complication according to cluster of location in 2002 patients with Crohn disease. (*From* Cosnes J, Cattan S, Blain A, et al. Long-term evolution of disease behavior of Crohn's disease. Inflamm Bowel Dis 2002;8:244–50. *With permission from* John Wiley and Sons (2002).)

with immunosuppressive agents, intestinal resection, or operation because of perianal disease.[58]

Natural history

CD is classically characterized by periods of remission and clinical relapse. A population-based cohort study from Scandinavia that analyzed an inception cohort of 373 patients with CD observed that none of the clinical factors such as age, sex, extent of disease at CD diagnosis, and treatment during the first year after initial disease diagnosis was predictive of the subsequent course of disease.[59] However, with time there was a rapid decrease in the probability of the relapse-free course of disease from 22% after 5 years to 12% after 10 years of CD duration.[59] There was a low probability (4% after 5 years and 1% after 10 years) of a continuously active disease course.[59] Markov model analysis determined that disease activity in the 1 year after diagnosis has an impact on disease activity in subsequent years with 70% to 80% of patients with active CD maintaining similar activity of CD during the following years and 80% of patients who were in remission maintaining remission during the subsequent years.[59] Of note, after 15 years of disease duration, disease "burnout" was observed with 29% and 14% of patients changing from active to inactive disease and inactive to active annually, respectively ($P<.04$).[59] The IBSEN study with a 10-year follow-up separated the clinical course of CD into four distinct categories: (a) decrease in the intensity of activity of disease with time (43%), (b) increase in the intensity of the disease with time (3%), (c) chronic continuous activity of disease (19%), and (d) chronic intermittent activity (32%).[60] It was observed that treatment with systemic corticosteroids during the first disease flare increased the risk twofold of chronic continuous disease activity in subsequent years (crude OR = 2.32, 95% CI 1.04–5.14, P = .35), whereas younger age at the time of diagnosis (less than 40 years) was associated with nearly threefold increased risk of chronic intermittent disease activity (crude OR = 2.63, 95% CI 1.18–5.88, P = .16).[60] Overall, the observed cumulative relapse rate at 1, 5, and 10 years of CD was 53%, 85%, and 90%, respectively.[60] Patients who were treated with systemic steroids at the time of initial diagnosis had significantly greater cumulative relapse rates during follow-up when compared with those who did not receive them.[60]

An observation study of a homogenous cohort of 480 patients with CD highlighted that disease activity in the year following diagnosis predicts future disease activity for over 10 years.[61] Patients with inactive disease within that year had a 77% probability of maintaining remission in the subsequent year with a further gradual decrease until reaching a plateau at 58% after 6 years of disease.[61] However, patients with active CD within the first year after diagnosis had only a 16% probability of having disease remission in the subsequent year with a gradual increase to a plateau at 38% after 6 years.[61]

Predictors of surgery and postsurgical recurrence
Although CD is primarily treated medically, in certain cases intestinal resection is necessary. A surgical approach is indicated in patients presenting with acute free perforation, subacute perforation with formation of abscess, chronic perforation with formation of internal fistula (perforating indications) or complete intestinal obstruction, medical intractability, dysplasia or cancer, hemorrhage, and toxic dilatation without perforation (nonperforating indications).[62] According to the IBSEN population-based study with 10 years of follow-up of 237 CD patients, the cumulative probability of surgery increased nearly threefold within 10 years from initial diagnosis (13.6%, 27%, and 37.9% at 1, 5, and 10 years following diagnosis of CD, respectively).[60] Multivariable logistic regression analysis determined that among several clinical variables at the time of disease diagnosis, age younger than 40 years (P = .03), location of disease in the terminal ileum (P = .001), stricturing (P = .004), and penetrating (P = .001) behavior of disease were factors predictive of surgery.[60] Patients with stricturing or penetrating behavior were two (HR = 2.3, 95% CI 1.3–4.1) or five times (HR = 5.4, 95% CI 3.0–9.9) more likely to undergo surgery than those with inflammatory behavior, respectively.[60] An analysis of data from a retrospective Swedish population-based cohort (n = 1936) showed that at 1, 5, and 10 years after disease diagnosis, 44%, 61%, and 71% of patients underwent their first surgery and that age at diagnosis between 45 and 59 years, any involvement of small bowel, and the presence of perianal fistulas at the time of diagnosis were independent predictors of the first intestinal resection.[63] Disease localization within small bowel had the highest risk (two- to threefold) of the first surgery when compared with disease involving only colon.[63] Postoperative recurrence was observed in nearly half the patients (48%), and the risk of relapse was independently associated with female sex (RR = 1.2, 95% CI 1.01–1.4), presence of perianal fistulas (RR = 1.4, 95% CI 1.2–1.7), and disease confined to small bowel (RR = 1.8, 95% CI 1.2–2.6) or continuously involving ileum and colon (RR = 1.5, 95% CI 1.1–2.0).[63] Recurrence of disease occurred in 33% and 44% of patients after 5 and 10 years following their initial surgery, respectively.[63] Data from an English population-based study of 341 CD patients from 1986 to 2003 showed a significant decrease in rates of surgery within 5 years of diagnosis of CD from 59% for patients diagnosed between 1986 and 1991 through 37% for patients diagnosed between 1992 and 1997 to 25% for patients diagnosed between 1998 and 2003.[63,64] It was determined that diagnosis of CD before 1998 (HR = 1.7, 95% CI 1.1–2.6) and use of oral corticosteroids within 3 months of diagnosis were associated (HR = 1.7, 95% CI 1.2–2.4) with nearly twofold increased risk of surgery, whereas use of thiopurines within the first year of diagnosis and colonic disease location at the time of diagnosis were associated with

significantly decreased risk of surgery (HR = 0.47, 95% CI 0.27–0.79 and HR = 0.39, 95% CI 0.26–0.56, respectively).[64] Retrospective analysis of a Hungarian referral cohort showed that among various clinical factors, only smoking was independently associated with an increased risk of the first surgery (OR 1.61, 95% CI 1.05–2.47), whereas use of azathioprine alone or in combination with biologic agents was independently predictive of decreased risk of first surgery with respective odds ratios of 0.26 and 0.22 (P<.001).[65] A recent metaanalysis of 16 studies that included 2962 patients with CD observed that smokers when compared with nonsmokers had twofold and 2.5-fold increased risk of clinical postoperative disease recurrence (OR = 2.07, 95% CI 1.25–3.44) and 10-year reoperation rates (OR = 2.56, 95% CI 1.79–3.67), respectively.[66] Of note, cessation of smoking had a beneficial effect on the recurrence rates. Patients who stopped smoking had nonsignificantly decreased risk of repeated surgery (OR 0.30, 95% CI 0.09–1.07) and nonsignificantly increased risk of clinical recurrence (OR 1.54, 95% CI 0.78–3.02) when compared with those who never smoked.[66] However, smokers had a significant twofold increased risk of both clinical recurrence (OR 2.01, 95% CI 1.06–3.80) and reoperation (OR 1.87, 95% CI 1.01–3.44) when compared with ex-smokers.[66]

Mortality

A recent metaanalysis of 9 population-based cohort studies with an overall SMR from 0.72 to 3.2 found a significant increase in overall mortality in unselected patients with CD when compared with general population with SMR of 1.39 (95% CI 1.30–1.49).[67] When CD-related deaths were excluded from the analysis, an overall SMR was not increased when compared with the general population (SMR 1.03, 95% CI 0.92–1.15).[67] The observed number of deaths related to CD caused by severe complicated CD (abscess, perforation, sepsis, cardiovascular complications, cancer, gastrointestinal hemorrhage, liver disease due to primary sclerosing cholangitis) and its treatment (postsurgical complications, short bowel syndrome) ranged from 26% to 50%.[67]

Women with CD were found to be at a greater risk of death than men (SMR 1.42, 95% CI 1.26–1.61 vs 1.22, 95% CI 1.05–1.42).[67] There was a significantly increased risk of death from nonmalignant gastrointestinal diseases including CD (SMR 6.76, 95% CI 4.37–10.45) that was reduced when CD was excluded (SMR 2.49, 95% CI 1.68–3.71) and diseases potentially associated with tobacco product use such as chronic obstructive pulmonary disease (SMR 2.55, 95% CI 1.19–5.47), pulmonary malignancy (SMR 2.72, 95% CI 1.35–5.45) and genitourinary tract diseases (SMR 3.24, 95% CI 1.69–6.35).[67] Although the overall risk of death from cancer was increased 1.5-fold (SMR 1.5, 95% CI 1.18–1.92), the risk of death from colon cancer was not significantly increased (SMR 1.34, 95% CI 0.54–3.33).[67]

Clinical Predictors of Aggressive/Disabling CD

Several retrospective referral center studies evaluated the clinical factors that might predict the aggressive course of CD[57,58,68–71] (**Table 2**). Loly and colleagues[68] used the same criteria for disabling CD proposed by Beaugerie and colleagues[58] that were described in the introduction to this section of this article. In these two studies, independent factors present at the time of disease diagnosis and predictive of aggressive disease course within 5 years of CD diagnosis were age below 40 years,[58] necessity of steroid use at initial presentation[58] or for the treatment of first flare,[68] presence of perianal lesions,[58,68] and ileocolonic location of disease.[68] Study by Cosnes and colleagues[57] with the mean follow-up of 8.6 years identified that development of penetrating complications was independently predicted at the time of disease diagnosis by age less than 40 years, nonwhite race, and presence of

Table 2
Clinical factors predictive of aggressive Crohn disease as determined by multivariable logistic regression analyses

Author and Year	Patients (n)	Risk Factors	Odds Ratio or Hazard Ratio (95% CI)	Comment
Beaugerie et al 2006[58]	1123	• Requirement for corticosteroids at CD dx	3.1[a] (2.2–4.4)	Factors predictive of disabling disease over 5-year follow-up
		• Age <40 y at CD dx	2.1[a] (1.3–3.6)	
		• Presence of perianal disease at CD dx	1.8[a] (1.2–2.8)	
Loly et al 2008[68]	361	• Perianal lesions at CD dx	2.6[a] (1.4–5.1)	Factors predictive of disabling disease over 5-year follow-up
		• Corticosteroids for the first CD flare	1.7[a] (1.02–2.7)	
		• Ileocolonic CD at dx	1.74[a] (1.06–2.8)	
		• Stricturing CD behavior at dx	2.11[b] (1.39–3.20)	Factors predictive of time to development of disabling disease
		• Weight loss >5 kg at CD dx	1.67[b] (1.14–2.45)	
Lakatos et al 2009[69]	340	• Duration of CD >10 y	4.37[a] (2.04–9.38)	Factors predictive for behavior change from B1 to B2 and/or B3
		• Perianal CD	3.86[a] (1.72–8.67)	
		• Smoking at CD	2.76[a] (1.29–5.89)	
		• Corticosteroids use	8.07[a] (1.64–39.7)	
		• Early azathioprine use	0.35[a] (0.16–0.74)	
		• CD of terminal ileum	2.13[b] (1.11–4.08)	Factors predictive of time to disease behavior change from B1 to B2 and/or B3
		• Perianal CD	3.26[b] (1.90–5.59)	
		• Corticosteroids use	7.48[b] (1.79–31.2)	
		• Early azathioprine use	0.46[b] (0.27–0.79)	
		• Smoking at CD	1.79[b] (1.05–3.05)	
Cosnes et al 2002[57]	2002	• Age <40 y at CD dx	1.3[b] (1.0–1.5)	Factors predictive of penetrating disease (B3)
		• Nonwhite	1.3[b] (1.1–1.6)	
		• Anoperineal lesions at CD dx	2.6[b] (2.3–3.0)	
		• Recent CD dx	1.3[b] (1.0–1.6)	Factors predictive of stricturing disease (B2)
		• Jejunal involvement at CD dx	3.2[b] (2.2–4.7)	
		• Ileal involvement at CD dx	2.5[b] (1.9–3.3)	
		• No colonic involvement at CD dx	2.0[b] (1.6–2.4)	
		• No anoperineal lesions at CD dx	1.4[b] (1.1–1.8)	

Study	N	Factor	Value (95% CI)	Notes
Cosnes et al 2001[70]	474	Current smoking	2.71[b] (1.67–4.41)	Predictors of flare-up. Flare up defined as Crohn Disease Activity Index >150 with 60-point increase from baseline
		Small bowel lesions	1.78[b] (1.08–2.95)	
		Recently active disease	2.70[b] (1.65–4.41)	
		Previous intestinal resection	0.39[b] (0.23–0.66)	
Seksik et al 2009[71]	2795	Female sex	1.16[a] (1.06–1.26)	Factors predictive of annual CD activity
		Age <36 y	1.43[a] (1.34–1.53)	
		Disease duration <96 mo	1.68[a] (1.56–1.79)	
		Smoking ≤10 cigarettes per day	1.30[a] 1.19–1.43	
		Smoking >10 cigarettes per day	1.68[a] (1.57–1.81)	
		Ulcerative colitislike endoscopic lesions	1.39[a] (1.27–1.52)	
		Use of oral contraceptives	0.90[a] (0.82–0.99)	
		High socioeconomic status	0.77[a] (0.72–0.82)	
		White	0.75[a] (0.69–0.82)	
		Prior intestinal resection	0.57[a] (0.53–0.60)	

Abbreviation: dx, diagnosis.
[a] Odds ratio.
[b] Hazard ratio.

anoperineal lesions, whereas development of stricturing complications was predicted by jejunal or ileal disease, absence of colonic disease, and absence of anoperineal disease.[57] Disease behavior change from nonstricturing and nonpenetrating to more complicated stricturing or penetrating was evaluated by Lakatos and colleagues[69] who determined that duration of CD greater than 10 years, perianal disease, smoking, use of steroids, and lack of early (at least 6 months prior to disease behavior change) treatment with azathioprine were independently associated with an increased risk of developing more aggressive disease behavior.[69]

Recent metaanalysis of 7 case-control and 2 prospective cohort studies found an increased risk of CD among current smokers (OR 1.76, 95% CI 1.40–2.22) and ever smokers (ex-smokers and current smokers) (OR 1.61, 95% CI 1.27–2.03) than never smokers versus non-IBD controls.[44] Active smoking has also been found to independently increase nearly threefold the risk of having a subsequent flare of CD that was further fivefold increased among patients who did not receive corticosteroids or immunosuppressive medications (adjusted HR 5.41, 95% CI 2.63–11.10).[70] Other independent predictors increasing two- to threefold risk of disease flare in the prospective referral-based cohort were small bowel lesions and recent activity of disease.[70] Another prospective referral-based center study determined that clinical factors present at the study baseline that were associated with increased risk of annual disease activity were female sex, age less than 36 years, shorter disease duration (<96 months), light and heavy smoking, and ulcerative colitislike lesions on endoscopy.[71] However, clinical factors such as prior intestinal resection, use of oral contraceptives, high socioeconomic status, and white race were independently associated with a decreased risk of annual disease activity.[71]

Summary

Many clinical factors predict the aggressive course of CD. Younger age at initial diagnosis, the presence of perianal lesions, ileal involvement, smoking, and the need for therapy with corticosteroids are the major predictors of disabling disease or change of behavior to a more aggressive disease. On the other hand, treatment with azathioprine and biologic agents and colonic localization of disease are the major factors that are predictive of less aggressive CD course. The problem we face with determining the factors that increase the risk of disabling disease is that there is no standardized and consistent definition of disabling or aggressive disease. Only two studies analyzed predictors using the same definition of aggressive disease.[58,68] Only Beaugerie and colleagues[58] developed the score predictive of disabling disease based on three independent factors associated with disabling course that were present at the time of initial diagnosis of CD (requirement of corticosteroids, age less than 40 years, and presence of perianal disease).[58] This score ranged from 0 to 3 points based on the presence of given parameters.[58] The positive predictive value was 0.91 and 0.93 in patients having two or three risk factors, 0.61 for no factors present, and 0.67 for one factor present.[58] In order to determine factors predictive of disabling CD there is a need to establish consistent definition of disabling disease with subsequent future studies on large group of patients to validate such definition and determine factors that may predict the aggressive course.

REFERENCES

1. Farrell RJ, Peppercorn MA. Ulcerative colitis. Lancet 2002;359:331–40.
2. Su C, Lichtenstein G. Ulcerative colitis. In: Feldman M, Friedman L, Brandt L, editors. Sleisenger and Fordtran's gastrointestinal and liver disease. 8th edition. Philadelphia: Saunders Elsevier; 2006. p. 2499–549.

3. Singleton JW, Law DH, Kelley ML Jr, et al. National Cooperative Crohn's Disease Study: adverse reactions to study drugs. Gastroenterology 1979;77:870–82.
4. Lichtenstein GR, Abreu MT, Cohen R, et al. American Gastroenterological Association Institute technical review on corticosteroids, immunomodulators, and infliximab in inflammatory bowel disease. Gastroenterology 2006;130:940–87.
5. Rutgeerts P, Sandborn WJ, Feagan BG, et al. Infliximab for induction and maintenance therapy for ulcerative colitis. N Engl J Med 2005;353:2462–76.
6. Farmer RG, Easley KA, Rankin GB. Clinical patterns, natural history, and progression of ulcerative colitis. A long-term follow-up of 1116 patients. Dig Dis Sci 1993;38: 1137–46.
7. Bitton A, Peppercorn MA, Antonioli DA, et al. Clinical, biological, and histologic parameters as predictors of relapse in ulcerative colitis. Gastroenterology 2001;120: 13–20.
8. Hoie O, Wolters F, Riis L, et al. Ulcerative colitis: patient characteristics may predict 10-yr disease recurrence in a European-wide population-based cohort. Am J Gastroenterol 2007;102:1692–701.
9. Lundqvist K, Broome U. Differences in colonic disease activity in patients with ulcerative colitis with and without primary sclerosing cholangitis: a case control study. Dis Colon Rectum 1997;40:451–6.
10. Kane SV. Systematic review: adherence issues in the treatment of ulcerative colitis. Aliment Pharmacol Ther 2006;23:577–85.
11. Menees S, Higgins P, Korsnes S, et al. Does colonoscopy cause increased ulcerative colitis symptoms? Inflamm Bowel Dis 2007;13:12–8.
12. Langholz E, Munkholm P, Davidsen M, et al. Course of ulcerative colitis: analysis of changes in disease activity over years. Gastroenterology 1994;107:3–11.
13. Langholz E, Munkholm P, Nielsen OH, et al. Incidence and prevalence of ulcerative colitis in Copenhagen county from 1962 to 1987. Scand J Gastroenterol 1991;26: 1247–56.
14. Hendriksen C, Kreiner S, Binder V. Long term prognosis in ulcerative colitis–based on results from a regional patient group from the county of Copenhagen. Gut 1985;26: 158–63.
15. Stonnington CM, Phillips SF, Zinsmeister AR, et al. Prognosis of chronic ulcerative colitis in a community. Gut 1987;28:1261–6.
16. Kornbluth A, Sachar DB. Ulcerative colitis practice guidelines in adults: American College Of Gastroenterology, Practice Parameters Committee. Am J Gastroenterol 2010;105:501–23 [quiz: 24].
17. Langholz E, Munkholm P, Davidsen M, et al. Colorectal cancer risk and mortality in patients with ulcerative colitis. Gastroenterology 1992;103:1444–51.
18. Travis SP, Farrant JM, Ricketts C, et al. Predicting outcome in severe ulcerative colitis. Gut 1996;38:905–10.
19. Leijonmarck CE, Persson PG, Hellers G. Factors affecting colectomy rate in ulcerative colitis: an epidemiologic study. Gut 1990;31:329–33.
20. Langholz E, Munkholm P, Davidsen M, et al. Changes in extent of ulcerative colitis: a study on the course and prognostic factors. Scand J Gastroenterol 1996;31:260–6.
21. Hoie O, Wolters FL, Riis L, et al. Low colectomy rates in ulcerative colitis in an unselected European cohort followed for 10 years. Gastroenterology 2007;132: 507–15.
22. Solberg IC, Lygren I, Jahnsen J, et al. Clinical course during the first 10 years of ulcerative colitis: results from a population-based inception cohort (IBSEN Study). Scand J Gastroenterol 2009;44:431–40.

23. Ananthakrishnan AN, Issa M, Beaulieu DB, et al. History of medical hospitalization predicts future need for colectomy in patients with ulcerative colitis. Inflamm Bowel Dis 2009;15:176–81.

24. Jess T, Gamborg M, Munkholm P, et al. Overall and cause-specific mortality in ulcerative colitis: meta-analysis of population-based inception cohort studies. Am J Gastroenterol 2007;102:609–17.

25. Sinclair TS, Brunt PW, Mowat NA. Nonspecific proctocolitis in northeastern Scotland: a community study. Gastroenterology 1983;85:1–11.

26. Ayres RC, Gillen CD, Walmsley RS, et al. Progression of ulcerative proctosigmoiditis: incidence and factors influencing progression. Eur J Gastroenterol Hepatol 1996;8: 555–8.

27. Powell-Tuck J, Ritchie JK, Lennard-Jones JE. The prognosis of idiopathic proctitis. Scand J Gastroenterol 1977;12:727–32.

28. Andres PG, Friedman LS. Epidemiology and the natural course of inflammatory bowel disease. Gastroenterol Clin North Am 1999;28:255–81, vii.

29. Moayyeri A, Daryani NE, Bahrami H, et al. Clinical course of ulcerative colitis in patients with and without primary sclerosing cholangitis. J Gastroenterol Hepatol 2005;20: 366–70.

30. Papatheodoridis GV, Hamilton M, Mistry PK, et al. Ulcerative colitis has an aggressive course after orthotopic liver transplantation for primary sclerosing cholangitis. Gut 1998;43:639–44.

31. Gurbuz AK, Giardiello FM, Bayless TM. Colorectal neoplasia in patients with ulcerative colitis and primary sclerosing cholangitis. Dis Colon Rectum 1995;38:37–41.

32. Broome U, Lofberg R, Veress B, et al. Primary sclerosing cholangitis and ulcerative colitis: evidence for increased neoplastic potential. Hepatology 1995;22:1404–8.

33. Faubion WA Jr, Loftus EV Jr, Harmsen WS, et al. The natural history of corticosteroid therapy for inflammatory bowel disease: a population-based study. Gastroenterology 2001;121:255–60.

34. Lindgren SC, Flood LM, Kilander AF, et al. Early predictors of glucocorticosteroid treatment failure in severe and moderately severe attacks of ulcerative colitis. Eur J Gastroenterol Hepatol 1998;10:831–5.

35. Elloumi H, Ben Abdelaziz A, Derbel F, et al. Predictive factors of glucocorticosteroid treatment failure in severe acute idiopathic colitis. Acta Gastroenterol Belg 2005;68: 226–9.

36. Cassinotti A, Actis GC, Duca P, et al. Maintenance treatment with azathioprine in ulcerative colitis: outcome and predictive factors after drug withdrawal. Am J Gastroenterol 2009;104:2760–7.

37. Evans JM, McMahon AD, Murray FE, et al. Non-steroidal anti-inflammatory drugs are associated with emergency admission to hospital for colitis due to inflammatory bowel disease. Gut 1997;40:619–22.

38. Felder JB, Korelitz BI, Rajapakse R, et al. Effects of nonsteroidal antiinflammatory drugs on inflammatory bowel disease: a case-control study. Am J Gastroenterol 2000;95:1949–54.

39. Meyer AM, Ramzan NN, Heigh RI, et al. Relapse of inflammatory bowel disease associated with use of nonsteroidal anti-inflammatory drugs. Dig Dis Sci 2006;51: 168–72.

40. Takeuchi K, Smale S, Premchand P, et al. Prevalence and mechanism of nonsteroidal anti-inflammatory drug-induced clinical relapse in patients with inflammatory bowel disease. Clin Gastroenterol Hepatol 2006;4:196–202.

41. Sandborn WJ, Stenson WF, Brynskov J, et al. Safety of celecoxib in patients with ulcerative colitis in remission: a randomized, placebo-controlled, pilot study. Clin Gastroenterol Hepatol 2006;4:203–11.
42. Bonner GF, Fakhri A, Vennamaneni SR. A long-term cohort study of nonsteroidal anti-inflammatory drug use and disease activity in outpatients with inflammatory bowel disease. Inflamm Bowel Dis 2004;10:751–7.
43. Kane S, Huo D, Aikens J, et al. Medication nonadherence and the outcomes of patients with quiescent ulcerative colitis. Am J Med 2003;114:39–43.
44. Mahid SS, Minor KS, Soto RE, et al. Smoking and inflammatory bowel disease: a meta-analysis. Mayo Clin Proc 2006;81:1462–71.
45. Rudra T, Motley R, Rhodes J. Does smoking improve colitis? Scand J Gastroenterol Suppl 1989;170:61–3 [discussion: 6–8].
46. de Castella H. Non-smoking: a feature of ulcerative colitis. Br Med J (Clin Res Ed) 1982;284:1706.
47. Abraham N, Selby W, Lazarus R, et al. Is smoking an indirect risk factor for the development of ulcerative colitis? An age- and sex-matched case-control study. J Gastroenterol Hepatol 2003;18:139–46.
48. Boyko EJ, Perera DR, Koepsell TD, et al. Effects of cigarette smoking on the clinical course of ulcerative colitis. Scand J Gastroenterol 1988;23:1147–52.
49. Beaugerie L, Massot N, Carbonnel F, et al. Impact of cessation of smoking on the course of ulcerative colitis. Am J Gastroenterol 2001;96:2113–6.
50. Nishio Y, Ando T, Maeda O, et al. Pit patterns in rectal mucosa assessed by magnifying colonoscope are predictive of relapse in patients with quiescent ulcerative colitis. Gut 2006;55:1768–73.
51. Fujiya M, Saitoh Y, Nomura M, et al. Minute findings by magnifying colonoscopy are useful for the evaluation of ulcerative colitis. Gastrointest Endosc 2002;56:535–42.
52. Watanabe C, Sumioka M, Hiramoto T, et al. Magnifying colonoscopy used to predict disease relapse in patients with quiescent ulcerative colitis. Inflamm Bowel Dis 2009;15:1663–9.
53. Froslie KF, Jahnsen J, Moum BA, et al. Mucosal healing in inflammatory bowel disease: results from a Norwegian population-based cohort. Gastroenterology 2007; 133:412–22.
54. Schirbel A, Fiocchi C. Inflammatory bowel disease: established and evolving considerations on its etiopathogenesis and therapy. J Dig Dis 2010;11:266–76.
55. Gasche C, Scholmerich J, Brynskov J, et al. A simple classification of Crohn's disease: report of the Working Party for the World Congresses of Gastroenterology, Vienna 1998. Inflamm Bowel Dis 2000;6:8–15.
56. Louis E, Collard A, Oger AF, et al. Behaviour of Crohn's disease according to the Vienna classification: changing pattern over the course of the disease. Gut 2001;49:777–82.
57. Cosnes J, Cattan S, Blain A, et al. Long-term evolution of disease behavior of Crohn's disease. Inflamm Bowel Dis 2002;8:244–50.
58. Beaugerie L, Seksik P, Nion-Larmurier I, et al. Predictors of Crohn's disease. Gastroenterology 2006;130:650–6.
59. Munkholm P, Langholz E, Davidsen M, et al. Disease activity courses in a regional cohort of Crohn's disease patients. Scand J Gastroenterol 1995;30:699–706.
60. Solberg IC, Vatn MH, Hoie O, et al. Clinical course in Crohn's disease: results of a Norwegian population-based ten-year follow-up study. Clin Gastroenterol Hepatol 2007;5:1430–8.
61. Veloso FT, Ferreira JT, Barros L, et al. Clinical outcome of Crohn's disease: analysis according to the vienna classification and clinical activity. Inflamm Bowel Dis 2001;7:306–13.

62. Greenstein AJ, Lachman P, Sachar DB, et al. Perforating and non-perforating indications for repeated operations in Crohn's disease: evidence for two clinical forms. Gut 1988;29:588–92.
63. Bernell O, Lapidus A, Hellers G. Risk factors for surgery and postoperative recurrence in Crohn's disease. Ann Surg 2000;231:38–45.
64. Ramadas AV, Gunesh S, Thomas GA, et al. Natural history of Crohn's disease in a population-based cohort from Cardiff (1986–2003): a study of changes in medical treatment and surgical resection rates. Gut 2010;59:1200–6.
65. Szamosi T, Banai J, Lakatos L, et al. Early azathioprine/biological therapy is associated with decreased risk for first surgery and delays time to surgery but not reoperation in both smokers and nonsmokers with Crohn's disease, while smoking decreases the risk of colectomy in ulcerative colitis. Eur J Gastroenterol Hepatol 2010;22:872–9.
66. Reese GE, Nanidis T, Borysiewicz C, et al. The effect of smoking after surgery for Crohn's disease: a meta-analysis of observational studies. Int J Colorectal Dis 2008;23:1213–21.
67. Duricova D, Pedersen N, Elkjaer M, et al. Overall and cause-specific mortality in Crohn's disease: a meta-analysis of population-based studies. Inflamm Bowel Dis 2010;16:347–53.
68. Loly C, Belaiche J, Louis E. Predictors of severe Crohn's disease. Scand J Gastroenterol 2008;43:948–54.
69. Lakatos PL, Czegledi Z, Szamosi T, et al. Perianal disease, small bowel disease, smoking, prior steroid or early azathioprine/biological therapy are predictors of disease behavior change in patients with Crohn's disease. World J Gastroenterol 2009;15:3504–10.
70. Cosnes J, Beaugerie L, Carbonnel F, et al. Smoking cessation and the course of Crohn's disease: an intervention study. Gastroenterology 2001;120:1093–9.
71. Seksik P, Nion-Larmurier I, Sokol H, et al. Effects of light smoking consumption on the clinical course of Crohn's disease. Inflamm Bowel Dis 2009;15:734–41.

The Promise and Pitfalls of Serologic Testing in Inflammatory Bowel Disease

Joseph H. Sellin, MD[a],*, Rashesh R. Shah[b]

KEYWORDS

- Inflammatory bowel disease • Crohn disease
- Ulcerative colitis • Serologic testing

Serologies have well-established roles in the diagnosis of a variety of immunologically driven diseases; rheumatologists rely on an alphabet soup of antibodies, hepatologists depend on serologic tests to diagnose primary biliary cirrhosis (PBC) and autoimmune hepatitis, and celiac experts have used a battery of tests for diagnosis, adherence, and a better understanding of pathophysiology. In these specialties, serologies provide a robust diagnostic accuracy either by themselves or with a minimum of other studies to establish a diagnosis or guide therapeutic decision making.

Serologic testing is a natural consideration in another immunologically driven disease, inflammatory bowel disease (IBD). If a relatively simple blood draw could provide an equally accurate but less expensive, less laborious, and less invasive test than the present gold standard of endoscopy, it would be a major advance in our approach to diagnosis and treatment of IBD. There is a 5-decade history of antibodies in ulcerative colitis; the first report of antibodies in human ulcerative colitis date from 1959.[1] Over the last 2 decades, there has been an intensification of the interest in IBD-related antibodies.

In this review, we examine 4 areas in which IBD serologies might be important: (1) to provide insight into the etiopathogenesis of IBD, (2) to establish the diagnosis of IBD, (3) to differentiate Crohn disease (CD) from ulcerative colitis (UC), and (4) to stratify risk of developing a complicated course that might dictate earlier more aggressive treatment.

There are considerable data to suggest that IBD serologies may provide important information in all of these areas. However, it is not clear that serologic testing can adequately replace endoscopy or other simpler clinical indicators or surrogate

The authors have nothing to disclose.
Division of Gastroenterology, Baylor College of Medicine, 1709 Dryden, Houston, TX 77030, USA
Department of Medicine, Baylor College of Medicine, Baylor Faculty Clinic, 1709 Dryden 8.20, Houston TX 77030, USA
* Corresponding author.
E-mail address: sellin@bcm.edu

Gastroenterol Clin N Am 41 (2012) 463–482
doi:10.1016/j.gtc.2012.01.001
0889-8553/12/$ – see front matter © 2012 Elsevier Inc. All rights reserved.
gastro.theclinics.com

markers of inflammation. If they can serve only a limited, adjunctive role in diagnosis and management of IBD, then one would need to carefully evaluate the specific circumstances and added value of additional testing.

Understandably, most studies have examined IBD serologies in well-defined IBD patient populations. Few studies attempt to characterize prospectively the utility of these serologies in patients who have yet to have IBD diagnosed or who are early in the course of IBD.

In 2011, there is limited evidence to recommend routine use of the current panels of serologic markers for diagnosing, stratifying, or monitoring IBD in clinical practice. However, this is a rapidly evolving field, and, perhaps, new findings may establish a role for IBD serologies in the future. As always, more studies are needed.

PATHOGENESIS

What is the connection between IBD antibodies and the pathophysiology of the disease? In some diseases, there is a strong link between an identified antibody and the underlying immunopathogenesis. For example, in celiac disease, antibodies directed against tissue transglutaminase provide insight into the molecular pathogenesis of the disease. Similarly, anti mitochondrial antibodies target a specific pathway important in the development of PBC.

The identification of an increasing number of diverse antimicrobial antibodies in IBD suggests that none of these are likely to be integral to the pathogenesis but are surrogate markers for a change in the interaction of the gut epithelium and the gut microbiome. Two possible changes that have been implicated in IBD are (1) a "leaky gut" with subsequent development of antibodies secondary to increased permeability, or (2) a generalized loss of tolerance to commensal organisms in the intestinal lumen in Crohn that may, for unknown reasons, lead to a more targeted microbial and auto antigen response.

If IBD-associated antibodies are a reflection of increased permeability, then one might expect an increased incidence of antibodies against dietary antigens. This does not appear to be the case.[2] The plethora of antibodies associated with CD suggests a more generalized immune response. However, there is no indication of what is specific about these antigens that would lead to IBD. A higher rate of multiple antibody production may indicate a more global loss of tolerance to intestinal flora. Indeed, Adams and colleagues[3] suggested that immunoglobulin (IgG) antibodies against common bacteria are more diagnostic for CD than IgG against mannan (anti-Saccharomyces cerevisiae antibody [ASCA]) or flagellin (CBir1).[3]

Although there has been a greater focus on antimicrobial antibodies associated with IBD, there are some less-characterized (auto) antibodies directed against components of the intestinal epithelium, including goblet cells and microfilament proteins. These might conceivably be more directed to the etiology of disease. Further studies are needed to clarify a possible connection.

The observations that there can be "preclinical seropositivity" in individuals in whom IBD develops years later and that there is a significant familial incidence of positive IBD-related antibodies in clinically unaffected, first-degree relatives of IBD patients raises questions about whether genetic factors may also play a role. To date there does not seem to be an IBD gene locus that predicts seropositivity. This is an important area for future investigation.

There is an interesting inverse relationship between IBD serologies and seroprevalence of *Helicobacter pylori* infection.[4] Although one might speculate whether *H pylori* may have a protective effect on IBD, it is more probable that both antibody responses

Table 1
IBD-associated antibodies, presumed targets, and select population prevalences

Antibody	Target	Prevalence (%)		
		Ulcerative Colitis	Crohn Disease	Healthy Controls
pANCA	Unidentified protein of the nuclear envelope of neutrophils	41–73	6–38	0–8
ASCAgASCA	Carbohydrate epitopes present in the phophopeptidomannan of the cell wall of Saccharomyces cerevisiae Covalently bound mannin	0–29	29–69	0–16
OmpC	Omp-C transport protein of E coli	2–24	24–55	5–20
I2	Pseudomonas-associated sequence I2	42	38–60	15
Cbir1	Bacterial flagellin CBir1	6	50–56	8
ALCA	Laminaribioside (Glc[b1,3]Glc[b])	3–8	19–27	2
ACCA	Chitobioside (GlcNAc[b1,4]GlcNAc[b])	5–7	8–25	0.5–12
AMCA	Mannobioside (Man[a1,3]Mana)	7	12–28	9
Anti-L	Laminarin (Glc[b 1,3])3n(Glc[b 1,6])n	3–7	18–26	1–10
Anti-C	Chitin (GlcNAc[b 1,4])n	2–11	10–25	2–12
Antigoblet cell	Goblet cells of the intestines			
Tropomyosin	Microfilament protein tropomyosin	79	12	
Pancreatic autoantibody	GP2 a major zymogen granule membrane glycoprotein		30	

Data from Prideaux L, De Crux P, Ng SC, et al. Serological antibodies in inflammatory bowel disease: a systematic review. Inflamm Bowel Dis 2011. DOI:10.1002/ibd.21903. [Epub ahead of print.]

may be linked to environmental effects during childhood that have been synthesized as the hygiene hypothesis.

CHARACTERISTICS OF IBD ANTIBODIES

Identification, description, and commercialization of 2 antibodies, antineutrophilic cytoplasmic antibody (ANCA) and ASCA invigorated research in IBD serologies. Over the last several years, there has been a steady increase in the number of IBD antibodies identified. Eventually, this range of antibodies should provide a better understanding of the etiopathogenesis of IBD and lead to more judicious clinical management of patients with ulcerative colitis and Crohn. However, at this point, the array of antibodies may leave the clinician more confused than enlightened.

We will classify these antibodies into 3 somewhat arbitrary groups: (1) what may be considered the first-generation of IBD-related antibodies that are widely available now through Prometheus Labs, (2) a group of antiglycan antibodies, and (3) a group of orphan autoantibodies with diverse targets in the gastrointestinal mucosa (**Table 1**).

First-Generation Antibodies

ANCA
ANCAs were first associated with IBD, specifically UC, in the 1980s. ANCAs describe a class of autoantibodies, typically of the IgG subclass, directed against antigens in the cytoplasm of neutrophils and monocytes. B cells, in the intestinal mucosa, produce p-ANCA presumably against a self epitope or resident pathogen.[5]

In 1983, Nielson and colleagues[6] described the presence of ANCA in the sera of patients with UC. They used an indirect immunofluorescence technique to identify a perinuclear pattern to the ANCA in UC.[6] Subsequently, numerous groups went on to further characterize p-ANCA in IBD, with groups noting a certain percentage of CD patient's would express ANCAs.

Vasiliauskas and coworkers[7] in 1996, performed a study comparing ANCA-positive CD patients with negative controls to further characterize clinical subtypes. They found that p-ANCA–positive CD patients more frequently have left-sided colitis and symptoms of left-sided inflammation than patients negative for p-ANCA.[7]

Sandborn and colleagues[8] showed in a study comparing the tests properties of p-ANCA and ASCA across several laboratories that the sensitivity of testing for p-ANCA varies between 0 and 63%. They attributed this variation to the tests potentially targeting different unidentified antigens.[8] Vidrich and coworkers[9] showed that the use of DNase with UC sera disrupts its reactivity to p-ANCA, potentially improving the sensitivity of detecting UC-specific p-ANCA.

Reese and coworkers[10] examined the diagnostic ability of p-ANCA and ASCA to identify UC and CD, respectively. They performed a meta-analysis of 60 studies, which included 3,841 UC patients and 4,019 CD patients. They found that p-ANCA positivity translated to a sensitivity and specificity of 55.3% and 88.5%, respectively, for the diagnosis of UC.[10]

Taylor and colleagues[11] in 2001 described the relationship between p-ANCA positivity and response to anti-tumor necrosis factor (TNF) therapy in a cohort of CD patients. They examined the response of 59 patients to anti-TNF therapy based on serologic and genetic factors. They found that patients with p-ANCA had a similar response to anti-TNF therapy as they did to placebo, with ASCA patients responding significantly better.[11] Ferrante and coworkers[12] found similar results when they examined the response of 100 UC patients to infusion with infliximab. The subgroup with pANCA+ and ASCA– serologies had a statistically lower response rate (55% vs 76%, $P = .049$).[12]

The relationship between surgical interventions for UC and p-ANCA was also examined. Aitola and colleagues[13] examined the sera of 15 UC patients before surgery and followed up with them for a median duration of 24 months postoperatively to study p-ANCA titers. They found that preoperatively, 13 of 15 patients had positive results for p-ANCA, and postoperatively titers decreased in 10 patients and became negative in 2.[13]

Mow and coworkers[14] examined the prognostic value of p-ANCA in a cohort of 303 CD patients, correlating phenotypes to serologic abnormalities. They found that p-ANCA–positive patients had a statistically significantly decreased risk of small bowel disease, fibrostenosing disease, and small bowel surgery. They did, however, have a higher risk of exhibiting UC-like features.[14]

ASCA

ASCAs are produced in response to yeast cell wall components, particularly mannan. It is commonly known as baker's or brewer's yeast and is common in diets. Main and colleagues[15] in 1988 described the presence of this antibody in a small cohort of IBD patients. They found that the sera of CD patients expressed a larger proportion of IgG and IgA antibodies directed against Saccharomyces cerevisiae when compared with UC and normal controls.[15]

Giaffer and colleagues[16] further characterized the antibody responses with particular strains of Saccharomyces cerevisiae yeast. They tested for IgG and IgA antibody levels in 49 CD patients, 43 UC patients and 21 controls through ELISA. Both IgG and

IgA levels were significantly increased in the CD cohort, versus both the UC cohort and the healthy controls.[16]

Vasiliauskas and colleagues[17] studied the ability of ASCA to define clinical phenotypes and natural history in CD. They studied the sera of 156 consecutive established CD patients for ASCA and then correlated sera to their clinical phenotype in a blinded fashion. They found that higher ASCA titers correlated with earlier age of onset, fibrostenosing, and internal penetrating disease.[17]

In the previously described study by Reese and coworkers,[10] ASCA was also examined for its sensitivity and specificity in diagnosing CD. They found positive ASCA combined with negative p-ANCA yielded a sensitivity and specificity of 54.6% and 92.8%, respectively. Mow and colleagues[14] also showed the presence of ASCA can be used to describe phenotype and possibly assist in prognosis, because these patients have a higher risk for small bowel surgery.

Recent literature has described gASCAs, which are antibodies against covalently immobilized mannan.[18] Although there may be some subtle differences between the 2 assays, they seem to perform basically the same in identification of patients with CD.

Outer membrane porin C

Outer membrane porin C (Omp-C) is a protein belonging to *Escherichia coli* that is used to regulate metabolite and toxin transport. It was first associated with IBD in 2000 through bacterial library screening, which identified *E coli*.[19] Further studies showed the Omp-C protein was immunogenic, with a proportion of UC patients generating antibodies to Omp-C. In CD, Omp-C has been correlated with increased risk of fibrostenosing disease, internal penetrating disease, and need for small bowel surgery.[14]

In a pilot study performed by Mow and coworkers,[20] they examined the possible role the presence of Omp-C may have in identifying CD patients with better chances of clinical response to antibiotic therapy. They compared patients taking budesonide with patients taking budesonide plus metronidazole and ciprofloxacin. They found that in patients expressing higher levels of Omp-C, patients responded better, defined as a decrease in the Crohn Disease Activity Index score of 150 or greater, with the addition of antibiotics. These results, however, did not reach statistical significance.[20]

I2

I2 was first discovered by cloning fragments of bacterial DNA recovered from lamina propria mononuclear cells present in active CD tissue but not uninvolved tissue or UC. Further genetic analysis showed this bacterial sequence belongs to *Pseudomonas fluorescens*.[21] I2 correlates, in CD patients, to small bowel disease, fibrostenotic disease, and small bowel surgery.[14] I2 was also shown, in the previously mentioned pilot study by Mow and colleagues,[20] to select CD patients, who might benefit from treatment with antibiotics.

Spivak and coworkers[22] found that I2 was a predictor of response to fecal diversion in CD. Seventeen of 27 (63%) patients achieved clinical response from fecal diversion; however, 15 of 16 patients who were I2 positive (94%) responded.[22]

CBir1

CBir1, a flagellin, is a microbial antigen that presumably induces colitis through an adaptive immune response. Targan and coworkers[23] evaluated serum responses to CBir1 in CD patients, compare this with other known IBD-related serologies and CD phenotypes. They tested sera from 484 CD patients and found CBir1 present in all

Table 2
IBD-associated antibodies, predominant disease location in Crohn disease patients, and disease behavior

Antibody	Predominant Disease Location	Disease Behavior/Significance
pANCA	Colon	Distal colitis (inflammatory phenotype)
ASCA	Small bowel	FS, IP
Omp-C	Small bowel (+/–) In combination with other Abs	FS, IP
I2	Small bowel	FS
CBir1	Small bowel	FS, IP DDx pANCA+ CD vs UC
ALCA	Small bowel in combination with other Abs	FS
ACCA	?Small bowel in combination with other antibodies	FS, IP
AMCA	?Small bowel in combination with other antibodies	FS
Anti-L	Small bowel	FS, IP
Anti-C	?Small bowel in combination with other Abs	FS, IP

Data on localization and disease phenotype are complicated by the fact that multiple antibody positivity is more common than isolated single antibodies. Additionally, not all antibodies are measured in all studies.
Abbreviations: FS, fibrostenosing; IP, internal penetration.
Data from Refs.[14,23,37]

previously described antibody subgroups. The expression of CBir1 increased with combinations of other IBD-related serologies. CBir1 was associated with small bowel disease, fibrostenotic disease, and internal penetrating disease.[23] **Tables 1** and **2** summarize the previously described antibodies in relation to their prevalences and clinical characteristics.

Antiglycan Antibodies

Glycan is a generic term for all molecules bearing glycosidic bonds, which are major constituents of cell surface components of, among others, immune cells and micro-organisms. Glycans may modulate the immune system through stimulation of cell proliferation, phagocytosis, and cytokine secretion.[24]

ASCA was the first antiglycan antibody identified. However, several novel antibodies have subsequently been demonstrated. Dotan and colleagues[18] first reported the association of these antibodies with CD.

The antibody targets are laminarbioside (ALCA), chitobioside (ACCA) and mannobioside (AMCA). Seroreactivity against oligosaccharides is common in patients with CD: ALCA 37.5% and ACCA 36%. Less than 10% of patients with UC or miscellaneous inflammatory conditions demonstrate seropositivity. However, another intestinal inflammatory process, celiac disease, has a high rate of ACCA positivity.[18]

Recently, 2 additional antiglycan antibodies have been described: anti-laminarin IgA (Glc[β1,3])3n(Glc[β1,6])n carbohydrate antibody (Anti-L) and anti-chitin GlcNAc(β1,4)n IgA carbohydrate antibody (Anti-C).

In general, the incidence of these antiglycan markers is a bit lower than the first-generation antibodies. However, much like the first-generation antibodies, when multiple antiglycan antibodies are positive, there is improved sensitivity and specificity for diagnosis of CD. Increasing titers of the antibodies appear to be associated with more complicated disease and earlier surgery, similar to the first-generation antibodies.[25,26]

Despite a lower rate of seropositivity in Crohn, they may have clinical relevance in that ALCA or ACCA may be positive in almost half of the ASCA-negative patients.[18]

The first-generation antibodies are generally stable over time. However, there may be an effect of increasing antiglycan antibody positivity with disease duration. This will be an important question to define carefully if they are to be used for disease stratification. Although not as commonly used in the United States, they are available commercially (http://www.ibdx.net/index.html).

Orphan Antibodies

Antibodies directed toward some specific intestinal epithelial antigens have been described. They have not been as widely tested as the more commercialized antibodies described above; therefore, their clinical role has yet to be defined. Antigoblet cell antibodies may occur in up to 40% of patients with IBD (both UC and CD) and in a significant number of first-degree relatives. Although healthy controls rarely exhibit antigoblet cell antibodies, inflammatory controls, such as celiac disease, may do so frequently. Given the obvious change in goblet cells and mucin in IBD, the existence of antigoblet cell antibodies suggests a potential pathogenic mechanism. Clinical applicability of anti goblet cell antibodies remains to be determined.[27–29]

Das and colleagues[30,31] isolated a UC-associated antibody and eventually identified its target, the microfilament protein, tropomsyoin. The major colonic tropomyosin isoform (hTm5) induces both humoral and T cell responses in UC patients. A higher percentage of patients with UC (79%) had an enhanced antibody response compared with 12% of Crohn. This tropomyosin isoform is expressed on colonic epithelium but not small bowel. If this autoantibody indeed does have a causative role in UC, this may explain why disease activity is restricted to the colon.[30,31]

Pancreatic autoantibodies (targeted to zymogen granule membrane glycoprotein) may occur in about 30% of patients with CD. They are not clearly correlated with clinical features but perhaps with early-onset disease.[32,33]

Sophisticated technologies such as protein microarrays may lead to the identification of novel autoantigens in IBD.[34] As the number of autoantibodies and antibodies directed against microbes continue to increase, it will be necessary to sort through which ones are clinically relevant and pathophysiologically important. Given the large gaps in our knowledge in IBD, this area of research may hold considerable promise.

IBD Serologies in Diagnosing IBD and Distinguishing UC From CD: Statistical Considerations

The diagnostic power of serologic testing in many diseases is well established. However, the promise of IBD serologies for screening in a general population, for distinguishing IBD from other gastrointestinal diseases, and for separating UC from CD has not been fully realized.

Sorting through the statistics on IBD serologies is akin to wandering through a labyrinthine maze. For the statistically challenged, some insights and guidance are provided by Austin and colleagues[35] in an informative evaluation of IBD serologic testing. Although sensitivity and specificity of an individual test are relatively fixed, the relevant clinical parameters are positive and negative predictive values (PPV, NPV, respectively). The PPV and NPV depend on the disease prevalence in the test population. If the disease prevalence is low, the positive predictive value falls.

An enabling calculation helps illustrate the dilemma of screening for a disease with low prevalence. If we assume that there are 1 million patients with CD in the United States and half are Omp-C positive, then there are perhaps 500,000 Omp-C–positive IBD patients. If the prevalence in a healthy population ("false-positive" rate) is only 1% and the US population is now 300,000,000, this would suggest there are 3 million Omp-C–positive people in the general population, a 6:1 ratio of non-IBD to IBD cases.

However, few studies start with a relatively undefined population to evaluate the role of serologies in individuals without an established diagnosis. Instead, they compare patients with known IBD and different control populations, already diagnosed. This may include healthy controls or individuals with a variety of gastrointestinal diseases; there may be changes depending on the comparator.[25]

IBD prevalence in most of these studies may range from 40% to 60%. In this range, the positive predictive value is high (>90%), but the negative predictive value is limited and less impressive, about 50%. The frequently quoted sensitivity (>80%) and positive predictive value (>90%) for the serologic markers for CD depend on a high prevalence of the disease in the tested population; this may be as high as 38%.[36] Austin and colleagues[35] point out that as more tests are added to a panel, the sensitivity of the overall test will increase as long as only 1 test needs to be positive. However, there will be a concomitant decrease in specificity. Thus, as we see panels of more antibodies added to serologic testing, it is important to keep in mind the impact on diagnostic accuracy.

In distinguishing between UC and CD, several studies have consistently shown that the pANCA+/ASCA− profile for UC and the pANCA-/ASCA+ pattern provide accurate discrimination between the two.[25,37]

This can serve to confirm the clinical diagnosis. Multiple studies have linked a specific antibody positivity to disease location or phenotype (see **Table 2**). Broad patterns hold true. For example, ASCA positivity is associated with small bowel location and fistulizing disease. However, untangling associations when multiple antibodies are positive has led to conflicting observations about whether 1 antibody is associated with fistulizing or penetrating disease.[37] In general, both the antiglycan and antimicrobial antibodies are associated with complicated small bowel disease and surgery (see Prognosis and Stratification). There have been no antibody associations with perianal disease. In the more clinically challenging matter of indeterminate colitis, the diagnostic capability is less helpful (or predictive; see below).

The interpretation of the Prometheus panel of IBD serologies has become somewhat opaque with the development of pattern recognition technology that is trained to recognize subtle patterns and relationships among serum biomarkers. This may increase the sensitivity of the assay but sometimes yields a diagnosis of IBD when all the individual biomarkers are normal.

Serologic testing is neither necessary nor sufficient for the primary diagnosis of IBD. The serologic markers cannot replace a conventional clinical evaluation. However, after a thorough clinical workup in cases of indeterminate differentiation of CD versus UC, the use of this antibody panel may be a potential method of discrimination.

FALSE-POSITIVE ANTIBODIES

What are reasonable considerations concerning seemingly false-positive IBD serologies? In our experience, it is not uncommon to have someone referred for an isolated positive serology that suggested CD, but an extensive workup, usually including upper, lower, and capsule endoscopies has been negative. Omp-C is the most common culprit, but it certainly may occur with other serologic tests.[38] Do they represent a *forme fruste* of IBD, a different disease, or a true false-positive? Consideration of these possibilities is critical to meaningful interpretation of IBD serologies.

Preclinical Antibodies

If IBD serologies may represent a preclinical marker of disease, then one might expect to find data to support this in family studies or blood specimens of general populations that have been saved for years or decades.

A small but very interesting study from banked sera from the Israeli Defense Force allowed a backward look at people with a recent diagnosis of CD. ASCA were present in 10 of 32 (31.3%) CD patients before clinical diagnosis compared with 0 of 95 (0%) controls ($P<.001$). None of the 8 patients with serum samples available before diagnosis of UC were ASCA positive. ASCA was positive in 54.5% of patients after diagnosis of CD. This provides some tantalizing data that will need corroboration in larger studies.[39]

Are relatives of IBD patients more likely to have positive serologies? And, does the presence of a positive IBD serology in family members of IBD patients represent a predictor of future disease?

In UC patients and families, probands had 68% to 86% positive ANCAs, whereas unaffected family members had 15% to 30% positive ANCAs. In a similar vein, first-degree relatives of patients with Crohn have a 25% incidence of positive ASCAs.[40] These studies are similar to studies of intestinal permeability in CD, in which a significant number of asymptomatic family members had abnormal permeabilities. Unfortunately, to our knowledge, there are few studies that follow family members prospectively to determine if CD does develop.

One small study from Germany, addressing this question, followed up with 102 first-degree relatives of IBD patients for 7 years. Thirty-three percent were seropositive, and, over the 7 years, IBD developed in 2 individuals (1 Crohn, 1 UC). However, neither of these 2 cases had initially been seropositive.[41] Does the familial incidence of seropositivity represent a yet-to-be-defined genetic factor or a common environmental etiology? Close follow-up of asymptomatic, first-degree seropositive relatives may eventually provide us with some insight into the temporal and perhaps also the causal relations between IBD antibodies and clinical diseae.[40–43]

IBD Serologies in Other Diseases

Although there has been a focus on the relationship between the first-generation antibodies and IBD, it is important to keep in mind that these antibodies may be positive in several different gastrointestinal and inflammatory diseases. Recognition of these other conditions is important when confronting an apparent false-positive IBD serology. Although for the most part, the serology-positive non-IBD diseases have been viewed as a confounding variable, they may also provide some clues as to the common links among these conditions.

Given the overlap in possible presenting symptoms, it is important to appreciate that almost two-thirds of patients with celiac disease may have positive serologies. In a series of 37 patients with biopsy-confirmed celiac disease, 8 were ANCA positive and 16 were ASCA positive. Antiglycan antibodies are also positive in patients with celiac disease. It is curious that celiac disease is associated with both UC- and CD-related antibodies. Because celiac disease is more common than IBD in many populations, this becomes an important consideration and perhaps should be incorporated into a diagnostic workup of seemingly false-positive IBD serologies. Therefore, in workup of diarrhea, positive IBD serologies may obscure rather than clarify a diagnosis.[44,45]

Clinically, Behcet's disease may have some features that mimic CD. Behcet's may also have ASCA positivity in approximately one-third of patients. Intriguingly, like IBD, family members are more likely to have a positive serology than healthy controls.[46]

At least 2 diseases considered classic extraintestinal manifestations of IBD also exhibit a significant IBD seropositivity. Patients with ankylosing spondylitis (AS) demonstrate seroreactivity to multiple IBD antibodies, including ASCA, ANCA, I2 and Omp-C. Although patients with UC and ankylosing spondylitis had a positive pANCA more frequently than AS alone, there was a significant ANCA positivity in isolated AS. It is interesting that in AS there did not appear to be a preponderance of UC- or CD-like antigen patterns.[47]

Patients with primary sclerosing cholangitis (PSC) exhibit a very high rate of ANCA positivity as do their relatives. Seibold and colleagues found pANCA in 82% of patients with PSC and in 25% of their relatives. In UC, 70% of the patients and 30% of their relatives had pANCA. pANCA positivity was found only in low titers in 27% of patients with CD and in 6% of their relatives. pANCA were not detected in members of healthy families. Only 16% of the patients with ulcerative colitis and their families and none of the patients with PSC and their families were completely negative for pANCA.[42]

Although it is not uncommon to find IBD antibodies in a liver disease closely linked to IBD, several other liver diseases may exhibit positive serologies, including autoimmune hepatitis and PBC (particularly AMA negative PBC). More unexpectedly, antimicrobial IBD antibodies were also found in cirrhosis of diverse etiology. Occurrence of antibodies seemed to increase in more advanced cirrhosis.[48,49]

Other diseases that also have a high seropositivity are cystic fibrosis (CF) and rheumatoid arthritis. CF patients have greater than 40% ANCA or ASCA antibodies. Approximately 33% of rheumatoid arthritis patients may be ANCA positive.[50,51]

Therefore, antibodies associated with IBD are not necessarily specific for IBD. This is relevant both for clinical interpretation of these tests and for understanding the underlying immune and pathophysiologic mechanisms that may lead to the development of these antibodies.

Seropositivity in Different Populations

Different populations appear to have a wide range of IBD seropositivity. This may be because of patient selection or variable assay methodologies. In general, population-based cohorts seem to have a lower incidence of both ANCAs and ASCAs than those drawn from tertiary referral centers. Alternatively, the differences in sensitivity may be because of some (unknown) genetic or environmental factor that affects on the rate of seropositivity. Specificity of both ANCAs and ASCAs are relatively consistent from study to study.

Several European studies of the first-generation antibody incidences are generally lower than those reported from tertiary care referral centers in the United States. ANCA positivity in Italian UC patients was fairly low (39.6%).[52] In a population-based Norwegian cohort with IBD, 27% of CD patients were ASCA positive and 31% of UC patients were pANCA positive. The healthy controls had an 11% ASCA positivity, much higher than most other studies.[53] In another European study, the prevalence of ASCA was low (28.5%). In this study, the positive serologies were associated with younger age and more severe disease.[54]

In contrast, in a Hispanic UC population in Texas, ANCA positivity was 100% compared with the white controls (40%, $P = .033$).[55] The incidence of IBD serologies may be high in First Nation (Inuit) populations without IBD. pANCAs in a control group were greater than 30%. Close to one-fourth of healthy controls had at least 1 positive CD-related antibody.[50]

The geographic variability of control seropositivity raises the possibility that there may be environmental factors that have an impact on the development of IBD-related antibodies. One might speculate on the impact of recurrent intestinal infections on the genesis of antimicrobial antigens in individuals without IBD. It would be interesting to determine the incidence of the IBD antibodies in other nonurbanized, non-Western populations.

IBD SEROLOGIES IN THE DIFFERENTIAL DIAGNOSIS OF GASTROINTESTINAL DISEASES
Do Serologies Help in a Differential Diagnosis of Individuals with Intestinal Symptoms?

Although IBD serologies have reasonable sensitivity and specificity for UC and Crohn, it is not clear where to place them in clinical practice. What role can they serve in diagnostic algorithms? Although they perform very well in well-defined groups of patients, it is less clear how useful they would be in the clinical arena. Very few studies have evaluated how IBD serologies might be useful prospectively in clinical practice.

In one series of 76 patients, the indications for obtaining serologies included evaluation of atypical signs of inflammation as detected by endoscopy/histology or radiology (50%), evaluation of chronic diarrhea (22%), differentiating UC from Crohn in established IBD (13%), differentiating pouchitis versus CD (4%), and evaluation of a family history of IBD (4%). The authors concluded that serologies had no significant impact on diagnosis or management in 46% of cases. The utility in evaluation of chronic diarrhea was very limited. Serologies (primarily ASCA) were positive in a group of patients with segmental colitis and diverticulitis (SCAD); whether this represents a variant of CD or "nonspecificity" of the tests is unclear.[56]

A frequent clinical conundrum is distinguishing IBD from IBS. Schoepfer and colleagues[57] found that IBD serologies were not useful in separating individuals with functional disease from those with IBD. In contrast, surrogates for fecal leukocytes, such as calprotectin and lactoferrin, proved highly accurate in discriminating between the 2 diagnoses.

In a group of 304 pediatric patients referred to an academic medical center for evaluation for possible IBD, the predictive value of the IBD 7 serologies was evaluated in the context of other diagnostic testing. A final diagnosis of IBD was established in 38% of these patients. (n = 115, 62 with CD). The sensitivity (67%), specificity (76%), PPV (63%), and NPV (79%) were lower than those in other studies. In particular, the specificity was much lower than that in other cohorts of patients. Routine laboratory tests to measure anemia, thrombocytosis, and an elevated sedimentation rate performed better at a much lower cost.[58] Whether these divergent results can be explained, in part, by the fact that these patients were early in the course of their disease is unclear.

IBD Undetermined

Approximately 10 % of IBD patients are left with a diagnosis of IBD undetermined (IBDU) after extensive evaluation to identify characteristic findings of either UC or Crohn. (Although many use the term *indeterminate colitis*, this is reserved for the situation in which a colectomy is done and CD versus UC cannot be distinguished on the pathology.) Are serologies useful in these diagnostic dilemmas? A European study followed up with 97 patients with the diagnosis of IBDU for almost 10 years. In a small minority, characteristic serologic patterns were able to establish a diagnosis of ASCA+/ANCA– Crohn or ASCA–/ANCA+ UC. In most cases, however, after serologic testing, there was insufficient information to change the diagnosis from IBDU. Adding Omp-C and I2 testing did not increase the diagnostic efficacy. Therefore, in most patients with IBDU, serologic testing did not prove useful.[59,60]

ASSOCIATION WITH DISEASE CHARACTERISTICS
Prognosis/Stratification

There has been considerable interest in applying IBD serologies for estimating prognosis and risk of complications in IBD to individualize treatment more effectively. In patients with confirmed IBD, there are 2 areas in which IBD serologies may be able to provide the clinician with information that will guide management decisions: (1) pouchitis and (2) complicated (penetrating or fistulizing) CD leading to surgery.

Top down therapy is a tantalizing strategy that holds promise to reverse the course of aggressive CD. However, clearly, not all patients with Crohn have aggressive disease; therefore, although this approach might prevent unfavorable outcomes in some patients, treating all patients with Crohn would lead to "overtreatment" of many patients. Individual patients would end up receiving biologics or immunomodulators that they may not have needed, with the associated risks and costs of "unnecessary" therapy.

Because of this, the ability to select out those destined for an unfavorable course may provide a semblance of rational selection of those who should receive top down therapy. Given the frequency of penetrating and fistulizing disease and the likelihood of surgery (29%–61% at 10 years), early identification of these patients may be important in clinical stratification. It is also clear that perhaps 50% of Crohn patients have a relatively benign course over 10 to 20 years that does not require aggressive therapy.[61]

There are well-defined clinical indicators of aggressive disease, as described by Beaugerie and coworkers[62] such as presentation at age less than 40, small intestinal disease, presence of perianal disease, and an initial requirement for steroids. Endoscopic severity may also be an indicator of aggressive disease. Over time there is trend for CD to evolve from inflammatory to fibrostenotic/perforating disease.

The addition of a laboratory study that also may provide a basis for assessing prognosis and stratifying patients for different treatment pathways would be a valuable management tool. At a minimum, such a test would have to (1) be present early in the course of the disease, for example, before complications have occurred; (2) be reproducible through the evolution of the disease, for example, not change after a complication has occurred; (3) provide information not available through more basic evaluation and testing; and (4) clearly differentiate those who do or do not require a specific treatment. For a test to prove clinically useful, it needs to not only identify statistically significant differences, but also change the pretest probability of a specific finding or outcome sufficiently to alter medical management and decision making. Stratification strategies have generally followed 2 overlapping quantification schemes: (1) the number of positive antibodies and (2) the titer levels of individual tests and the composite of the panel. The composite is frequently expressed as a quartile sum score (QSS), derived from dividing the range of titers for each test into quarters, and then assigning a numerical value to each quartile (1, 2, 3, 4). In this approach, some antibody test may be more "positive" than another.

Obviously, decisions on stratification of presumed complicated disease and development of treatment strategies based on those calculations depend on a predictable consistency of antibody titer levels. Most reports of ANCA/ASCA titers appear to be stable over time and do not necessarily change with the vicissitudes of disease activity. ANCA titers persist after colectomy in UC. ASCA titers do not predictably decrease during remission in CD.[63] However, at least 2 studies suggest that there may be an effect of increasing antiglycan antibody positivity with disease duration.[26,64]

A longitudinal study by Rieder and colleagues[65] demonstrated that although antibody status (+/-) remained relatively stable over time, some patients demonstrated variability in titer levels and QSS in CD. UC patients, in contrast, did not exhibit significant changes in antibody status or levels. As with other studies, this one demonstrates a QSS relation with clinical phenotype in Crohn. But it was unable to address the issue of QSS predicting clinical course. The overwhelming number of patients in this study had already demonstrated aggressive Crohn: 87.7% of the Crohn patients with at least 4 available samples already had a complication before first sample procurement, a proportion that increased to 90.8% (second sample), and 93.3% (third and fourth sample) during follow-up. Eighty-five percent of the Crohn patients already underwent surgery once at time of first sample, which increased during follow-up to 90% for the other 3 time points.[65]

In CD, many studies have documented that the finding of higher titers of multiple antibodies is associated with a more complicated course, with an increased incidence of fibrotic/fistulizing disease and surgery. Mow and colleagues[14] stratified the clinical spectrum of disease in correlation with both the number of antibodies (ASCA, anti–Omp-C, and anti-I2) and the titer levels of antibodies to these microbial antigens calculated as a quartile sum score. Patients with I2 reactivity were more likely to have fibrostenosing Crohn and require small bowel surgery. Anti–Omp-C patients were more likely to have perforating disease and require small bowel surgery. The combination of 3 positive antibodies was 8 times more likely to have had surgery than the antibody negative patients. In the quartile analysis of titers, those in the highest quartiles clearly had the most frequent surgery. Additionally, there was no significant change in the serologic profile after surgery.[14] Several other studies have shown a similar pattern using an overlapping panel of antibody tests.[66]

Rieder and coworkers[25] used a similar strategy of quartile analysis for a panel of antiglycan antibodies that yielded comparable results in characterizing Crohn phenotypes. Several single markers as well as increasing antibody response were associated with a more severe disease phenotype represented by complications, surgery, and early-onset disease.[25,64]

Many studies that show a relationship between IBD serologies and clinical phenotype are cross sectional rather than prospective; therefore, they can prove an association, but are not truly predictive of the evolution of the disease. Therefore, recent reports looking prospectively at the ability of panels of IBD serologies to predict clinical course is of great interest.

In a recent single center study of 149 German Crohn patients who had experienced neither complications or surgery, antiglycan antibodies including gASCA, AMCA, ACCA, and anti-L were predictive of progression to complications or surgery. The risk increased with greater number of positive antibodies. Interestingly, the antibody panels were not as effective in predicting a second complication.[25]

Studies of pediatric IBD patients may provide better insight into the prognostic capacity of IBD serologies. Markowitz and colleagues[67] showed a different antibody profile in very young patients (<8 years old) than older children. Younger children were more likely to be ASCA negative and CBir1 positive than the older patients. These age-associated differences suggest that there may be a temporal evolution of serology or that there may be novel genetic, immunologic, or microbial factors involved in very young individuals with Crohn.[67]

Dubinsky and coworkers[68] focused on a subset of pediatric patients in whom IBD serologies were available before the development of complications or surgery. Longitudinal analysis of this group showed that, in general, those with more antibodies positive and a higher QSS were more likely to progress to surgery or fistulizing/stricturing disease. Not unexpectedly, only a small minority had early significant complications. However, there was not a clear correlation between antibody sum or QSS and unfavorable outcomes.[68]

In a preliminary study of 116 pediatric patients followed up with for more than 5 years after initial diagnosis, most continued with an inflammatory phenotype, but 25 had complicated Crohn (6 stricturing, 19 penetrating, 24 within 5 years). The investigators assayed banked blood from the time of presentation for the Prometheus Crohn Prognostic Test (ASCA, Omp-C, CBir1, I2, pANCA, and nucleotide-binding oligomerization domain containing 2 [NOD2] single nucleotide polymorphism). In the subgroup of 79 patients who were followed up for more than 5 years and those in whom complications developed earlier than 5 years, the test poorly predicted the rate of complicated CD.[69]

The reasons for these discordant results are unclear. Does the fact that these individuals were tested very early in the course of the disease matter? Or, perhaps treatment altered the natural history of the disease. Further information on the effects of time and treatment will help clarify the predictive power of serologic testing.

Although these studies clearly show a meaningful association between antibody profiles and IBD phenotype, several factors need to be considered before routinely adopting this information for clinical decision making. For example, it would be important to compare antibody profiles with simpler and less expensive clinical indicators described by Beaugerie and colleagues[62] in predicting complicated Crohn. Individuals with colonic Crohn, especially UC like Crohn, are less likely to have a complicated course of fistulizing and penetrating disease; antibody profiles may not be helpful in guiding therapeutic decisions. Excluding this group from antibody profile analysis might alter the discriminate power of the serologic profiles.

This may be particularly important with the quartile analysis approach, in that there appears to be a nonlinear distribution of titers among the 4 quartiles. The highest quartile had titer values several-fold greater than the other 3. The range of titers in the 3 lower quartiles huddled very close to each other and, thus, may have less prognostic acumen. Therefore, it would be important to analyze the antibody profiles in limited, more relevant groups (eg, small bowel Crohn).

One would also need to determine how much of a prognostic difference will be required to impact clinical decision making. For example, in the study by Mow and coworkers[14] if one focused solely on those patients with small bowel disease, even those within the lowest quartile of response to I2, Omp-C or ASCA required surgery 42% to 47% of the time. Although there clearly was an increasing frequency of surgery as the titers increase, the fact that nearly half of the cases involving the small bowel required surgery may limit clinically meaningful stratification and decision making.

Does the addition of genetic analysis improve the ability to predict and stratify clinical course? The literature does not provide a consistent answer. Patients with NOD2 mutations have a similar clinical pattern as those with positive IBD serologies, such as, fibrostenosis, small bowel disease and surgery. Ippoliti and colleagues[70] found that, although there was no association between individual IBD serologies and NOD2 status, using an integrative approach, there was a relationship with a profile of multiple positive antibodies. However, several other investigators not have found a convincing relationship. A thorough analysis of this evolving topic is beyond the scope of the current discussion.

Pouchitis

The frequency of pANCA in chronic pouchitis (100%) was significantly greater than in UC (50%) or familial polyposis (0%) without pouchitis and colitis with an ileostomy (70%); P = .00, .00, and .01, respectively. The finding that pANCA occurs more frequently in patients with chronic pouchitis raises the possibility that this antibody may mark a genetically distinct subset of UC patients.[71] However, it will be important to determine whether the presence of this antibody before ileal pouch-anal anastomosis is predictive for later development of chronic pouchitis. And, if so, would it truly alter the decision of what type of surgery a patient with UC should undergo?

SUMMARY

The role of IBD serologies is still evolving. However, as that evolution progresses, it will continue to provide important insights into the etiology of IBD and help define individualized treatment strategies for patients.

The presence of multiple IBD antimicrobial antibodies and increased reactivity form a useful heuristic model to understand the evolution of CD. The role of ANCAs and

Table 3
When should IBD serologies be ordered?

Indication	Utility	Comment
Diarrhea/abdominal pain. Unusual gastrointestinal symptoms	0	High probability of false-positives. Surrogate markers of inflammation more helpful
Diagnosis of IBD	+	Serologies should not (cannot) replace conventional diagnostic modalities
Diagnosis of pediatric IBD	+++	Threshold for endoscopy may be higher in pediatric population, but fecal markers may be preferred
Diagnosis of Crohn vs UC	++	May be helpful in differentiating UC from Crohn.
IBDU	++	In a minority of cases of IBDU, serologies may be diagnostic
First-degree relatives of IBD patients	0	High percentage of first-degree relatives may have positive results, but never have disease, contributing to needless testing and anxiety
Risk of pouchitis	++	Serologies may identify those with high risk of pouchitis after IPAA, but unclear whether that would preclude surgery
Prognosis/risk stratification in Crohn disease	+++	Panel of IBD antibodies may identify those at greater risk for progression to fistulizing/penetrating disease or surgery. Not clear if it significantly exceeds clinical predictive factors. Statistically significant, but clinically significant?

Utility graded on a 0 (not indicated) to ++++ (clearly necessary) scale.

autoantibodies in pathogenesis of UC is an area that requires further investigation. Although IBD serologies exhibit considerable diagnostic accuracy, it is unclear whether they will supplant simpler and more direct evaluations in making an initial diagnosis of UC or Crohn (**Table 3**). The utility of panels of IBD serologies to stratify and predict the course of CD has been an arena of fertile investigation. Developing individual treatment strategies based on the probability of developing complicated aggressive disease would be a significant advance in medical management of CD. However, if major clinical decisions are to be made based on these serologies, we will need more prospective critical studies from the time of diagnosis to define their clinical applicability and to demonstrate a true difference in outcomes.

REFERENCES

1. Broberger O, Perlmann P. Autoantibodies in human ulcerative colitis. J Exp Med 1959;110:657–74.
2. Konrad A, Rutten C, Flogerzi B, et al. Immune sensitization to yeast antigens in ASCA positive patients with Crohn's disease. Inflamm Bowel Dis 2004;10:97–105.
3. Adams RJ, Heazlewood SP, Gilshenan KS, et al. IgG antibodies against common bacteria are more diagnostic for Crohn's disease than IgG against mannan or flagellin. Am J Gastroneterol 2008;103:386–96.
4. Vare PO, Heikius B, Silvennoinen JA. Seroprevalence of Helicobacter pylori infection in inflammatory bowel disease: is Helicobacter pylori infection a protective factor? Scand J Gastroenterol 2001;36:1295–300.
5. Abreu MT, Vasiliauskas EA, Kam LY, et al. Use of serologic tests in Crohn's disease. Clin Gastroenterol Hepatol 2001;4:158–64.
6. Nielsen H, Wiik A, Elmgreen J. Granulocyte-specific antinuclear antibodies in ulcerative colitis. APMIS 1983;91:23–6.
7. Vasiliauskas EA, Plevy SE, Landers CJ, et al. Perinuclear antineutrophil cytoplasmic antibodies in patients with Crohn's disease define a clinical subgroup. Gastroenterology 1996;110:1810–9.
8. Sandborn WJ, Loftus EV, Colombel, JF et al. Evaluation of serologic disease markers in a population-based cohort of patients with ulcerative colitis and Crohn's disease. Inflamm Bowel Dis 2001;7:192–201.
9. Vidrich A, Lee J, James E, et al. Segregation of pANCA antigenic recognition by DNase treatment of neutrophils: ulcerative colitis, type 1 autoimmune hepatitis, and primary sclerosing cholangitis. J Clin Immunol 1995;15:293–9.
10. Reese GE, Constantinides VA, Simillis C, et al. Diagnostic precision of anti-Saccharomyces cerevisiae antibodies and perinuclear antineutrophil cytoplasmic antibodies in inflammatory bowel disease. Am J Gastroenterol 2006;101:2410–22.
11. Taylor KD, Plevy SE, Yang H, et al. ANCA pattern and LTA haplotype relationship to clinical responses to anti-TNF antibody treatment in Crohn's disease. Gastroenterology 2001;120:1347–55.
12. Ferrante M, Vermeire S, Katsanos K, et al. Predictors of early response to infliximab in patients with ulcerative colitis. Inflamm Bowel Dis 2007;13:123–8.
13. Aitola P, Miettinen A, Mattila A, et al. Effect of proctocolectomy on serum antineutrophil cytoplasmic antibodies in patients with chronic ulcerative colitis. J Clin Pathol 1995:48:645–7.
14. Mow WS, Vasiliauskas EA, Lin YC, et al. Association of antibody responses to microbial antigens and complications of small bowel Crohn's disease. Gastroenterology 2004;126:414–24.
15. Main J, McKenzie H, Yeaman GR, et al. Antibody to Saccharomyces cerevisiae (bakers' yeast) in Crohn's disease. BMJ 1988;297:1105–6.

16. Giaffer MH, Clark A, Holdsworth CD. Antibodies to Saccharomyces cerevisiae in patients with Crohn's disease and their possible pathogenic importance. Gut 1992; 33:1071–5.

17. Vasiliauskas EA, Kan LY, Karp LC, et al. Marker antibody expression stratifies Crohn's disease into immunologically homogeneous subgroups with distinct clinical characteristics. Gut 2000;47:487–96.

18. Dotan I, Fishman S, Dgani Y, et al. Antibodies against laminaribioside and chitobioside are novel serologic markers in Crohn's disease. Gastroenterology 2006;131:366–78.

19. Cohavy O, Bruckner D, Gordon LK, et al. Colonic bacteria express an ulcerative colitis pANCA-related protein epitope. Infect Immunol 2000;68:1542–8.

20. Mow WS, Lander CJ, Steinhart AH, et al. High-level serum antibodies to bacterial antigens are associated with antibiotic-induced clinical remission in Crohn's disease: a pilot study. Dig Dis Sci 2004;49:1280–6.

21. Wei B, Huang T, Dalwadi H, et al. Pseudomonas fluorescens encodes the Crohn's disease-associated I2 sequence and T-cell superantigen. Infect Immunol 2002;70: 6567–75.

22. Spivak J, Landers CJ, Vasiliauskas EA, et al. Antibodies to I2 predict clinical response to fecal diversion in Crohn's disease. Inflamm Bowel Dis 2006;12:1122–30.

23. Targan SR, Landers CJ, Yang H, et al. Antibodies to CBir1 flagellin define a unique response that is associated independently with complicated Crohn's disease. Gastroenterology 2005;128:2020–8.

24. Pang Z, Otaka M, Maoka T, et al. Structure of beta-glucan oligomer from laminarin and its effect on human monocytes to inhibit the proliferation of U937 cells. Biosci Biotechnol Biochem 2005;69:553–8.

25. Rieder F, Schleder S, Wolf A, et al. Association of the novel serologic anti-glycan antibodies anti-laminarin and anti-chitin with complicated Crohn's disease behavior. Inflamm Bowel Dis 2010;16:263–74.

26. Ferrante M, Henckaerts L, Joossens M, et al. New serological markers in inflammatory bowel disease are associated with complicated disease behavior. Gut 2007;56: 1394–403.

27. Hibi T, Ohara M, Kobayashi K, et al. Enzyme linked immunosorbent assay (ELISA) and immunoprecipitation studies on anti-goblet cell antibody using a mucin producing cell line in patients with inflammatory bowel disease. Gut 1994;35:224–30.

28. Folwaczny C, Noehl N, Tschop K, et al. Goblet cell autoantibodies in patients with inflammatory bowel disease and their first-degree relatives. Gastroenterology 1997; 113:101–6.

29. Ardesjö B, Portela-Gomes GM, Rorsman F, et al. Immunoreactivity against goblet cells in patients with inflammatory bowel disease. Inflamm Bowel Dis 2008;14: 652–61.

30. Das KM, Bajpai M. Tropomyosins in human diseases: ulcerative colitis. Adv Exp Med Biol 2008;644:158–67.

31. Das KM, Vecchi M, Sakamaki S. A shared and unique epitope on human colon, skin and biliary epithelium detected by a monoclonal antibody. Gastroenterol 1990;98: 464–9.

32. Seibold F, Mork H, Tanza S, et al. Pancreatic autoantibodies in Crohn's disease: a family study. Gut 1997;40:481–4.

33. Roggenbuck D, Hausdorf G, Martinez-Gamboa L, et al. Identification of GP2, the major zymogen granule membrane glycoprotein, as the autoantigen of pancreatic antibodies in Crohn's disease. Gut 2009;58:1620–8.

34. Vermeulen N, de Beeck KO, Vermeire S, et al. Identification of a novel autoantigen in inflammatory bowel disease by protein microarray. Inflamm Bowel Dis 2011:17:1291–300.

35. Austin GI, Shaheen NJ, Sandler RS. Positive and negative predictive values: use of inflammatory bowel disease serologic markers. Am J Gastroenterol 2006;101:413–6.

36. Abreu MT. Serologies in Crohn's disease: can we change the gray zone to black and white. Gastroenterol 2006;131:664–7.

37. Prideaux L, De Crux P, Ng SC, et al. Serological antibodies in inflammatory bowel disease: a systematic review. Inflamm Bowel Dis 2011. DOI:10.1002/ibd.21903. [Epub ahead of print].

38. Davis MK, Andres JM, Jolley CD, et al. Antibodies to Escherichia coli outer membrane porin C in the absence of anti-Saccharomyces cerevisiae antibodies and anti neutrophil cytoplasmic antibodies are an unreliable marker of Crohn's disease and ulcerative colitis. J Pediat Gastroenterol Nutr 2007;45:409–13.

39. Israeli E, Grotto I, Gilburd B, et al. Anti-Saccharomyces cerevisiae and antineutrophilic cytoplasmic antibodies as predictors of inflammatory bowel disease. Gut 2005;54:1232–6.

40. Shanahan F, Duerr RH, Rotter JI, et al. Neutrophil autoantibodies in ulcerative colitis: familial aggregation and genetic heterogeneity. Gastroenterology 1992;103:456–61.

41. Torok HP, Glas J, Hollay HC, et al. Serum antibodies in first-degree relatives of patients with IBD: a marker of disease susceptibility? A follow-up pilot-study after 7 years. Digestion 2005;72:119–23.

42. Seibold F, Slametschka D, Gregor M, et al. Neutrophil autoantibodies: a genetic marker in primary sclerosing cholangitis and ulcerative colitis. Gastroenterology 1994;107:532–6.

43. Seibold F, Stich O, Hufnagl R, et al. Anti-Saccharomyces cerevisiae antibodies in inflammatory bowel disease: a family study. Scand J Gastroenterol 2001;36:196–201.

44. Damoiseaux JG, Bouten B, Linders AM, et al. diagnostic value of anti Saccharomyces cerevisiae and anti neutrophil cytoplasmic antibodies for inflammatory bowel disease: high prevalence inpatients with celiac disease. J Clin Immunol 2002;22:281–8.

45. Desplat-Jego S, Johanet C, Escande A, et al. Update on anti-Saccharomyces cerevisiae, anti-nuclear associated anti-neutrophil antibodies and antibodies to exocrine pancreas detected by indirect immunofluorescence as biomarkers in chronic inflammatory bowel diseases: results of a multicenter study. World J Gastroenterol 2007;13:2312–8.

46. Monselise A, Weinberger A, Monselise Y, et al. Anti-Saccharomyces cerevisiae antibodies in Behcet's disease—a familial study. Clin Exp Rheumatol 2006;24:S87–90.

47. de Vries M, van der Horst-Bruinsma I, van Hoogstraten I, et al. pANCA, ASCA and OmpC antibodies in patients with ankylosing spondylitis without inflammatory bowel disease. J Rheumatol 2010;37:2340–4.

48. Murtori P, Muratori L, Guidi M, et al. Anti-Saccharomyces cerevisiae antibodies (ASCA) and autoimmune disease. Clin Exp Immunol 2003;132:473–6.

49. Papp M, Norman GL, Vitalis Z, et al. Presence of anti-microbial antibodies in liver cirrhosis—a tell-tale sign of compromised immunity? PLoS One 2010;23:e12957.

50. Bernstein CN, El-Gabalway H, Sargent M. Assessing inflammatory bowel disease associated antibodies in Caucasian and First Nation cohorts. Can J Gastroenterol 2011;25:269–73.
51. Lachenal F, Nkana K, Nove-Josserand R, et al. Prevalence and clinical significance of auto-antibodies in adults with cystic fibrosis. Eur Respir J 2009;34:1079–85.
52. Siabeni S, Folli C, de Franchis R, et al. Diagnostic role and clinical correlates of anti Saccharomyces cerevisiae antibodies (ASCA) and anti-neutrophil cytoplasmic antibodies (p-ANCA) in Italian patients with inflammatory bowel disease. Dig Liver Dis 2003;35:862–8.
53. Solberg IC, Lygren I, Cvancarova M, et al. Predictive value of serologic markers in a population-based Norwegian cohort with inflammatory bowel disease. Inflamm Bowel Dis 2009;15:406–14.
54. Riis L, Vind I, Vermeire S, et al. The prevalence of genetic and serologic markers in an unselected European population based cohort of IBD patients. Inflamm Bowel Dis 2007;13:24–32.
55. Basu D, Lopez I, Kulkarni A, et al. Impact of race and ethnicity on inflammatory bowel disease. Am J Gastroenterol 2005;100:2254–61.
56. Gupta A, Derbes C, Sellin J. Clinical indications of the use of antineutrophil cytoplasmic antibodies and anti Saccharomyces cerevisiae antibodies in the evaluation of inflammatory bowel disease in an Academic Medical Center. Inflamm Bowel Dis 2005;11:898–902.
57. Schoepfer AM, Trummier M, Seeholzer P, et al. Discriminating IBD from IBS: comparison of the Test Performance of Fecal Markers, Blood Leukocytes, CRP and IBD Antibodies. Inflamm Bowel Dis 2008;14:32–9.
58. Benor S, Russel GH, Silver M, et al. Shortcoming of the Inflammatory Bowel Disease Serology 7 Panel. Pediatrics 2010;125:1230–6.
59. Joossens S, Reinisch W, Vermeire S, et al. The value of serologic markers in indeterminate colitis: a prospective follow-up study. Gastroenterology 2002;122:1242–7.
60. Joossens S, Colombel JF, Landers C, et al. Anti-outer membrane of poric C and anti-I2 antibodies in indeterminate colitis. Gut 2006;55:1667–9.
61. Lewis JD. The utility of biomarkers in the diagnosis and therapy of inflammatory bowel disease. Gastroenterology 2011;140:1817–26.
62. Beaugerie L, Seksik P, Nion-Larmurier I, et al. Predictors of Crohn's disease. Gastroenterol 206;130:650-6.
63. Seibold F. ASCA genetic markers, predictor of disease, or marker of a response to an environmental antigen. Gut 2005;54:1212–3.
64. Arnott ID, Landers CJ, Nimmo EJ, et al. Sero-reactivity to microbial components in Crohn's behavior is associated with disease severity and progression, but not NOD2/CARD12 genotype. Am J Gastroenterol 2004;99:2376–84.
65. Rieder F, Lopez R, Franke A, et al. Characterization of changes in serum anti-glycan antibodies in Crohn's disease—a longitudinal analysis. PLoS One 2011;6:e18172.
66. Amre DK, Lu SE, Costea F, et al. Utility of serologic markers in predicting the early occurrence of complications and surgery in pediatric Crohn's disease. Am J Gastroenterol 2006;101:645–52.
67. Markowitz J, Kugathasan S, Dubinsky M, et al. Age of diagnosis influences serologic responses in children with Crohn's disease: a possible clue to etiology. Inflamm Bowel Dis 2009;15:714–9.
68. Dubinsky M, Kugasthasan S, Mei L, et al. Increased immune reactivity predicts aggressive complicating Crohn's disease. Clin Gastroenterol Hepatol 2008;6:1105–11.

69. Markowitz J, Lileiko NS, Keljo DJ, et al. The Prometheus Crohn's prognostic test does not reliably predict complicated Crohn's disease in children. Presentation at a National Meeting. DDW. Chicago (IL), 2011 [abstract #935].

70. Ippoliti A, Devlin S, Mei L, et al. combination of innate and adaptive immune alterations increased the likelihood of fibrostenosis in Crohn's disease. Inflamm Bowel Dis 2010;16:1279–85.

71. Sandborn WJ, Landers CJ, Tremaine WJ, et al. Antineutrophilic cytoplasmic antibody correlates with chronic pouchitis after ileal pouch-anal anastomosis. Am J Gastroenterol 1995;90:740–7.

Fecal Markers: Calprotectin and Lactoferrin

Bincy P . Abraham, MD, MS[a],*, Sunanda Kane, MD, MSPH[b]

> **KEYWORDS**
> - Calprotectin • Lactoferrin • Fecal markers
> - Crohn disease • Ulcerative colitis
> - Inflammatory bowel disease

CLINICAL SIGNIFICANCE OF FECAL BIOMARKERS

Differentiating patients with inflammatory disease from those with functional disorders may be difficult in patients with nonspecific symptoms, such as diarrhea and abdominal pain. Most often, invasive procedures, such as endoscopy, with biopsies are required. A marker or a set of markers that can accurately detect inflammation and monitor disease activity would be useful clinically.

Although serum inflammatory markers are helpful in determining active inflammation, they are not specific and can be elevated in other nongastrointestinal conditions. Fecal biomarkers, because of their direct contact with the intestinal mucosa, may be more accurate in determining gastrointestinal inflammation. If fecal markers are specific for mucosal inflammation, invasive and expensive endoscopic examinations could potentially be avoided.

The mucosa of actively inflamed colon contains a large number of neutrophils. Fecal proteins derived from neutrophils have the potential to be ideal markers of intestinal inflammation. Two of these fecal proteins, calprotectin and lactoferrin, have been studied extensively.

Fecal Calprotectin

Fecal calprotectin, a calcium- and zinc-binding neutrophilic cytosolic protein, is found in proportion to the degree of inflammation present. Fecal calprotectin is resistant to colonic bacterial degradation, is evenly distributed and stable in stool for up to 1 week at room temperature, and can be measured by a commercially available enzyme-linked immunosorbent assay (ELISA) with less than 5 g of stool.[1] Calprotectin plays a

The authors have nothing to disclose.

[a] Section of Gastroenterology and Hepatology, Baylor College of Medicine, 1709 Dryden Street, Suite 800, Houston, TX 77030, USA
[b] Section of Gastroenterology and Hepatology, Mayo Clinic College of Medicine, 200 First Street SW, Rochester, MN 55905, USA
* Corresponding author.
E-mail address: bincya@bcm.edu

Gastroenterol Clin N Am 41 (2012) 483–495
doi:10.1016/j.gtc.2012.01.007
0889-8553/12/$ – see front matter © 2012 Elsevier Inc. All rights reserved.

regulatory role in the inflammatory process and is a very sensitive marker for detection of inflammation in the gastrointestinal tract. Unfortunately, results from the ELISA test take 5 to 7 days to process, which obviates the ability to make a bedside diagnosis or make timely management decisions. Recently, however, Calpro,™ has developed a rapid test (not yet US Food and Drug Administration approved) that can be done within minutes and correlates well ($r=0.92$, $P<.001$) with its conventional ELISA equivalent.[2]

Insurance coverage for fecal calprotectin may not always occur, depending on specific policies, and out-of-pocket cost can run about $340. For example, Blue Cross and Blue Shield[3] as well as United Healthcare[4] consider this testing to be "investigative." Current procedural terminology (CPT) code for ordering this test is 83520.

Fecal Lactoferrin

Fecal lactoferrin is an iron-binding protein that is similar to fecal calprotectin in that it is neutrophil derived, has antimicrobial properties, and is available through commercial ELISA testing.[5,6] Lactoferrin is a major component of neutrophil secondary granules, released upon neutrophil activation and degranulation,[5] and is resistant to proteolysis in the feces.[7] Insurance coverage is slightly better, and out-of-pocket costs are lower compared with calprotectin, running around $90 to $180.[8] For example, Cigna Healthcare considers fecal lactoferrin testing as medically necessary as part of an evaluation of diarrhea but does not cover it because it considers the testing "experimental, investigational, or unproven."[9] CPT codes for ordering this test include 83630 and 83631.

DIAGNOSIS OF INFLAMMATORY BOWEL DISEASE
Differentiating Inflammatory Bowel Disease from Irritable Bowel Syndrome

In a patient presenting with abdominal pain and diarrhea, it can be difficult to ascertain if the etiology is organic or functional. It is common for some symptoms of inflammatory bowel disease (IBD) and irritable bowel syndrome (IBS) to overlap, and endoscopic evaluation is used to distinguish between the two. A biomarker that is specific for IBD can prevent those patients with IBS from undergoing unnecessary endoscopic evaluation.

Lactoferrin concentrations have been shown to be increased in active ulcerative colitis (UC) and Crohn disease (CD) with 93% correlation of levels to disease activity; lactoferrin level was also elevated in inactive IBD, above levels from IBS patients and healthy controls.[6,10–12] Overall, sensitivity of fecal lactoferrin for IBD was 78% (95% confidence interval [CI], 69%–83%), and the specificity was 90% (95% CI, 83%–96%), correlating well with endoscopic and histologic grading of disease activity.[12,13] Moreover, elevated fecal lactoferrin was 100% specific in ruling out IBS.[12]

Lactoferrin tested in 177 patients was significantly higher in those with active IBD compared with those with inactive disease, IBS patients, those with enteric infection, and healthy volunteers. The sensitivity and specificity of fecal lactoferrin were 92% and 88%, respectively, for UC, and 92% and 80%, respectively, for CD.[14]

Another comparison study of 139 patients (54 with IBS, 42 with UC, and 43 with CD), found that UC and CD patients with active inflammation had significantly higher levels of lactoferrin and calprotectin compared with those with inactive disease ($P<.05$) and with IBS ($P<.05$).[15] This study, however, found an overall diagnostic accuracy in IBD of 80.0% for lactoferrin greater than 7.05 μg/mL and 80.0% for calprotectin greater than 48 μg/mL, for the respective clinical disease scores.

Calprotectin had the highest diagnostic accuracy in CD (81.4%), whereas lactoferrin was superior in UC (83.3%).

Both fecal calprotectin and lactoferrin have been found to be quite accurate in diagnosing inflammatory disease. In discriminating IBS, Schoepfer and colleagues[16] found that calprotectin and lactoferrin were 89% and 91% accurate, respectively. Overall accuracy for discrimination of IBS from patients with Crohn disease in remission (Crohn Disease Activity Index [CDAI]<150) was 90% for both lactoferrin and calprotectin. Calprotectin and lactoferrin were significantly elevated in patients with Crohn disease with CDAI greater than 150 compared with those in remission. In a comparison study, both fecal calprotectin and lactoferrin had similar sensitivity (78%, 80%), specificity (83%, 85%), PPV (86%, 87%), and accuracy (80%, 81%), respectively.[17]

In yet another study, fecal calprotectin was found to be 95% sensitive (95% CI, 0.93–0.97) and 91% specific (95% CI, 0.86–0.91) for discriminating IBD from functional disorders.[18] Tibble and coworkers[19] found that an abnormal calprotectin test had an odds ratio (OR) for organic disease confirmed by imaging or endoscopic examination of 27.8 (95% CI, 17.6–43.7; $P<.0001$) compared with an odds ratio of 4.2 (95% CI, 2.9–6.1; $P<.0001$) and 3.2 (95% CI, 2.2–4.6; $P<.0001$) for elevated C-reaction protein (CRP) and erythrocyte sedimentation rate. This test also supports the utility of the fecal maker and Rome criteria for differentiating organic disease from functional disorder 1.[19]

A meta-analysis by von Roon and colleagues[18] found that the precision of fecal calprotectin for the diagnosis of IBD was superior to serologic markers such as CRP, erythrocyte sedimentation rate, anti- *Saccharomyces cerevisiae* antibody, perinuclear antineutrophil cytoplasmic antibody, and anti-*Escherichia coli* outer membrane porin C antibody.

A meta-analysis of 13 prospective studies (6 adult and 7 pediatric) found fecal calprotectin a useful screening tool for identifying patients who are most likely to need endoscopy for suspected inflammatory bowel disease.[20] Screening by measuring fecal calprotectin levels would result in a 67% reduction in the number of adults requiring endoscopy and a lower, albeit still beneficial, 35% reduction in children to safely exclude IBD with 93% sensitivity and 96% specificity for adults, and 92% sensitivity and 76% specificity for children and teenagers.

Other Etiologies of Elevated Fecal Markers

Although fecal markers are good indicators of IBD compared with IBS, they are not specific for IBD; elevated levels have been found in other diseases (**Table 1**).[20–22] Studies showing elevations in fecal calprotectin have found, however, that levels in these other conditions are typically much lower (especially in noninfectious etiologies) than those found in active inflammatory bowel disease. Thus, the fecal markers are still useful, especially if the absolute levels are taken into consideration.

Differentiating Between Crohn Disease and Ulcerative Colitis

Currently, endoscopy, histology, imaging, and serologic testing are used to help differentiate between CD and UC. Although fecal markers are useful to differentiate between IBD and IBS, they have not been found to be useful to differentiate between CD and UC. One study of 48 patients found no statistical difference between Crohn and non-Crohn patients (ulcerative colitis [UC], indeterminate colitis [IC]) in the levels of fecal calprotectin (median, 760 μg/g; interquartile range [IQR], 325–1251 vs 419 μg/g; IQR, 91–1355, respectively, $P = .64$).[23] Quail and colleagues[23] also found no difference in gender (male vs female, 714 μg/g vs 1032.5 μg/g, $P = .74$) or age at IBD

Table 1
Non-IBD causes of abnormal fecal markers (*most studies in calprotectin*)

Infections	Bacterial enteritis
	Viral gastroenteritis
	Helicobacter pylori gastritis
	Giardia lamblia
	Diverticulitis
Malignancies	Colorectal cancer
	Gastric carcinoma
	Intestinal lymphoma
Drugs	Nonsteroidal anti-inflammatory drugs
	Proton pump inhibitors
Other gastrointestinal diseases	Gastroesophageal reflux disease
	Cystic fibrosis
	Celiac disease (untreated)
	Diverticular disease
	Protein-losing enteropathy
	Colorectal adenoma
	Juvenile polyposis
	Autoimmune enteropathy
	Microscopic colitis
	Liver cirrhosis
	Food allergy (untreated)
	Nonspecific abdominal pain (in children)
Other	Young age (<5 years)
	Older age
	Obesity
	Immunodeficiency (in children)

Adapted from van Rheenen PF, Van de Vijver E, Fidler V. Faecal calprotectin for screening of patients with suspected inflammatory bowel disease: diagnostic meta-analysis. BMJ 2010;341.

diagnosis with the calprotectin levels (Kruskal-Wallis test, $P = .26$). Unlike calprotectin, fecal lactoferrin may differentiate those with UC, which had significantly higher levels (mean, 1125 μg/g) than those with CD (mean, 440 μg/g; $P = .04$) in one study.[24] However, another study showed similar fecal lactoferrin levels in patients with active CD (1035.25 μg/g) versus active UC (1126.29 μg/g).[14]

Small Bowel Inflammation Versus Colon Inflammation

No significant data were found in the use of fecal markers to distinguish location of disease. However, the likelihood of differentiating between small bowel and colonic inflammation appears to be low, especially because these fecal markers appear unlikely to distinguish CD from UC patients.[14,23]

PREDICTOR OF DISEASE ACTIVITY
Active versus Quiescent Disease: Associations Between Activity Indices

Activity indices have traditionally been used for research purposes. However, these may be subject to bias of functional symptoms in patients with IBD. Despite this, they are inexpensive and have been considered the standard of evaluating patient response and remission rates to treatment in clinical trials. Several studies have evaluated the association between these indices and fecal markers.

In a study of 164 patients with Crohn disease undergoing colonoscopy, no significant associations between the CDAI scores and the fecal concentrations of calprotectin and lactoferrin were found. However, in this same study, the fecal markers were found to be associated with endoscopic activity, as will be described in a following section.[25]

In a later study of 78 patients presenting with IBD, a total of 52 patients' samples demonstrated histologic inflammation.[26] Of these, 49 were lactoferrin positive, and 40 were calprotectin positive ($P<.0001$). Lactoferrin and calprotectin findings correlated in both the CD and UC groups with the CDAI values ($P = .043; 0.010$) and with Mayo Disease Activity Index values in UC cases ($P<.0001$).

The fecal calprotectin concentration in the patients with active UC (determined by the Sutherland criteria) was significantly higher than that in the inactive UC and controls (402.16 ± 48.0 μg/g vs 35.93 ± 3.39 μg/g vs 11.5 ± 3.42 μg/g; $P<.01$). The fecal calprotectin concentration in the inactive UC group was significantly higher than that in the control group ($P<.05$). A significant difference was also found in the patients with active UC of mild, moderate, and severe degrees. The sensitivity for fecal calprotectin was 91.9% and specificity was 79.4%.[27]

PREDICTION OF RESPONSE TO TREATMENT

Fecal markers have been used to evaluate for response to medications. In an evaluation of 27 patients with UC and 11 with CD, 97% had elevated calprotectin levels (defined as >94.7 μg/g). After treatment, a normalized calprotectin level predicted a complete response in 100% of patients, whereas elevated calprotectin predicted incomplete response in 30%.[28] A similar study using fecal lactoferrin found elevated lactoferrin levels had 94% sensitivity and 100% specificity for the diagnosis of UC from those without UC (healthy controls). After treatment, on follow-up, a significant decrease in levels occurred corresponding to a decrease in Mayo scores.[29]

Monitoring Anti–Tumor Necrosis Factor Therapy

Palmon and colleagues[30] showed that both calprotectin and lactoferrin decrease significantly from baseline values at week 2 and week 4 after an infliximab dose, suggesting that these markers may help guide infliximab dosing and frequency. Compared with pretreatment values, a significant decrease in concentrations of fecal calprotectin (median concentration pretreatment 1173 μg/g to posttreatment 130 μg/g [$P<.001$]) and fecal lactoferrin (median concentration pretreatment from 105.0 μg/g to posttreatment 2.7 μg/g; $P<.001$) occurred after initiation of anti–tumor necrosis factor (TNF) therapy, which correlated closely with improvement in Crohn Disease Endoscopic Index of Severity (CDEIS) scoring. Although this study evaluated only 15 patients undergoing ileocolonoscopy, the early data suggest that these might be used as surrogate markers of mucosal healing on anti-TNF therapy.[31]

PREDICTION OF DISEASE RELAPSE

Fecal calprotectin levels have been used to predict those patients at risk of relapse. In a prospective study of 44 IBD patients, those with quiescent disease monitored over 12 months with a calprotectin level of 50 μg/g or more had a similar 13-fold increased risk of relapse, with a sensitivity of 90%, but higher specificity of 83% for predicting relapse compared with only 43% specificity in the Costa study.[32]

For patients in remission for an average of 5 months, a larger study of 163 patients found that a baseline fecal calprotectin level greater than 150 μg/g had a sensitivity for predicting relapse within the next year of 89% in UC and 87% in CD. The specificity in UC was 82% but only 43% in CD, yielding a 2-fold increased risk in CD and a 14-fold higher probability of relapse in UC.[33] In a retrospective chart review of 32 CD patients, 90% of patients with a clinical relapse had calprotectin levels more than 400 μg/g in CD, whereas 89% remained in clinical remission if they had calprotectin levels less than 400 μg/g.[34]

Among 10 of 53 patients with CD of comparable clinical features, such as disease duration, smoking, location of disease, history of ileocecal resection, and baseline CDAI scores, median fecal calprotectin level was significantly higher in patients that had relapse compared with those in the nonrelapse group (380.5 vs 155 μg/g, $P<.001$). A cutoff value of 340 μg/g fecal calprotectin gave sensitivity of 80% and specificity of 90.7% in predicting clinical relapse. Patients with a baseline calprotectin level greater than 340 μg/g had an 18-fold higher risk of relapse ($P<.001$).[35]

Relapse risk was higher in IBD patients with high (>150 μg/g) calprotectin concentrations (30% vs 7.8%; $P<.001$) or positive lactoferrin (25% vs 10%; $P<.05$). Fecal lactoferrin had a 46% sensitivity and 61% specificity to predict relapses in UC patients and 77% sensitivity and 68% specificity to predict relapses in CD. Predicting IBD relapse in the first 3 months of follow-up had improved sensitivity of 100%, specificity of 62%, positive predictive value 6%, and negative predictive value 100%.[36]

In patients tapering off steroids, persistent elevations in fecal lactoferrin predicted an increased risk of early clinical relapse and suggested its use in guiding the rapidity of the steroid taper as well as in predicting subsequent IBD flares.[11]

The ability of calprotectin to predict relapse may stem from capturing ongoing active disease that may be asymptomatic to the individual patient. Finding elevated levels of this marker in patients can guide the clinician in monitoring and treating them more aggressively to prevent relapse.

Predictor of Colectomy

In a study of 90 patients with severe UC, those who required colectomy had significantly higher calprotectin levels than those that did not undergo colectomy (1200.0 vs 887.0; $P = .04$), yielding a sensitivity of 24.0% and specificity of 97.4% for predicting colectomy.[37] At a cutoff point of 1922.5 μg/g a Kaplan-Meier analysis for a median follow-up of 1.10 years found 87% of patients needed subsequent colectomy. They also found a trend toward significance when comparing corticosteroid nonresponders and responders (1100.0 μg/g vs 863.5 μg/g; $P = .08$) as well as between infliximab nonresponders and responders (1795.0 μg/g vs 920.5 μg/g; $P = .06$).

PREDICTION OF MUCOSAL HEALING

Although endoscopy and histologic findings are the standard for assessing clinical activity, less-invasive methods are available. Capsule endoscopy is still invasive, and certain imaging studies can place patients at risk of radiation exposure. Clinical symptoms may not always correlate to the actual amount of inflammation, and may be related to an IBS component of the symptoms. Thus, mucosal healing has become a gold standard in the definition of "remission" in IBD. Although clinical trials have traditionally used activity indices for both UC and CD, more recent studies also evaluate with a more stringent criteria of endoscopic scores. Besides clinical practice, a biomarker for endoscopic and histologic healing can also be useful in clinical trials in reducing cost and improving recruitment of patients. Several studies show that both fecal calprotectin and lactoferrin correlated well with endoscopic and histologic inflammation.

Overall, fecal calprotectin concentrations correlate well with endoscopic and histologic grading of disease activity at a suggested cutoff value of 50 μg/g for adults and 100 μg/g for children based on a meta-analysis of 30 studies (5983 patients).[18]

CD

In Crohn disease, a study of 164 patients undergoing colonoscopy found fecal calprotectin and lactoferrin concentrations were significantly higher in patients with more severe endoscopic disease activity defined by the Simple Endoscopic Score for Crohn Disease (SES-CD) greater than 7 points ($P<.001$ for all comparisons).[25]

In an another prospective study of 140 ileocolonoscopies done in CD patients compared with controls, SES-CD correlated closest with fecal calprotectin levels (Spearman's rank correlation coefficient $r = 0.75$), followed by CRP ($r = 0.53$), blood leukocytes ($r = 0.42$), and the CDAI ($r = 0.38$). The overall accuracy for the detection of endoscopically active disease was 87 % for calprotectin (at a cutoff of 70 μg/g), 66% for elevated CRP, 54% for blood leukocytosis, and 40% for the CDAI $\geq$150. Moreover, calprotectin could discriminate inactive endoscopic disease from mild activity, mild from moderate activity, and moderate from high activity (SES-CD defined as: inactive, 0–3; mild, 4–10; moderate, 11–19; and high, $\geq$20).[38]

Sipponen and colleagues[31] also evaluated CDEIS scores in 77 CD patients undergoing ileocolonoscopies. Both fecal calprotectin and lactoferrin correlated significantly with CDEIS (Spearman's $r = 0.729$ and $r = 0.773$, $P<.001$). With a cutoff level of 200 μg/g for a raised fecal calprotectin concentration, sensitivity was 70%, specificity 92%, PPV 94%, and NPV 61% in predicting endoscopically active disease (CDEIS>3). A fecal lactoferrin concentration of 10 μg/g as the cutoff value gave a sensitivity, specificity, PPV, and NPV of 66%, 92%, 94%, and 59%, respectively, whereas the sensitivity of CDAI greater than150 to detect endoscopically active disease was only 27%, specificity 94%, PPV 91%, and NPV 40%. A raised serum CRP (>5 mg/L) gave a sensitivity, specificity, PPV, and NPV of 48%, 91%, 91%, and 48%, respectively.[31]

UC

Strong correlation between the fecal calprotectin concentration and the endoscopic gradings for UC ($r = 0.866$, $P<.001$) was found in a study by Xiang and colleagues.[27] A subsequent prospective study of endoscopic activity based on Rachmilewitz score in UC patients, endoscopic disease activity correlated closest with calprotectin (Spearman's rank correlation coefficient $r = 0.834$). Fecal calprotectin levels were significantly lower in UC patients with inactive disease (endoscopic score 0–3, calprotectin 42 $\pm$ 38 μg/g), compared with patients with mild (score 4–6, calprotectin 210 $\pm$ 121 μg/g; $P<.001$), moderate (score 7–9, calprotectin 392 $\pm$ 246 μg/g; $P<.002$), and severe disease (score 10–12, calprotectin 730 $\pm$ 291 μg/g; $P<.001$), correlating well with endoscopic severity. The overall accuracy for the detection of endoscopically active disease (score $\geq$4) was 89% for calprotectin at a cutoff value of 50 μg/g, which did not improve accuracy at a higher cutoff value of 100 μg/g (86%).[16]

PREDICTION OF HISTOLOGIC REMISSION

In a study of 72 patients undergoing colonoscopy, patients with abnormal histologic findings had significantly higher calprotectin levels (218 $\pm$ 125 μg/g) than patients with

Table 2
Summary of use of calprotectin and lactoferrin

	Calprotectin	Lactoferrin
Distinguish IBD vs IBS	+	+
Distinguish UC vs CD	–	–
Determine active disease vs remission	+	+
Sensitivity	78–100%	66–80%
Specificity	44–100%	67–100%
Assess mucosal healing	+	+
Correlation coefficient	0.48–0.83	0.19–0.87
Predict relapse	+	+
Predict response to treatment	+	+

Symbols: +, yes; –, no
Adapted from Lewis JD. The utility of biomarkers in the diagnosis and therapy of inflammatory bowel disease. Gastroenterology 2011;140(6):1817–26.

normal colonoscopy (77 ± 100 μg/g). On multivariate analysis, calprotectin was a significant predictor of abnormal colonic histology (P = .005; OR, 1.007; 95% CI, 1.002–1.012). A fecal calprotectin concentration of 150 mg/mL had a sensitivity of 75%, specificity of 84%, PPV of 80%, and NPV of 75% in predicting abnormal colonic histology.[39]

In Sipponen and colleague's study[31] of 87 patients with CD undergoing ileocolonoscopies, both fecal calprotectin and lactoferrin correlated significantly with colon SES-CD (P<.001) and colon histology (P<.001) in those with ileocolonic or colonic disease. In patients with normal calprotectin or lactoferrin levels, endoscopic and histologic scores were significantly lower than in those with elevated concentrations (P<.001). However, in ileal CD, ileal SES-CD correlated with histology (P<.001) but not with fecal calprotectin (P = .161) or lactoferrin (P = .448).[31] See **Table 2** for summary of use of calprotectin and lactoferrin.[40]

ASSESSMENT AFTER SURGERY

In a study evaluating the use of fecal markers after ileocolonic resection for surgical remission of CD, fecal calprotectin concentrations remained high with mean levels of 247 ng/mL ± 22.7 ng/mL at long-term follow-up, even in those patients who remained in clinical remission.[24] Although the reason for the continuously elevated levels is unclear, this would make calprotectin less useful for follow-up of patients after surgery. Possible explanations from the authors included that surgery does not remove all active disease or the possibility of postoperative recurrences.[24]

Other studies, however, have found that fecal calprotectin can be a useful marker of endoscopic recurrence. In a prospective longitudinal study evaluating the role of calprotectin as a predictive marker of endoscopic recurrence at 1 year, 50 consecutive CD patients with ileocecal resection underwent measurement of fecal calprotectin and abdominal ultrasound scan (US) at 3 months, followed by colonoscopy at 1 year. The sensitivity and specificity of calprotectin and US as predictive markers of recurrence were 26% and 60% versus 75% and 90%, respectively. The authors concluded that at 3 months, US is more specific than calprotectin in predicting endoscopic recurrence. However, fecal calprotectin values greater than 200 mg/L show a higher sensitivity than US, suggesting that these levels may be an indication for colonoscopy in CD patients with negative US to detect early recurrence.[41]

In a prospective study of 13 patients, fecal calprotectin as well as lactoferrin normalized within 2 months after surgery in patients with an uncomplicated postoperative course.[42] Higher levels of fecal calprotectin and lactoferrin were found to be more accurate in predicting clinical disease activity measured by Harvey Bradshaw Index ($P<.001$) and relapse after surgery than CRP, platelet count, or endoscopic appearance. They suggested that in symptomatic postoperative patients, a single fecal calprotectin or lactoferrin measurement 2 months or more after resection could identify genuine disease recurrence and help target immunosuppressant therapy.

In a follow-up study of 36 Crohn patients in clinical remission after bowel resection, fecal lactoferrin levels were significantly correlated with interleukin-6 (IL-6; $r = 0.431$, $P = .025$) and CRP ($r = 0.507$, $P = .007$), whereas no correlation was observed between lactoferrin and the following cytokines: IL-1β, IL-12, TNF-α, or transforming growth factor–β1.[43] Reoperation for anastomotic recurrence tended to occur significantly more frequently in patients with higher IL-6 ($P = .10$) suggesting that subclinical intestinal inflammation expressed by elevated fecal lactoferrin levels occurred through the IL-6-CRP cascade.

POUCHITIS

Pouchitis is a common complication of ileal pouch anal anastomosis in patients who have undergone restorative proctocolectomy for medically refractory UC, Crohn colitis, or IBD-associated dysplasia. Because of a poor correlation between macroscopic and histologic assessments of inflammation, endoscopic evaluation often is required. However, fecal markers have been studied in this group of patients showing possible benefit with accurate diagnosis and management of pouch disorders as well as cost reduction in their utility.

Significantly elevated calprotectin levels were found in all 9 patients with endoscopic and histologic evidence of pouch inflammation in this small study compared with patients without pouch inflammation. The first-morning calprotectin levels correlated well ($r = 0.91$, $P \leq .0001$) with 24-hour stool collection, with endoscopic and histologic scores, and also with the percentage of CD15+ mature neutrophils and CD14+ macrophages within the lamina propria.[44]

Similar findings were also confirmed in a larger study showing significantly higher calprotectin concentrations in inflamed pouches compared with those obtained from noninflamed pouches (Mann-Whitney, $P<.0001$) in stool samples collected from 46 UC patients and 8 familial adenomatous polyposis patients who had undergone restorative proctocolectomy.[45] Using a threshold of 92.5 μg/g, calprotectin levels correlated closely with the Objective Pouchitis Score, the Pouch Disease Activity Index, and endoscopic and histological inflammatory scores (Spearman rank test, $P<.0001$) with a sensitivity of 90% and a specificity of 76.5%.

In pediatric-onset ulcerative colitis, fecal calprotectin levels after restorative proctocolectomy also correlated positively with frequency of pouchitis ($r = 0.468$, $P<.01$), with mean calprotectin levels of 71 $\pm$ 50 μg/g among patients with no history of pouchitis, 290 $\pm$ 131 μg/g among patients with a single episode of pouchitis, and highest level 832 $\pm$ 422 μg/g among those with recurrent pouchitis ($P=.019$ between recurrent pouchitis and no pouchitis).[46] A history of recurrent pouchitis was a significant predictor of fecal calprotectin greater than 300 μg/g (OR, 51; 95% CI, 1.2–2200; $P<.040$). Sensitivity, specificity, PPV, and NPV for fecal calprotectin concentration over 300 μg/g to detect recurrent pouchitis were 57%, 92%, 67%, and 89%, respectively.

At a cutoff of 7 μL/mL using ELISA, fecal lactoferrin levels correlated with pouchitis disease activity index scores and had a sensitivity and specificity of 100% and 85%, respectively, in diagnosing pouchitis.[47] In another study of 11 patients using a modification of the quantitative ELISA lactoferrin, the test had a sensitivity of 100% and a specificity of 86% with a positive predictive value of 76% in diagnosing pouchitis.[48] Lactoferrin was also found to be cost effective in comparison with endoscopic evaluation for the diagnosis of pouchitis.[49]

Both fecal markers lactoferrin and calprotectin were found to be useful in distinguishing inflammatory from noninflammatory pouch disorders. Because of the small numbers of patients in these studies, larger studies may be required before using these fecal markers in place of conventional endoscopic testing for this diagnosis. However, these markers could be a useful tool for initial evaluation of symptomatic patients with ileal pouch anal anastomosis. No studies have evaluated the use of these markers in follow-up of patients with pouchitis.

MICROSCOPIC COLITIS

Very few studies have evaluated the use of fecal markers in microscopic colitis. Tibble and colleagues[50] had only 6 patients with microscopic colitis—too small a sample size to be useful. The study by Limburg and coworkers[51] of 11 patients with microscopic or collagenous colitis found elevated fecal calprotectin levels (median value of 266 μg/g of stool) compared with subjects without colorectal inflammation but lower than those with CD or UC (median value of 1722 μg/g of stool).[51]

In the largest study of fecal markers in patients with collagenous colitis, those with active disease had higher median levels of fecal calprotectin (80 μg/g) compared with patients with quiescent collagenous colitis (26 μg/g, P = .025), and controls (6.25 μg/g, P = .002).[52] However, 8 of 21 patients (38%) with active collagenous colitis had normal levels of calprotectin, making this an unpredictable marker for monitoring or diagnosing active microscopic colitis. Only 1 of the 21 patients with active collagenous colitis had elevated lactoferrin levels.

SUMMARY

Overall, fecal markers have been found to be more accurate than serum markers. However, fecal markers are not specific for IBD and may be elevated in a range of organic conditions.

Fecal calprotectin and lactoferrin can still differentiate inflammatory disease from functional bowel disorders. Comparison studies have found an overall diagnostic accuracy in IBD of 80% to 100% for both calprotectin and lactoferrin. Elevated levels are found in both CD and UC making it difficult to distinguish between these 2 diagnoses from these biomarkers alone. Both markers correlated well to mucosal healing and histologic improvement. Hence, they may be useful in monitoring response to treatment and predicting endoscopic and clinical relapse. Overall, patients with elevated markers were at higher risk of postoperative recurrence than those with normal levels. Fecal markers are useful in predicting pouchitis as well.

Fecal markers are helpful as an adjunctive tool in overall evaluation of patients with nonspecific symptoms and as a management tool in those with inflammatory disease to monitor disease activity and possibility of relapse. They are less invasive than colonoscopy and can help guide management in a more cost-effective manner.

REFERENCES

1. Roseth AG, Fagerhol MK, Aadland E, et al. Assessment of the neutrophil dominating protein calprotectin in feces. A methodologic study. Scand J Gastroenterol 1992;27:793–8.

2. Available at: http://www.calpro.no. Accessed November 3, 2011.
3. Medical and Behavioral Health Policy Manual, Section: Laboratory, Policy Number: VI-39, Effective Date: 09/26/2011. Under: Fecal calprotectin Testing. Available at: http://notes.bluecrossmn.com/web/medpolman.nsf/8178b1c14b1e9b 6b8525624f0062fe9f/072d5feb5cf55550862579170066d6a1/$FILE/Fecal% 20Calprotectin%20Testing.pdf. Accessed November 10, 2011.
4. Available at: https://www.unitedhealthcareonline.com/ccmcontent/ProviderII/ UHC/en-US/Assets/ProviderStaticFiles/ProviderStaticFilesPdf/Tools%20and%20 Resources/Policies%20and%20Protocols/Medical%20Policies/Medical%20Policies/ fecal_calprotectin_testing.pdf. Accessed November 10, 2011.
5. Buderus S, Booner J, Lyerly D, et al. Fecal lactoferrin: a new parameter to monitor infliximab therapy. Dig Dis Sci 2004;49(6):1036–9.
6. Sugi K, Saitoh O, Hirata I, et al. Fecal lactoferrin as a marker for disease activity in inflammatory bowel disease: comparison with other neutrophil-derived proteins. Am J Gastroenterol 1996;91:927–34.
7. Angriman I, Scarpa M, D'Incì R, et al. Enzymes in feces: useful markers of chronic inflammatory bowel disease. Clin Chim Acta 2007;381:63–8.
8. Available at: http://www.enterolab.com/StaticPages/TestInfo.aspx. Accessed November 10, 2011.
9. Available at: https://secure.cigna.com/health/provider/medical/procedural/ coverage_positions/medical/mm_0414_coveragepositioncriteria_lactoferrin_ test.pdf. Accessed November 10, 2011.
10. van der Sluys VA, Biemond I, Verspaget HW, et al. Faecal parameters in the assessment of activity in inflammatory bowel disease. Scand J Gastroenterol 1999; S230:106–10.
11. Walker TR, Land ML, Cook TM, et al. Serial fecal lactoferrin measurements are useful in the interval assessment of patients with active and inactive inflammatory bowel disease. Gastroenterology 2004;126:A215.
12. Kane SV, Sandborn WJ, Rufo PA, et al. Fecal lactoferrin is a sensitive and specific marker in identifying intestinal inflammation. Am J Gastroenterol 2003;98:1309–14.
13. Uchida K, Matsuse R, Tomita S, et al. Immunochemical detection of human lactoferrin in feces as a new marker of inflammatory gastrointestinal disorders and colon cancer. Clin Biochem 1994;27:259–64.
14. Dai J, Liu WZ, Zhao YP, et al. Relationship between fecal lactoferrin and inflammatory bowel disease. Scand J Gastroenterol 2007;42(12):1440–4.
15. Langhorst J, Elsenbruch S, Koelzer J, et al. Noninvasive markers in the assessment of intestinal inflammation in inflammatory bowel diseases: performance of fecal lactoferrin, calprotectin, and PMN-elastase, CRP, and clinical indices. Am J Gastroenterol 2008;103:162–9.
16. Schoepfer AM, Trummler M, Seeholzer P, et al. Discriminating IBD from IBS: comparison of the test performance of fecal markers, blood leukocytes, CRP, and IBD antibodies. Inflamm Bowel Dis 2008;14:32–9.
17. D'Incà R, Dal Pont E, Di Leo V, et al. Calprotectin and lactoferrin in the assessment of intestinal inflammation and organic disease. Int J Colorectal Dis 2007;22(4):429–37.
18. von Roon AC, Karamountzos L, Purkayastha S, et al. Diagnostic precision of fecal calprotectin for inflammatory bowel disease and colorectal malignancy. Am J Gastroenterol 2007;102:803–13.
19. Tibble JA, Sigthorsson G, Foster R, et al. Use of surrogate markers of inflammation and Rome criteria to distinguish organic from nonorganic intestinal disease. Gastroenterology 2002;123(2):450–60.

20. van Rheenen PF, Van de Vijver E, Fidler V. Faecal calprotectin for screening of patients with suspected inflammatory bowel disease: diagnostic meta-analysis. BMJ 2010; 341.

21. Guerrant RL, Araujo V, Soares E, et al. Measurement of fecal lactoferrin as a marker of fecal leucocytes. J Clin Microbiol 1992;30:1238–42.

22. Berni Canani R, Rapacciuolo L, Romano MT, et al. Diagnostic value of faecal calprotectin in paediatric gastroenterology clinical practice. Dig Liver Dis 2004;36: 467–70.

23. Quail MA, Russell RK, Van Limbergen JE, et al. Fecal calprotectin complements routine laboratory investigations in diagnosing childhood inflammatory bowel disease. Inflamm Bowel Dis 2009;15(5):756–9.

24. Scarpa M, D'Incà R, Basso D, et al. Fecal lactoferrin and calprotectin after ileocolonic resection for Crohn's disease. Dis Colon Rectum 2007;50:861–9.

25. Jones J, Loftus EV Jr, Panaccione R, et al. Relationships between disease activity and serum and fecal biomarkers in patients with Crohn's disease. Clin Gastroenterol Hepatol 2008;6(11):1218–24.

26. Vieira A, Fang CB, Rolim EG, et al. Inflammatory bowel disease activity assessed by fecal calprotectin and lactoferrin: correlation with laboratory parameters, clinical, endoscopic and histological indexes. BMC Res Notes 2009;29:2:221.

27. Xiang JY, Ouyang Q, Li GD, et al. Clinical value of fecal calprotectin in determining disease activity of ulcerative colitis. World J Gastroenterol 2008;14(1):53–7.

28. Wagner M, Peterson CG, Ridefelt P, et al. Fecal markers of inflammation used as surrogate markers for treatment outcome in relapsing inflammatory bowel disease. World J Gastroenterol 2008;14(36):5584–9.

29. Masoodi I, Kochhar R, Dutta U, et al. Fecal lactoferrin, myeloperoxidase and serum C-reactive are effective biomarkers in the assessment of disease activity and severity in patients with idiopathic ulcerative colitis. J Gastroenterol Hepatol 2009;24(11): 1768–74.

30. Palmon R, Brown S, Ullman TA, et al. Calprotectin and lactoferrin decrease with maintenance infliximab administration [abstract]. Gastroenterology 2006;130(Suppl S2):A–212.

31. Sipponen T, Savilahti E, Kärkkäinen P, et al. Fecal calprotectin lactoferrin and endoscopic disease activity in monitoring anti-TNF-alpha therapy for Crohn's disease. Inflamm Bowel Dis 2008;14:1392–8.

32. Tibble JA, Sigthorsson G, Bridger S, et al. Surrogate markers of intestinal inflammation are predictive of relapse in patients with inflammatory bowel disease. Gastroenterology 2000;119:15–22.

33. Costa F, Mumolo MG, Ceccarelli L, et al. Calprotectin is a stronger predictive marker of relapse in ulcerative colitis than in Crohn's disease. Gut 2005;54:364–8.

34. Walkiewicz D, Werlin SL, Fish D, et al. Fecal calprotectin is useful in predicting disease relapse in pediatric inflammatory bowel disease. Inflamm Bowel Dis 2008;14:669–73.

35. Kallel L, Ayadi I, Matri S, et al. Fecal calprotectin is a predictive marker of relapse in Crohn's disease involving the colon: a prospective study. Eur J Gastroenterol Hepatol 2010;22(3):340–5.

36. Gisbert JP, Bermejo F, Pérez-Calle JL, et al. Fecal calprotectin and lactoferrin for the prediction of inflammatory bowel disease relapse. Inflamm Bowel Dis 2009;15(8): 1190–8.

37. Ho GT, Lee HM, Brydon G, et al. Fecal calprotectin predicts the clinical course of acute severe ulcerative colitis. Am J Gastroenterol 2009;104:673–8.

38. Schoepfer AM, Beglinger C, Straumann A, et al. Fecal calprotectin correlates more closely with the Simple Endoscopic Score for Crohn's disease (SES-CD) than CRP, blood leukocytes, and the CDAI. Am J Gastroenterol 2010;105(1):162–9.
39. Shitrit AB, Braverman D, Stankiewics H, et al. Fecal calprotectin as a predictor of abnormal colonic histology. Dis Colon Rectum 2007;50(12):2188–93.
40. Lewis JD. The utility of biomarkers in the diagnosis and therapy of inflammatory bowel disease. Gastroenterology 2011;140(6):1817–26.
41. Orlando A, Modesto I, Castiglione F, et al. The role of calprotectin in predicting endoscopic postsurgical recurrence in asymptomatic Crohn's Disease: a comparison with ultrasound. Eur Rev Med Pharmacol Sci 2006;10:17–22.
42. Lamb CA, Mohiuddin MK, Gicquel J, et al. Faecal calprotectin or lactoferrin can identify postoperative recurrence in Crohn's disease. Br J Surg 2009;96(6):663–74.
43. Ruffolo C, Scarpa M, Faggian D, et al. Subclinical intestinal inflammation in patients with Crohn's disease following bowel resection: a smoldering fire. J Gastrointest Surg 2010;14(1):24–31.
44. Thomas P, Rihani H, Røseth A, et al. Assessment of ileal pouch inflammation by single stool calprotectin assay. Dis Colon Rectum 2000;43:214–20.
45. Johnson MW, Maestranzi S, Duffy AM, et al. Fecal calprotectin: a noninvasive diagnostic tool and marker of severity in pouchitis. Eur J Gastroenterol Hepatol 2008;20:174–9.
46. Pakarinen MP, Koivusalo A, Natunen J, et al. Fecal calprotectin mirrors inflammation of the distal ileum and bowel function after restorative proctocolectomy for pediatric-onset ulcerative colitis. Inflamm Bowel Dis 2010;16(3):482–6.
47. Parsi M, Shen B, Achkar J, et al. Fecal lactoferrin for diagnosis of symptomatic patients with ileal pouch-anal anastomosis. Gastroenterology 2004;126:80–6.
48. Lim M, Gonsalves S, Thekkinkattil D, et al. The assessment of a rapid noninvasive immunochromatographic assay test for fecal lactoferrin in patients with suspected inflammation of the ileal pouch. Dis Colon Rectum 2008;51:96–9.
49. Parsi MA, Ellis JJ, Lashner BA. Cost-effectiveness of quantitative fecal lactoferrin assay for diagnosis of symptomatic patients with ileal pouch-anal anastomosis. J Clin Gastroenterol 2008;42:799–805.
50. Tibble J, Teahon K, Thjodleifsson B, et al. A simple method for assessing intestinal inflammation in Crohn's disease. Gut 2000;47:506–13.
51. Limburg PJ, Ahlquist DA, Sandborn WJ, et al. Fecal calprotectin levels predict colorectal inflammation among patients with chronic diarrhea referred for colonoscopy. Am J Gastroenterol 2000;95:2831–7.
52. Wildt S, Nordgaard-Lassen I, Bendtsen F, et al. Metabolic and inflammatory faecal markers in collagenous colitis. Eur J Gastroenterol Hepatol 2007;19:567–74.

Imaging for Luminal Disease and Complications: CT Enterography, MR Enterography, Small-Bowel Follow-Through, and Ultrasound

David J. Grand, MD[a],*, Adam Harris, MD[b], Edward V. Loftus Jr, MD[c]

KEYWORDS

- Inflammatory bowel disease • Crohn disease
- Magnetic resonance enterography
- Computed tomography enterography • Imaging

In the past decade, there has been a seismic shift in the use of imaging for Crohn disease (CD) away from small-bowel follow-through (SBFT) to cross-sectional techniques, most commonly computed tomography enterography (CTE) and magnetic resonance enterography (MRE). Because of rapid advances in CT and MRI hardware, as well as routine use of oral contrast agents designed to distend the lumen of the small bowel, cross-sectional techniques have become a first-line imaging modality, promising accurate assessment of the mucosa as well as the extraintestinal manifestations of penetrating disease. In most situations, the choice of cross-sectional modality (clinically) is essentially a tradeoff between the ease and cost of the study (which favor CTE) and the desire to minimize radiation exposure (which favors MRE).

In this new era, fluoroscopic studies, including SBFT, have been relegated to a more focused, problem-solving role including evaluation of possible obstruction and road mapping of complex fistulae. Ultrasound of the small bowel currently does not

The authors have nothing to disclose.

[a] Diagnostic Imaging, Warren Alpert School of Medicine, Brown University, 593 Eddy Street, Providence, RI 02903, USA

[b] Department of Gastroenterology, Warren Alpert School of Medicine, Brown University, 110 Lockwood Street, Providence, RI 02903, USA

[c] Division of Gastroenterology & Hepatology, Mayo Clinic, 200 First Street, SW, Rochester, MN 55905, USA

* Corresponding author.

E-mail address: dgrand@lifespan.org

Gastroenterol Clin N Am 41 (2012) 497–512

doi:10.1016/j.gtc.2012.01.015

provide the comprehensive assessment of cross-sectional techniques. It is limited in the United States by the lack of Food and Drug Administration (FDA)-approved intravenous contrast agents.

Imaging of CD remains an active and evolving research topic as investigators hope to reliably differentiate active from chronic disease, predict disease response to medical therapy, and potentially assess bowel motility, while simultaneously reducing exposure to ionizing radiation. The next decade promises great steps forward.

CROSS-SECTIONAL ENTEROGRAPHY: CTE AND MRE
What is Enterography?

Enterography refers to the use of oral contrast agents designed to distend the lumen of the small bowel, without being reabsorbed. Although water may distend the upper tract, it does not provide adequate distension of the terminal ileum, the most commonly affected bowel segment in CD.

Adequate distention of the small bowel is critical for reliable and reproducible diagnostic enterography, as it facilitates evaluation of both mucosal enhancement and bowel wall thickening. If the lumen is not distended, the mucosa cannot be evaluated accurately, and collapsed bowel segments are too easily mistaken for pathologic bowel wall thickening.

In addition to distending the small bowel, oral contrast agents should be hypoattenuating ("dark") on CT and hypointense ("dark") on T1-weighted MRI images to allow evaluation of the adjacent, brightly enhancing mucosa. Contrast agents that are hypointense on both T1- and T2-weighted images may be additionally helpful, but are not in widespread use.

Unfortunately, in daily practice, the distention achieved by oral contrast agents is variable. This variation is in part due to physiologic differences in bowel motility, but successful bowel distension is also dependent on the patient's ability and willingness to drink the contrast. Overall, however, routine use of oral agents has been shown to be reliable and better tolerated than enteroclysis.[1,2] Although CT or MR enteroclysis may still have a role for detection of low-grade small-bowel obstruction, neither is routinely performed at our institutions.

There is no shortage of effective oral contrast preparations for enterography. As a general rule, as the osmolality of the agent increases, the palatability decreases and side effects (nausea, diarrhea, and flatulence) increase.[3,4] At our institutions, we routinely use 0.1% low-density barium sulfate suspension (VoLumen, E-Z-EM, NY) for both CTE and MRE.

The volume and timing of oral contrast also vary among institutions. We currently ask patients to drink 450 mL of VoLumen (one bottle) over 15 minutes, beginning 45 minutes before imaging. They are then given a second bottle to drink over the next 15 minutes and finally 450 mL of water 15 minutes before imaging begins. We use water immediately before imaging because it is intended only to distend the proximal small bowel and we can therefore reduce the amount of hyperosmolar fluid administered and its subsequent side effects (**Fig. 1**).

Intravenous contrast should be administered for CTE or MRE whenever possible. Standard dosing varies slightly between institutions, but whatever agent and volume is typically used for a routine abdominal CT or MRI at a given institution may be used. CT is typically performed during the "enteric" phase, approximately 50 seconds after injection (although a more standard portal venous phase will also suffice),[5] whereas MR should be performed dynamically; that is, imaging should be performed at multiple time points (or phases) after contrast administration.

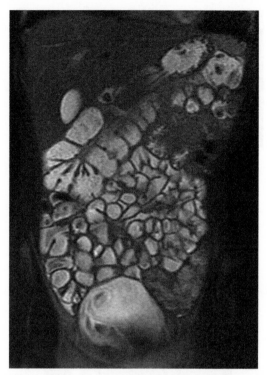

Fig. 1. Excellent small distension. Coronal single-shot fast-spin-echo image demonstrating excellent small-bowel distension after oral administration of contrast. This is what we hope to achieve in all patients.

The technique outlined in the preceding, and discussed in more detail later, is how we perform enterography under ideal circumstances. Careful attention to technique results in the best chance of obtaining high-quality images and reliable, useful diagnostic information. However, one practical consideration is worth noting. What if the patient will not or cannot drink the oral contrast? In these situations, the study should be performed without it. Most patients who refuse to drink the oral contrast do so because they are too sick to tolerate it. Anecdotally, the findings in these patients will often be significant enough that they will be detected without the additional sensitivity provided by good bowel distension.

CT Enterography

The efficacy of CTE has been repeatedly proven in clinical trials and the technique has gained widespread acceptance. Mayo Clinic, for example, reported a nearly 10-fold increase in its use between 2001 and 2004.[6] This marked increase has occurred in parallel to decreased use of the fluoroscopic SBFT, which CTE has largely replaced. Using the technique described previously, high-quality images allowing for robust small-bowel evaluation are routinely obtained with this quick, well tolerated exam.

The findings of CD on CTE have been well described and include bowel wall thickening, abnormal mural enhancement and stratification, and the "comb sign."[7] Mural hyperenhancement may be symmetric (nonspecific) or asymmetric (more

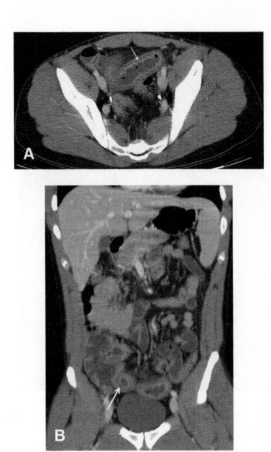

Fig. 2. Target sign. Axial (*A*) and coronal (*B*) images from CTE. Arrows indicate thickening of the terminal ileum with differential enhancement of the mucosa (*bright*), submucosa (*dark*), and serosa (*bright*).

suggestive of CD). Mural stratification, or the "target" sign, refers to the differential enhancement of the bowel wall layers: enhancing mucosa (bright), submucosal edema (dark), and enhancing serosa (bright).[8] Bowel wall thickening is diagnosed when the small-bowel wall exceeds 3 mm in thickness in a well distended bowel loop. The presence of bowel wall thickening in conjunction with asymmetric mural hyperenhancement is essentially pathognomonic for CD.[5] Finally, the "comb sign" refers to engorgement of the vasa recta and is highly suggestive of active inflammation[9] (**Figs. 2** and **3**).

There is a wide range of reported accuracy of CTE within the literature, owing in part to technologic changes/advances that often occur faster than the latest literature can reach press. But it is also due to routine use of inadequate reference standards, most commonly ileocolonoscopy. When ileocolonoscopy is used as the sole gold standard, patients with small-bowel inflammation detected on CTE (or MRE) may be misclassified as falsely positive simply because the endoscope did not reach the diseased segment. This is of particular concern in the CD population because of the prevalence of stenotic ileocecal valves, skipping of the terminal ileum, and intramural CD inflammation. In one large series of patients with suspected CD and normal

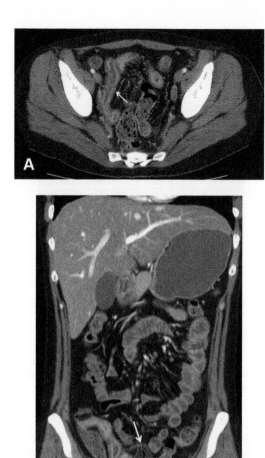

Fig. 3. Active CD, "comb" sign. Axial (*A*) image from CTE demonstrates stratified enhancement and asymmetric, mural thickening (*arrow*). Arrow on coronal reformatted image (*B*) demonstrates prominence of the vasa recta, the "comb" sign.

endoscopic examination of the terminal ileum, 54% actually had active small-bowel disease when radiologic, serologic, and clinical factors were used as the reference standard.[10] When the difficulties related to adequate reference standards are taken into consideration, the sensitivity of CTE for detection of CD is approximately 90%.[11]

In addition to this impressive sensitivity for detecting mucosal disease, CTE reliably detects sequelae of penetrating disease, such as fistula and abscess formation, with an accuracy of approximately 94%[12] (**Fig. 4**). Anecdotally, the low-density oral contrast routinely administered for CTE occasionally complicates the diagnosis of interloop abscess, as both normal bowel and abscess will contain low-density fluid (as opposed to routine abdominal–pelvic CT, in which bowel contents are "bright" due to barium-containing oral contrast and abscesses are "dark" because they contain unopacified fluid). If there is difficulty deciding whether a fluid-containing structure is

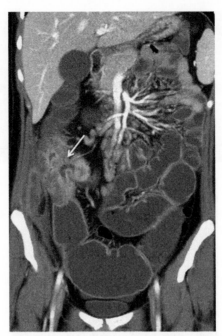

Fig. 4. Complications of CD. Coronal CTE image demonstrating marked thickening of the terminal ileum with dilated, fluid-filled, proximal small bowel compatible with obstruction. Arrow indicates entero-entero fistula.

an abscess or a bowel loop, high-attenuation oral contrast can be administered and the study repeated. Because CTE is exquisitely sensitive for detecting active CD, it may also have a role in monitoring response to increasingly powerful (and potentially toxic) medical treatments. Persistent inflammation is a risk factor for disease progression and complications. Unfortunately, clinical symptoms do not necessarily correspond with biological activity. Subjecting a patient to repeated invasive colonoscopies increases both cost and risk, and may not be practical depending on disease location. A recent retrospective study illustrated that radiologic improvement did not correlate closely with clinical symptoms, serum biomarkers, or endoscopic appearance; however, 60% of patients did show radiologic improvement after infliximab therapy.[13] This suggests that CTE may be an important biomarker for early disease response.

Radiation

The potential negative consequences of exposure to diagnostic radiation warrant brief discussion, as they are now in the forefront of the minds of clinicians, radiologists, and patients alike.[14] Two recent studies evaluated the radiation dose associated with commonly ordered CT scans as well as the potential risk of radiation-induced cancer due to CT scans alone.[15,16] The authors calculated a projected rate of CT-induced cancer of 1/250 20-year-old women and 1/330 20-year-old men who underwent multiphase CT abdomen/pelvis scans. The risk of CT-induced cancer decreased as the age of the patients increased. It is critical to remember, though, that these risks are theoretical and are based on principles that are at least questioned, if not rejected, by many medical physicists.[17] However, regardless of whether we can quantify the specific risk(s) of medical radiation, we can all agree that we should strive to limit exposure to the lowest possible dose necessary for diagnosis—the so-called ALARA principle (As Low As Reasonably Achievable).[18]

CTE exposes patients to up to five times the ionizing radiation of the typical SBFT, the test it has largely replaced.[19] That said, the radiation dose from a single CTE is not high enough to be particularly concerning. Newer CT techniques have demonstrated a significant decrease in radiation dose using modified protocols and reconstruction algorithms.[20,21] One recent study demonstrated that a 50% reduction in dose could be achieved without sacrificing sensitivity for acute inflammation.[22] Certainly, advances in scanner hardware and software technology will continue to lower the radiation dose of CTE.

However, the inflammatory bowel disease (IBD) population has two important characteristics that should alert physicians to use radiation judiciously. Patients are typically young at the time of diagnosis, and they will often require numerous examinations throughout their lives. Indeed, the increased lifetime radiation exposure of IBD patients compared to the general population has been well documented; the majority of this exposure is due to repeated CT exams.[23]

All medical decisions should be informed by analyzing the potential risks and benefits of any course of action as well as the potential risks and benefits of inaction. Coordination between emergency room, primary care, and gastrointestinal physicians is critical to helping minimize unnecessary radiation in the young IBD patients. Radiation exposure should not be a concern in the elderly (in whom the risk is very small) or in patients who are acutely ill (in whom the potential benefit is very high). Overall, CTE is too useful clinically and cost effective[24] to avoid based on radiation concerns. When used appropriately, it is a powerful tool to aid in the diagnosis and management of CD. Undoubtedly, investigators will continue to develop new ways to lower radiation dose while maintaining diagnostic efficacy.

MRE

In this relatively new era of radiation awareness, what dose is acceptable? There is no doubt that the organ and effective doses of CT will decrease significantly in the next decade. But, as discussed previously, patients with IBD are unique in their youth and need for serial exams. In this population, the option of MRE, which is free of ionizing radiation, is compelling.

Evaluation of the small bowel with MRE faces one major hurdle: bowel motion. Although MR pulse sequences have become increasingly fast, a single series can require greater than 20 seconds of imaging time, during which any bowel motion blurs the resulting image. This is an issue only for the contrast-enhanced images, as the remainder of the commonly used pulse sequences for MRE (single-shot fast-spin-echo and steady-state free-precession) are sufficiently rapid. Unfortunately, although the contrast-enhanced images are the most susceptible to motion, they are also the most critical.

Most centers therefore administer pharmacologic bowel paralytics to minimize small-bowel motion. Specific techniques vary between institutions; however, 1 mg of glucagon is most commonly used whether injected intravenously or intramuscularly, in a single dose or in split doses. These agents are not necessary for CTE because of the speed of acquisition of modern multidetector CT scanners. However, just as the radiation dose of CTE is certain to decrease, the speed of MR pulse sequences will certainly increase in the near future, which may render this problem irrelevant.

The findings indicative of CD on MRE are essentially the same as CTE, including wall thickening, abnormal enhancement, and engorgement of the vasa recta, with the

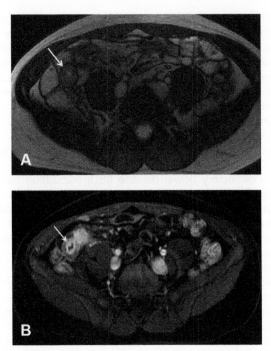

Fig. 5. Mild terminal ileitis. Axial SSFP (*A*) demonstates thickening of the terminal ileum (*arrow*). Corresponding axial post-contrast enhanced image (*B*) demonstrates stratified, layered enhancement (*arrow*).

addition of elevated T2 signal within or adjacent to the bowel wall.[25] Elevated T2 signal is caused by the presence of fluid and is indicative of an active inflammatory process.[26] When present, this finding is highly specific (**Figs. 5–7**).

Because of its inherent, exquisite soft tissue contrast, MRI is the gold-standard for detection and characterization of perianal fistulae. Accurate characterization is critical for surgical planning, and MRE easily depicts the relationship of fistulae to the sphincter complexes. MRE is clearly superior to CTE in this regard and has also been shown to be more effective than clinical examination and endosonography.[27,28]

As discussed earlier, multiple studies have been performed that show excellent accuracy of MRE compared to CTE and colonoscopy.[29,30] In addition to providing this diagnostic information without ionizing radiation, MRE has at least two distinct potential advantages compared to CTE.

One reason MRE may be more difficult/time consuming to interpret is the large number of images generated. However, the inherent redundancy of MRE is a significant potential advantage as it provides multiple images of each bowel segment at different time points. Thus, a collapsed loop of bowel seen on one pulse sequence (which could be mischaracterized as a stricture if imaged at a single time point) may be seen to open on a subsequent pulse sequence. This ability to image bowel segments over time is a critical component of SBFT that is lost on CTE and regained with MRE (**Fig. 8**).

In addition, MRE will likely prove more effective in distinguishing active inflammatory disease from chronic fibrostenotic disease, the "holy grail" of IBD imaging. If we can accurately make this distinction, gastroenterologists can more effectively triage

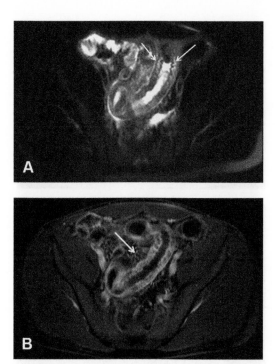

Fig. 6. Severe, active terminal ileitis. Axial HASTE (*A*) shows marked thickening of the terminal ileum. Arrows indicate fluid within the bowel wall compatible with active inflammation. Axial post–contrast-enhanced image (*B*) shows a thickened, enhancing terminal ileum. Note the arrow on the "comb" sign.

patients to potent medical versus surgical therapies and avoid the morbidity inherent in misclassification in either direction. MRE as a means of guiding patient therapy has been shown to be highly effective in small studies.[31]

Elevated T2 signal in or adjacent to the bowel wall is a specific indicator of active disease, as is a stratified enhancement pattern on dynamic, contrast-enhanced images, whereas dark T2 signal and homogeneous mural enhancement suggest fibrostenotic disease.[32–34] The ability to evaluate the T2 signal of the bowel wall is unique to MRE. Practically, however, dynamic contrast-enhanced imaging, performing imaging at multiple time points after administration of contrast, is also unique to MRE, as the additional radiation dose this would require for CTE is prohibitive.

More recent investigations have gone beyond simply detecting active CD to true quantitative assessment of disease severity. Rimola and colleagues have developed one such classification (based on wall thickness, degree of enhancement, T2 signal, and presence of ulceration) that in a study of 48 patients demonstrated excellent correlation with the Crohn Disease Endoscopic Index of Severity (CDEIS).[35] Accurate categorization of disease severity is critical to guide treatment choices and may be helpful in monitoring response to treatment, a powerful and exciting application of this noninvasive, radiation-free technique.

Nephrogenic Systemic Fibrosis

Nephrogenic systemic fibrosis (NSF) is a poorly understood syndrome characterized by progressive organ fibrosis that was first linked to gadolinium-based contrast

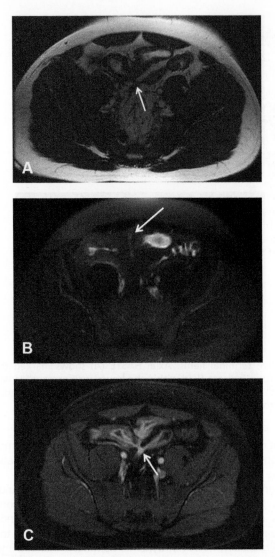

Fig. 7. Entero–entero fistula. Axial SSFP (*A*) demonstrates abnormal tethering of bowel loops connected by inflammation (*arrow*). Axial HASTE (*B*) shows a channel of bright signal (*arrow*), compatible with fluid, connecting the abnormal loops. Post–contrast-enhanced image (*C*) shows inflammation and abnormal kinking of the tethered bowel loops (*C*).

agents in 2006.[36] To the best of our knowledge, this potentially fatal syndrome occurs exclusively in patients with renal dysfunction. The precise degree of renal dysfunction at which gadolinium administration remains safe, measured by the estimated glomerular filtration rate (eGFR), is not known, but most institutions begin to *consider* the potential risk when the eGFR is less than 60 mL/min/m^2. That said, a recently published study involving 52,954 injections of gadolinium-based contrast agents reported not a single case of NSF despite injection of 6490 patients with an eGFR of less than 60 mL/min/m^2, including 36 patients with an eGFR less than 30 mL/min/m^2.[37]

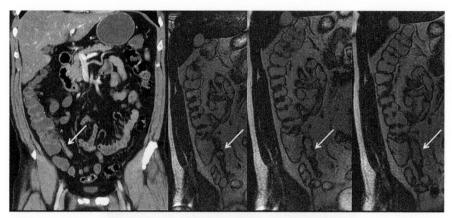

Fig. 8. Normal terminal ileum. First image (*far left*) from a CTE demonstrating collapsed TI mistakenly interpreted as a stricture (*arrow*). Three images from same-day MRE demonstrate normal motility of the TI (*arrows*).

The sudden appearance of a potentially fatal syndrome linked to what was thought to be an innocuous contrast agent appropriately shocked and frightened the medical community. The critical "take-home" message about NSF, however, is that it occurs only in patients with significant renal dysfunction. Given that the population that is best served by MRE is young and otherwise healthy, referring clinicians should not let fear of NSF affect their choice of imaging modality. In patients with normal renal function, gadolinium-based contrast agents are regarded as safer than the iodine-based agents used in CT, which have been shown to be directly nephrotoxic.

CTE versus MRE: How to Choose?

The algorithm for deciding between CTE and MRE to evaluate known or suspected CD varies between institutions. Numerous studies have been published that, despite minimal variation, generally suggest that MRE and CTE are essentially equivalent diagnostically for detection of CD.[38–41] CTE is more widely available. It is faster, easier for the patient, and probably easier to interpret. MRE involves no radiation. It may provide additional information based on T2 signal, dynamic contrast enhancement, and the ability to image bowel segments over time, but it is more expensive and more difficult on the patient. In our departments:

- **For young patients with known or suspected IBD, we recommend MRE.** We do so knowing that if they have IBD they will likely require numerous exams and if they later present to the ER with abdominal pain they will almost certainly undergo a CT scan.
- **When perianal disease is suspected, we recommend MRE.** Our routine MRE protocol allows confident assessment of the entire bowel as well the anus. Small perianal fistulae are simply too difficult to see on CT.
- **When the clinical question is active versus chronic disease in a patient with known IBD, we recommend MRE.** We are more confident assessing disease activity with the additional information of T2 signal and dynamic contrast enhancement than a single phase of injection.
- **In patients older than 50 years or with any indication other than known or suspected IBD, we recommend CTE.** CTE is fast, reliable, and easy to

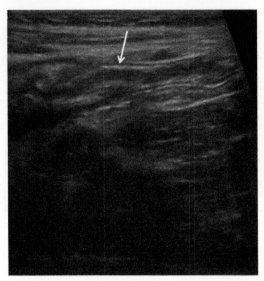

Fig. 9. Thickened terminal ileum. Sagittal ultrasound image of the right lower quadrant demonstrating a thickened terminal ileum (*arrow*) at the level of the ileocecal valve.

interpret. In older patients, or in patients with questionable symptoms, it is the test of choice.

Ultrasound

Ultrasound is an intriguing and compelling imaging option for IBD owing to its widespread availability, speed, relatively low cost, and lack of ionizing radiation. Although it has demonstrated efficacy in multiple studies,[42,43] its routine use has been limited, particularly in the United States (**Fig. 9**). Ultrasound is highly operator dependent, which limits its reproducibility. In addition, it rarely demonstrates the entire small bowel, particularly in patients with an elevated body mass index or large quantities of bowel gas.[44]

Finally, the studies reporting the most impressive performance of ultrasound have all used intravenous contrast agents, which are not FDA approved in the United States. With the addition of intravenous contrast, the sensitivity, specificity, and accuracy of ultrasound may reach 94%, 97%, and 94%, respectively.[45] In addition, at least two studies show that contrast-enhanced ultrasound has the potential to accurately differentiate active, inflammatory stenoses from chronic, fibrostenotic strictures.[46,47]

Despite its potential, ultrasound evaluation of IBD is unlikely to gain in popularity in the United States owing to the aforementioned limitations. It must also overcome the ubiquity of multidetector CT scanners, which provide comprehensive examination of the entire abdomen and pelvis in less than 1 minute.

SBFT

Although the mainstay of CD imaging for decades, the role of SBFT, and fluoroscopy in general, has diminished in parallel to the rise of CTE and MRE. However, despite the dramatic decrease in the number of fluoroscopic studies performed, SBFT maintains a small but important niche in imaging of IBD.

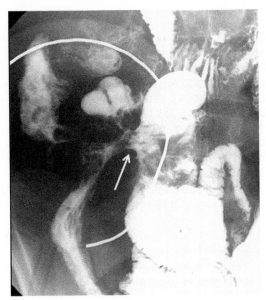

Fig. 10. Entero–entero fistulae (*arrow*). Spot-compression image from SBFT demonstrating abnormal tethering of bowel loops with complex entero–entero fistulae. SBFT remains an excellent test for mapping of complex fistulae.

Interestingly, the SBFT remains the most sensitive imaging test for the diagnosis of aphthous ulcers, the earliest macroscopic changes of CD.[48]

Findings of CD on SBFT include narrowing of the bowel lumen, ulceration, "cobblestoning" of the mucosa, and fistula formation.[49] However, in the era of CTE and MRE, it is most commonly used to assess bowel motility, to differentiate pseudo-obstruction from true anatomic obstruction, and to delineate complex fistulae that can be difficult to "road-map," particularly with the single time point provided by CTE (**Fig. 10**).

FUTURE DIRECTIONS

Despite great strides made in the last decade, there is extensive ongoing research in small-bowel imaging. Topics of interest include improving and refining the differentiation of active from chronic disease, perhaps using MR perfusion,[50] as well as evaluation of mucosal healing after medical therapy, which has recently been accepted as an important prognostic marker. Evaluation of mucosal healing is in the early stages of study with both CTE and MRE.[51,52] Finally, MRE may prove useful as functional imaging modality, identifying diseased bowel segments based on abnormal motility.

SUMMARY

The advent of cross-sectional enterography has revolutionized small-bowel imaging, providing comprehensive, reproducible evaluation of CD and its complications. Continued collaboration between radiologists and gastroenterologists is critical to ensure further progress toward the common goals of classifying disease activity, predicting response to treatment, and appropriate triage to medical versus surgical therapy.

REFERENCES

1. Negaard A, Sandivik L, Berstad AE, et al. A prospective randomized comparison between two MRI studies of the small bowel in Crohn's disease, the oral contrast method and MRE enteroclysis. Eur Radiol 2007;17:2294–301.
2. Negaard A, Sandvik L, Berstad AE, et al. MRI of the small bowel with oral contrast or nasojejunal intubation in Crohn's diseae: randomized comparison of patient acceptance. Scand J Gastroenterol 2008;43:44–51.
3. Ajaj W, Goyen M, Schneeman, et al. Oral contrast agents for small bowel distension in MRI: influence of the osmolarity for small bowel distension. Eur Radiol 2005;15:1400–6.
4. Borthne AS, Abdelnoor M, Hellund JC, et al. MR imaging of the small bowel with increasing concentrations of an oral osmotic agent. Eur Radiol 2005;15:667–71.
5. Fletcher JG, Fidler JL, Bruining DH, et al. New concepts in intestinal imaging for inflammatory bowel diseases. Gastroenterology 2011;140:1795–806.
6. Paulson SR, Huprich JE, Fletcher JG, et al. CT enterography as a diagnostic tool in evaluating small bowel disorders: review of clinical experience with over 700 cases. Radiographics 2006;26:641–62.
7. Paulsen SR, Huprich JE, Fletcher JG, et al. CT enterography as a diagnostic tool in evaluating small bowel disorders: review of clinical experience with over 700 cases. Radiographics 2006;26:641–62.
8. Bernstein CN, Boult IF, Greenberg HM, et al. A prospective randomized comparison between small bowel enteroclysis and small bowel follow-through in Crohn's disease. Gastroenterology 1997;113:390–8.
9. Lee S, Ha H, Yang S, et al. CT of prominent pericolic or perienteric vasculature in patients with Crohn's disease: correlation with clinical disease activity and findings on barium studies. AJR Am J Roentgenol 2002;179:1029–36.
10. Samuel S, Bruining DH, Loftus EV, et al. Skipping of distal terminal ileum in Crohn's disease. Gastroenterology 2011;140(5 Suppl 1):S72–3.
11. Lee SS, Kim AY, Yang SK, et al. Crohn disease of the small bowel: comparison of CT enterography, MR enterography, and small-bowel follow-through as diagnostic techniques. Radiology 2009;251:751–61.
12. Vogel J, da Luz Moreira A, Baker M, et al. CT enterography for Crohn's disease: accurate preoperative diagnostic imaging. Dis Colon Rectum 2007;50:1761–9.
13. Bruining DH, Loftus E, Ehman E, et al. Computed tomography enterography detects intestinal wall changes and effects of treatment in patients with Crohn's disease. Clin Gastroenterol Hepatol 2011;9(8):679-83.e1.
14. Brenner DJ, Hall EJ. Computed tomography—an increasing source of radiation exposure. N Engl J Med 2007;357:2277–84.
15. Smith-Bendman R, Lipson J, Marcus R, et al. Radiation dose associated with common computed tomographic examinations and the associated lifetime attributable risk of cancer. Arch Intern Med. 2009;169(22):2078–86.
16. Berrington de Gonzalez A, Mahadevappa M, Kwang-Pyo K, et al. Projected cancer risks from computed tomographic scans performed in the United States in 2007. Arch Intern Med 2009;169(22):2071–7.
17. Tubiana M, Feinendegen LE, Yang C, et al. The linear no-threshold relationship is inconsistent with radiation biologic and experimental data. Radiology 2009;251:13–22.
18. Title 10, Section 20.1003, Code of Federal Regulations.
19. Jaffe TA, Gaca AM, Delaney S, et al. Radiation doses from small-bowel follow-through and abdominopelvic MDCT in Crohn's disease. AJR Am J Roentgenol 2007;189:1015–22.

20. Silva AC, Lawder HJ, Hara A, et al. Innovations in CT dose reduction strategy: application of the adaptive statistical iterative reconstruction algorithm. AJR Am J Roentgenol 2010;194(1):191–9.

21. Siddiki H, Fletcher JG, Hara AK, et al. Validation of a lower radiation computed tomography enterography imaging protocol to detect Crohn's disease in the small bowel. Inflamm Bowel Dis 2011;17(3):778–86.

22. Lee SJ, Park SH, Kim AY, et al. A prospective comparison of standard-dose CT enterography and 50% reduced-dose CT enterography with and without noise reduction for evaluating Crohn's disease. AJR Am J Roentgenol 2011;197:50–7.

23. Peloquin JM, Pardi DS, Sandborn WJ, et al. Diagnostic ionizing radiation exposure in a population-based cohort of patients with inflammatory bowel disease. Am J Gastroenterol 2008;103(8):2015–22.

24. Cipriano L, Levesque BG, Zaric GS, et al. Cost-effectiveness of imaging strategies to reduce radiation-induced cancer risk in Crohn's disease. Inflamm Bowel Dis 2011. DOI: 10.1002/ibd.21862. [Epub ahead of print].

25. Siddiki H, Fidler J. MR imaging of the small bowel in Crohn's disease. Eur J Radiol 2009;69:409–17.

26. Maccioni F, Bruni A, Viscido A, et al. MR imaging in patients with Crohn disease: value of T2-versus T1-weighted gadolinium-enhanced MR sequences with use of an oral superparamagnetic contrast agent. Radiology 2006;238(2):517–30.

27. Buchanan GN, Halligan S, Bartram CI, et al. Clinical examination, endosonography, and MR imaging in preoperative assessment of fistula in ano: comparison with outcome-based reference standard. Radiology 2004;233(3):674–81.

28. Morris A, Spencer JA, Ambrose NS. MR imaging classification of perianal fistulas and its implications for patient management. RadioGraphics 2000;20:623–35.

29. Siddiki HA, Fidler JL, Fletcher JG, et al. Prospective comparison of state-of-the-art MR enterography and CT enterography in small-bowel Crohn's disease. AJR Am J Roentgenol 2009;193:113–21.

30. Lee SS, Kim AY, Yang SK, et al. Crohn disease of the small bowel: comparison of CT enterography, MR enterography, and small-bowel follow-through as diagnostic techniques. Radiology 2009;251(3):751–61.

31. Messaris E, Chandolias N, Grand DJ, et al. Role of magnetic resonance enterography in the management of Crohn disease. Arch Surg 2010;145(5):471–5.

32. Koh DM, Miao Y, Chinn RJS. MR imaging evaluation of the activity of Crohn's disease. AJR Am J Roentgenol 2001;177:1325–32.

33. Sempere GAJ, Sanjuan VM, Chulia EM, et al. MRI evaluation of inflammatory activity in Crohn's disease. AJR Am J Roentgenol 2005;184:1829–35.

34. Rimola J, Rodriguez S, Garcia-Bosch O, et al. Magnetic resonance for assessment of disease activity and severity in ileocolonic Crohn's disease. Gut 2009;58:1113–20.

35. Rimola J, Ordas I, Rodriguez S, et al. Magnetic resonance imaging for evaluation of Crohn's disease: validation of parameters of severity and quantitative index of activity. Inflamm Bowel Dis 2011;17:1759–68.

36. Grobner T. Gadolinium: a specific trigger for the development of nephrogenic fibrosing dermopathy and nephrogenic systemic fibrosis? Nephrol Dial Transplant 2006; 21(4):1104–8.

37. Wang Y, Alkasab TK, Narin O, et al. Incidence of nephrogenic systemic fibrosis after adoption of restrictive gadolinium-based contrast agent guidelines. Radiology 2011; 260:105–11.

38. Grand DJ, Beland MD, Machan JT, et al. Detection of Crohn's disease: comparison of CT and MR enterography without anti-peristaltic agents performed on the same day. Eur J Radiol 2011. [Epub ahead of print].

39. Lee SS, Kim AY, Yang SK, et al. Crohn disease of the small bowel: comparison of CT enterography, MR enterography, and small-bowel follow-through as diagnostic techniques. Radiology 2009;251(3):751–61.

40. Rimola J, Rodriguez S, Garcia-Bosch O, et al. Magnetic resonance for assessment of disease activity and severity in ileocolonic Crohn's disease. Gut 2009;58:1113–20.

41. Siddiki HA, Fidler JL, Fletcher JG, et al. Prospective comparison of state-of-the-art MR enterography and CT enterography in small-bowel Crohn's disease. AJR Am J Roentgenol 2009;193:113–21.

42. Bozkurt T, Richter F, Luz G. Ultrasonography as a primary diagnostic tool in patients with inflammatory disease and tumors of the small intestine and large bowel. J Clin Ultrasound 1994;22:85–91.

43. Tarjan Z, Toth G, Gyorke T, et al. Ultrasound in Crohn's disease of the small bowel. Eur J Radiol 2000;35:176–82.

44. Allen PB, DeCruz P, Lee WK, et al. Noninvasive imaging of the small bowel in Crohn's disease: the final frontier. Inflamm Bowel Dis 2011;17:1987–99.

45. Migaleddu V, Scanu AM, Quaia E, et al. Contrast-enhanced ultrasonographic evaluation of inflammatory activity in Crohn's disease. Gastroenterology 2009;137:43–52.

46. Kunihiro K, Hata J, Manabe N, et al. Predicting the need for surgery in Crohn's disease with contrast harmonic ultrasound. Scand J Gastroenterol 2007;42:577–85.

47. Lenze FW, Bremer J, Ullerich H, et al. Detection and differentiation of inflammatory versus fibromatous Crohn's disease strictutres—results of a prospective comparison of ^{18}F-FDG-PET/CT, MR-enteroclysis and transabdominal ultrasound vs endoscopic/histologic evaluation. Gastroenterology 2009;136:654.

48. Maglinte DD. Capsule imaging and the role of radiology in the investigation of diseases of the small bowel. Radiology 2005;236:763–7.

49. Marshak RH. Granulomatous disease of the intestinal tract (Crohn's disease). Radiology 1975;144:3–22.

50. Knuesel PR, Kubic RA, Crook DW, et al. Assessment of dynamic contrast enhancement of the small bowel in active Crohn's disease using 3D MR enterogrpahy. Eur J Radiol 2010;73:607–13.

51. Bruning DH, Loftus EV, Ehman EC. Computed tomography enterography detects intestinal wall changes and effects of treatment in patients with Crohn's disease. Clin Gastroenterol Hepatol 2011;9:679–83.

52. Rimola J, Rodriguez S, Garcia-Bosch O, et al. Magnetic resonance for assessment of disease activity and severity in ileocolonic Crohn's disease. Gut 2009;58:1113–20.

Genetics in Diagnosing and Managing Inflammatory Bowel Disease

Jacob L. McCauley, PhD[a],*, Maria T. Abreu, MD[b]

KEYWORDS

• Genomic medicine • Pharmacogenomics
• Next-generation sequencing • Gene chips

EPIDEMIOLOGY OF INFLAMMATORY BOWEL DISEASE

Although inflammatory bowel disease (IBD) is found worldwide, the majority of studies have focused on white populations in North America and Europe. The incidence (or number of new cases per year) and prevalence (total number of cases in the population) rates of IBD vary across populations and geographic locations. A number of publications have reviewed the differences in observed rates that have historically been attributed to social and economic development, industrialization, and a general conversion to the Western lifestyle.[1,2] Although individual studies suggest different outcomes with regard to the incidence of IBD (from rates having hit a plateau to others suggesting both increases and decreases), collectively, these reports suggest that rates are increasing or at the very least stable across the populations that have been studied.[2]

The differences in these incidence and prevalence rates are in part because of genetic differences across populations. A recent review by Molodecky and colleagues[2] showed the highest prevalence of IBD in Canada and Europe, with the lowest prevalence in Asia. These prevalence rates indicate that IBD affects as many as 1 in 200 individuals across Europe and as many as 1 in 300 individuals in North America (1 in 400 for ulcerative colitis [UC] and 1 in 300 for Crohn disease [CD]). The incidence rates in North America were among the highest reported (0 to 19.2 per 100,000 for UC and 0 to 20.2 for CD).[2] While the incidence of IBD continues to be highest in whites and individuals of Jewish descent, the rates across Hispanic and

The authors have nothing to disclose.

[a] John P. Hussman Institute for Human Genomics, Dr John T. Macdonald Foundation Department of Human Genetics, University of Miami Miller School of Medicine, 1501 NW 10th Avenue (BRB-307), Miami, FL 33136, USA

[b] Division of Gastroenterology, Department of Medicine, University of Miami Miller School of Medicine, 510 Gautier Medical Research Building, Miami, FL 33101, USA

* Corresponding author.

E-mail address: jmccauley@med.miami.edu

Asian populations appear to be on the rise.[3] Additional studies across populations of developing countries are needed to further understand these rates the world over.

Additional factors, such as age and gender, must also be considered when discussing the incidence and prevalence of IBD and the overall influence of genetic factors. IBD is generally considered a disease of early adulthood with a primary peak incidence range between 15 and 30 years of life, creating a substantial impact on a patient's long-term productivity and general well being.[2,4] There have also been reports of a secondary incidence peak in 50- to 70-year-olds, but these findings have much less broad support across populations.[4] The earlier age of onset seen in familial forms of both CD and UC when compared with sporadic cases provides further suggestive evidence of a strong genetic component.[5] Taken on the whole, reports are inconsistent on whether there is a significant gender difference seen in IBD.[2] In CD there seems to be a greater prevalence in females, particularly in familial cases, whereas in UC there may be a slight increase in males.[5–7] Although these gender ratios may at some level represent an epigenetic effect on IBD pathology, they appear to be highly dependent on age, population, and geographic region.

THE COMPLEX LANDSCAPE OF IBD GENETICS

There is overwhelming evidence for the role of genetics in IBD as evidenced by initial reports of familial clustering. An early report by Orholm and colleagues[8] noted a 10-fold increased risk of CD to first-degree relatives of CD, and an 8-fold increased risk of UC to first-degree relatives of UC. Furthermore, this group noted the likely genetic overlap between CD and UC, as relatives of CD or UC probands were at increased risk for both diseases when compared with the general population.[8,9] Another clear measure of the strong genetic influence in IBD stems from numerous twin studies. The most recent review combines data from previous studies and highlights the possibility that genetics may play a stronger role in CD (monozygotic twin [MZ] concordance rate ~30% vs dizygotic [DZ] twin concordance rate ~4%) when compared with UC (MZ ~15% vs DZ ~4%).[9] Though these concordance rates implicate a robust genetic component, the fact that they are not absolute indicates that genes alone are not sufficient to cause disease.

As we understand from numerous studies across complex genetic disorders, genetic background is not independent of environmental influences. Environmental factors (eg, gut flora, dietary changes, pollution exposure, microbial exposures, lifestyle changes, smoking, and geography) are likely to have a strong influence on the underlying genetic susceptibility.

Even though there is considerable evidence for genetic influence, IBD does not typically follow a simple Mendelian model of inheritance within a family. The only exception is that rare, autosomal recessive mutations found in the interleukin-10 (IL-10) receptor and IL-10 cytokine have been shown to be sufficient to cause severe forms of CD in infants.[10,11]

The last 15 years have seen a tremendous degree of progress regarding the identification of genetic loci involved in IBD. This has happened in part because of technological advances and growth in the genetic approaches used to identify these genes. Multiple linkage studies in the mid to late 1990s, utilizing multiple affected families, identified a handful of genomic regions of interest. One of these regions on chromosome 16, when combined with candidate gene approaches, led to the identification of the first IBD susceptibility gene, namely, NOD2 (nucleotide oligomerization domain 2).[12] As the genetic aspect continues to evolve, the last 5 years have seen the largest growth in the number of genetic loci identified in IBD. This is largely because of the expanse of large consortia using genome-wide association study

(GWAS) approaches. These so-called GWASs have been performed almost exclusively in North American and European white populations and have used genotyping arrays of hundreds of thousands of single-nucleotide polymorphisms (SNPs), which are spread throughout the genome. Combined, these studies have identified approximately 100 genetic regions (71 CD, 47 UC, and 28 across both) demonstrating a level of genome-wide significant association to IBD.[13–17] The large overlap of genetic loci seen across CD and UC are consistent with expectations based on clinical and epidemiologic predictions and will likely provide key insight into disease pathophysiology. The genetic loci identified for IBD point to a number of relevant biological pathways, including the IL-23 pathway suggesting a role in the maintenance of intestinal immune homeostasis, IL-10 signaling, and overall leukocyte trafficking. Despite the apparent overlap, there do appear to be some distinctions that are emerging. The genetic variation relevant in CD continues to point toward the body's mismanagement of microbe recognition and processing of intracellular bacteria by the innate immune system with a more specific focus on regulation of autophagy.[17,18] Meanwhile, the story for UC has a slightly different focus. UC continues to have a noticeably stronger association to the human leukocyte antigen class II genes compared with CD, suggesting that genes across the major histocompatibility complex confer a stronger risk in UC. Genes identified thus far for UC appear to focus on intestinal barrier integrity and function.[17–19]

Despite this vast expanse in the number of known loci from just a few years early, NOD2 continues to have the strongest individual effect on risk of IBD.[15] Moreover, these approximately 100 genes collectively account for a very small proportion of the genetic heritability of either CD or UC, with only about 23% and about 16%, respectively, of the genetic contribution defined.[17]

Although it is clear that GWASs have provided invaluable insight into the genetic contributions to IBD, they fall short of their initial promise to identify strong genetic effects through genetic tagging via common variation. The hallmark of these large commercial genome-wide screening arrays, now at the level of 2 to 5 million SNPs, has been to provide the most common (based on allele frequency) markers that best tag the known variation across the genome. These panels have implicitly focused on testing the "common-disease common-variant" hypothesis, which predicts that common alleles will be found to be in and of themselves disease causing.

Recent technologic advances in genomic sequencing, so-called "next-generation sequencing," have helped pave the way for the identification of rarer genetic variation that may manifest itself in common diseases. The identification and characterization of these variants will help to test the "common-disease multiple rare-variant" hypothesis, which states that susceptibility to common diseases is determined by a large number of rare variants of stronger effect. Franke and colleagues[15] highlight the relevance of this hypothesis in IBD as it relates to rare genetic variation of stronger effect within NOD2. They note that the most associated SNP within their analysis only explains just 0.8% of genetic variance, whereas the 3 NOD2 coding mutations (noted as mutations because these variants have shown functional effects) themselves account for nearly 5% of the heritability of CD.[15] They further highlight that if this same situation were relevant to even a portion of the nearly 100 genes, there would be a much more significant portion of the overall heritability explained. These findings help to highlight the need to characterize further the genetic regions that we have already identified. The latest work by Rivas and colleagues[20] further emphasizes the benefit to deep resequencing of currently known IBD loci. They find a number of additional independent risk factors in known IBD genes (including NOD2, IL23R, CARD9) and additional associations to coding variants in other previously identified IBD risk loci that are predictive of direct functional consequence.

Because technologic advances are allowing for whole-genome sequencing at a near cost-effective level, the future of genetics and genomics is now a reality that most researchers and clinicians could not imagine just a few years ago. Although the technology and our current genetic approaches have by many accounts been very successful, we still have quite a way to go to explain the complex genetic landscape of IBD.

GENETIC OVERLAP AMONG AUTOIMMUNE DISEASES

Ongoing genomic studies of human diseases, including IBD, contain ever-increasing sample sizes and phenotypic measures to help elucidate the genetic underpinnings of these complex disease traits. Evidence and GWAS performed over the last couple of years begin to point rather strongly to a genetic overlap among different autoimmune disease phenotypes. Numerous meta-analyses and reports of autoimmune diseases, including IBD, rheumatoid arthritis, type 1 diabetes, celiac disease, multiple sclerosis, systemic lupus erythematosus, and ankylosing spondylitis indicate a significant overlap in genes involved in immune cell signaling, T-cell differentiation, and innate immune response.[17,21,22]

The genetic overlap across these diseases is the focus of current efforts by the large international Immunochip Consortium. This group is comprised of the large international disease-specific consortia investigating the genetics of not only CD and UC, but also celiac disease, psoriasis, lupus, ankylosing spondylitis, rheumatoid arthritis, and multiple sclerosis. These consortia have come together to create a customized genotyping array or "gene-chip" (the so-called Immunochip), which contains nearly 200,000 SNPs. These SNPs were selected as a means to provide deep replication and fine mapping of the established genomic regions identified across these diseases via the large GWAS and subsequent meta-analyses that have been performed. The nearly 100 associated regions, demonstrating clear statistical evidence for involvement in IBD, in most cases have yet to clearly uncover the causative gene or the functional allele involved. The level of depth this gene-chip provides at these established loci is expected to help further elucidate the individual variants conferring the greatest risk and protection at these previously associated regions. This, in turn, will help narrow the focus and provide for clearer genetic targets for functional study. Collectively, this endeavor seeks to further understand the interconnection between the immune pathways across these devastating diseases and, in turn, provide substantial insights into IBD.[17,23]

GENOMIC MEDICINE

The completion of the human genome project and the wave of research studies, in particular GWAS, over the last decade have reinvigorated and redefined the use of genetic information in medicine. At its basic level, "genomic medicine" is simply the application of our knowledge of genomic and nongenomic factors that affect health and disease to the practice of clinical medicine. The review by Feero and colleagues[24] illustrates the current and practical knowledge to be applied in the clinical setting as this ever evolving landscape of genomic information becomes commonplace in our society. One of the primary goals of genomic medicine is to enable us to take research findings from "bench to bedside." Furthermore, the application of genomic findings will eventually help usher in personalized medicine, as everything from specific drug selection (pharmacogenomics), to preventative measures and individual risk-reduction strategies, to tailored treatments and therapeutics will be informed by readily available genomic information.

In the not too distant future, we can anticipate the use of genetic data generated from gene-chip technologies followed by entire genomic data generated through whole-genome sequencing to be a standard of care for disease diagnosis and management in diseases such as IBD. Currently, there are a handful of companies that offer direct-to-consumer genome-wide profiling, which provides individuals with some genetic data via the genotyping of their DNA on one of these common genome-wide panels used for the aforementioned GWAS experiments. By most accounts, these current data, as illustrated above, provide little to no clinical utility. Not only are the majority of genetic findings across complex disease in their infancy, they offer essentially no predictive value in disease risk or outcome. Thankfully, studies of the effect this information has had on individuals appears to be benign as measured by levels of anxiety, intake of dietary fat, and exercise behavior after election to purchase this information from private companies.[25] Although this can be seen as a positive outcome, the effect this type of genetic testing has on the population as a whole is not yet understood. As researchers and clinicians can fully appreciate, the current availability of this information (namely genotypes of variants demonstrating association to different complex diseases) can lead to mistrust, confusion, and frustration for the consumer.

Several things must occur before genomic information can be of value to clinical practice. One of the most important aspects of capitalizing on the use of genomic information at a clinical level is the thorough training of clinicians on the true utility of this information. Educational workshops and continuing medical education programs are a good mechanism, but in the future we would predict more of an emphasis on genomic information during formal medical school training. However, before a clinical practice can be prepared to order genomic testing, there is a host of issues that must be resolved, including, but not limited to, the establishment and maintenance of electronic medical records and means by which to catalogue this vast amount of data (especially at the level of whole-genome sequence data), protections and guidelines for patient privacy (patient's often are concerned about how this information might affect their health insurance), and, arguably one of the most important needs, to have proper genetic counseling in place to help the patients interpret the meaning of any findings.

DIAGNOSTIC AND THERAPEUTIC GENETICS IN IBD

As noted above, there have now been multiple generations of large genome-wide association studies conducted by large IBD consortia. These studies have identified numerous loci that show convincing evidence for involvement in IBD risk. Combined, these studies account for only a mere fraction of the heritability of IBD and at this current stage have yet to yield definitive genetic variation that is predictive of diagnosis, disease course, or severity. Although the future potential remains strong, these findings will remain in the research setting for the time being.

The most worthwhile use of genetic information in the treatment of IBD at this stage lies in the use of pharmacogenomic information. This type of genetic information is used to help predict drug treatment intervention, with a specific focus on limiting adverse drug effects that could cause significant harm to patients. In IBD, the only genetic test approved for clinical practice lies in this arena. Testing of thiopurine analogues before starting immunomodulatory treatments (including azathioprine and 6-mercaptopurine [6-MP]) is recognized as an important predictor of potential drug-induced toxicity and may influence responsiveness to antimetabolite therapy.

Azathioprine and 6-MP are metabolized by the enzyme thiopurine methyl transferase (TPMT). Genetic variation in the TPMT gene results in decreased enzyme activity, which has been associated with increased cytotoxicity.[26] Measuring TPMT enzyme activity in red blood cells or genotyping of common *TPMT* variants can be used clinically to predict patient outcomes using this therapy. Patients with high TPMT enzyme activity metabolize 6-MP into 6-methyl-MP and, in turn, may be resistant to treatment with thiopurine drugs. Patients with low TPMT enzyme activity shunt 6-MP metabolism toward increased production of 6-thioguanine nucleotides (6-TG) and are at increased risk of cytotoxicity. Monitoring levels of these metabolites and adjusting the dose of either azathioprine or 6-MP has been shown to optimize therapeutic effects and minimize the chance of toxicity. It can therefore be argued that any IBD patient placed on immunomodulatory therapy should be monitored carefully at the outset of therapy.[27,28] However, there is insufficient evidence to suggest the effectiveness of pretesting IBD patients.[29] Although the genotypic measures can be easier, they do not show complete correlation with enzyme activity and are currently less desirable compared with measures of these metabolties.[28,29] We suspect that further refinement and characterization of genetic variation at the *TPMT* gene will allow for more direct and better clinical application to thiopurine treatment in IBD.

As reviewed by Vermeire and coworkers,[28] a host of other genetic variations are associated with therapy outcomes; however, they are less well characterized with results lacking confirmatory evidence. They include variants in *ITPA* as it relates to azathioprine toxicity; variants across a number of genes including *AP-1*, *IκBα*, and *MDR1*, *TNF*, and *MIF* genes related to corticosteroid therapy; variants in *CARD15*, the tumor necrosis factor and tumor necrosis factor receptor pathway for monoclonal antibody treatment; and variants in apoptotic genes (FasL and Caspase) as a measure of induction of apoptosis to measure efficacy; just to name a few.

Other noteworthy studies have sought to further explore the predictive value of currently identified IBD genes. Candidate gene studies in a Dutch CD cohort suggest that an increase in the number of risk alleles (examining genetic variants in *NOD2*, the IBD5 locus [chr5q31], *DLG5*, *ATG16L1*, and *IL23R*) is associated with both increased risk and a more severe course of CD.[30] Others have used similar approaches to combine purely genetic data (from established CD-associated genetic variation) with clinical measures to establish a meaningful disease course prediction model.[31] Although the goal of such a study has extreme merit with regard to risk stratification, given the current limitation in our understanding of the precise causal variant at the identified genetic loci, these models are still premature. Overall, these results help strengthen the argument that genetic research findings combined with biologic therapies will provide meaningful clinical utility in the near future and help reduce the number of hospitalizations and surgeries.[32]

One of the more interesting developments warranting further study is the use of gene expression arrays (so-called microarray technology) to help predict outcomes in IBD. Arijs and colleagues[33] studied mucosal gene expression patterns in infliximab-naïve IBD patients and found that *IL-23Rα2* expression was predictive of responders and nonresponders with 100% sensitivity and 91% specificity. In a similar study, Lee and coworkers[34] performed whole-genome transcriptional analyses on CD4+ and CD8+ T cells. They identified a transcriptional signature in CD8+ T cells that predicts prognosis in both CD and UC patients, which consequently is analogous to a prognostic transcriptional signature identified in other unrelated autoimmune diseases. This evidence further highlights the likely overlap of common biological pathways across seemingly different autoimmune diseases and the usefulness of large genetic studies that analyze multiple autoimmune diseases together.

BIOMARKERS AND GENETICS

Although one can argue that biomarkers in IBD are either directly or indirectly related to the underlying genetic architecture (as highlighted in the examples above), on their own they provide a powerful tool for assessment of IBD patients. Biomarkers can potentially distinguish between whether a patient has CD or UC, predict disease course, determine prognosis, or predict treatment responses. In general, it is important to assess the predictive value, sensitivity, and specificity of any and all biomarkers when compared across studies, particularly recognizing the patient population used in the study.

Fecal biomarkers (calprotectin and lactoferrin), antibodies against *Saccharomyces cerevisiae* (ASCA) and anti-neutrophil cytoplasmic (pANCA) proteins, tests for C-reactive protein (CRP), and, as noted above, other drug metabolites can aid in disease management, distinguishing between CD and UC cases, assessment of disease activity, prediction of relapse, and prediction of response to specific therapies.[35,36] Calprotectin and lactoferrin, and serologic markers (CRP, ASCA, and pANCA) are useful in helping to determine if a patient has IBD-given IBD symptoms but are best used to determine whether a patient should undergo further evaluation via endoscopy or radiology. Evidence reviewed by Tamboli and colleagues[36] suggest that the fecal markers currently outperform the serologic markers. Serologic tests to differentiate CD and UC are much less accurate and vary greatly. In comparisons of quiescent versus active diseases, current literature suggests again that fecal markers provide increased sensitivity and specificity when compared with serologic markers. However, there is some evidence suggesting that the combined use of serologic and genetic data may prove useful in predicting whether a patient is likely to experience complications over time. Lichtenstein and coworkers[37] have suggestive evidence that combining serologic and *NOD2* variant data may help to predict disease complications.

Across other outcome measures it quickly becomes obvious that results vary wildly. In the end, one must determine if the biomarker data add to the predictive value of the thorough clinical examination. Taken together, current findings in the use of biomarkers suggest a degree of usefulness but leave a lot be desired to allow for more robust and efficient clinical evaluation. Ongoing research hopes to bring better biomarkers to the forefront for use in IBD. Ultimately, as shown by Lichtenstein and colleagues,[37] the utility of biomarker data can be further refined and augmented through additional investigations incorporating biomarker and genomic data.

SUMMARY

We believe the future clinical application of genomic information in IBD will lie in the use of a combination of "gene-chips" designed specifically for variation relevant to IBD and ultimately in the cataloging of an individual's entire collection of genomic variation through whole-genome sequencing. In the short term, the expansion of pharmacogenomic tests and biomarker assessments are likely to have the most significant influence on prescribed IBD treatment therapies and disease management. Moreover, these pharmacogenomic and biomarker data are likely to benefit greatly from the ongoing genomic analyses, as they can begin to put these data in the proper genetic context as they relate to monitoring and assessing these effects across different ethnic and racial populations. Although mentioned only briefly in this review, a clearer understanding of environmental triggers of IBD will be of utmost importance to furthering our understanding of the genetic factors and the complex interactions that are likely to exist between genes and environment.[38]

The successful identification of genetic factors influencing IBD risk has been accelerating over the last few years and is likely to continue. Currently, these genetic factors provide no direct bearing on clinical treatments or therapies. Instead, these findings aid in our understanding of disease pathogenesis and indirectly to potential for development of novel therapeutics. In the near term, they may be able to provide some additional utility in distinguishing CD cases from UC cases. Future use of genomic information and its role in diagnosing and managing IBD patients is promising but not yet mature. The search for the so-called missing heritability in IBD will undoubtedly continue to uncover novel genes, biological pathways, and the likely interplay between genetic variation and environmental factors. The creation of a customized gene-chip (allowing for the creation of a patient-specific cataloging of IBD relevant genetic information), for use in clinical practice, is an almost certainty. Although this information will likely provide significant aid to diagnostics and treatment, it is doubtful that it could ever fully stand alone. It must be accompanied by thorough clinical evaluation and data, a more complete characterization of a patient's potential environmental triggers, and integration with other known pharmacogenomic and molecular biomarker information.

REFERENCES

1. Menon R, Riera A, Ahmad A. A global perspective on gastrointestinal diseases. Gastroenterol Clin North Am 2011;2:427–39, ix.
2. Molodecky NA, Soon IS, Rabi DM, et al. Increasing incidence and prevalence of the inflammatory bowel diseases with time, based on systematic review. Gastroenterology 2012;142(1):46–54.
3. Hou JK, El-Serag H, Thirumurthi S. Distribution and manifestations of inflammatory bowel disease in Asians, Hispanics, and African Americans: a systematic review. Am J Gastroenterol 2009;8:2100–9.
4. Johnston RD, Logan RF. What is the peak age for onset of IBD? Inflamm Bowel Dis 2008;14(Suppl 2):S4–5.
5. Ishihara S, Aziz MM, Yuki T, et al. Inflammatory bowel disease: review from the aspect of genetics. J Gastroenterol 2009;11:1097–108.
6. Peeters M, Cortot A, Vermeire S, et al. Familial and sporadic inflammatory bowel disease: different entities? Inflamm Bowel Dis 2000;4:314–20.
7. Brant SR, Nguyen GC. Is there a gender difference in the prevalence of Crohn's disease or ulcerative colitis? Inflamm Bowel Dis 2008;S2–3.
8. Orholm M, Munkholm P, Langholz E, et al. Familial occurrence of inflammatory bowel disease. N Engl J Med 1991;2:84–8.
9. Brant SR. Update on the heritability of inflammatory bowel disease: the importance of twin studies. Inflamm Bowel Dis 2011;1:1–5.
10. Glocker EO, Kotlarz D, Boztug K, et al. Inflammatory bowel disease and mutations affecting the interleukin-10 receptor. N Engl J Med 2009;21:2033–45.
11. Glocker EO, Frede N, Perro M, et al. Infant colitis—it's in the genes. Lancet 2010; 9748:1272.
12. Hugot JP, Chamaillard M, Zouali H, et al. Association of NOD2 leucine-rich repeat variants with susceptibility to Crohn's disease. Nature 2001;6837:599–603.
13. Barrett JC, Hansoul S, Nicolae DL, et al. Genome-wide association defines more than 30 distinct susceptibility loci for Crohn's disease. Nat Genet 2008;8:955–62.
14. Xavier RJ, Podolsky DK. Unravelling the pathogenesis of inflammatory bowel disease. Nature 2007;7152:427–34.

15. Franke A, McGovern DP, Barrett JC, et al. Genome-wide meta-analysis increases to 71 the number of confirmed Crohn's disease susceptibility loci. Nat Genet 2010;12: 1118–25.

16. Anderson CA, Boucher G, Lee CW, et al. Meta-analysis identifies 29 additional ulcerative colitis risk loci, increasing the number of confirmed associations to 47. Nat Genet 2011;3:246–52.

17. Lees CW, Barrett JC, Parkes M, et al. New IBD genetics: common pathways with other diseases. Gut 2011;60(12):1739–53.

18. Cho JH, Brant SR. Recent insights into the genetics of inflammatory bowel disease. Gastroenterology 2011;6:1704–12.

19. Thompson AI, Lees CW. Genetics of ulcerative colitis. Inflamm Bowel Dis 2011;3: 831–48.

20. Rivas MA, Beaudoin M, Gardet A, et al. Deep resequencing of GWAS loci identifies independent rare variants associated with inflammatory bowel disease. Nat Genet 2011;11:1066–73.

21. Gregersen PK, Olsson LM. Recent advances in the genetics of autoimmune disease. Annu Rev Immunol 2009;27:363–91.

22. Zhernakova A, van Diemen CC, Wijmenga C. Detecting shared pathogenesis from the shared genetics of immune-related diseases. Nat Rev Genet 2009;1:43–55.

23. Cortes A, Brown MA. Promise and pitfalls of the Immunochip. Arthritis Res Ther 2011;1:101.

24. Feero WG, Guttmacher AE, Collins FS. Genomic medicine—an updated primer. N Engl J Med 2010;21:2001–11.

25. Bloss CS, Schork NJ, Topol EJ. Effect of direct-to-consumer genomewide profiling to assess disease risk. N Engl J Med 2011;6:524–34.

26. Weinshilboum RM, Sladek SL. Mercaptopurine pharmacogenetics: monogenic inheritance of erythrocyte thiopurine methyltransferase activity. Am J Hum Genet 1980;5: 651–62.

27. Cuffari C. The genetics of inflammatory bowel disease: diagnostic and therapeutic implications. World J Pediatr 2010;3:203–9.

28. Vermeire S, Van Assche G, Rutgeerts P. Role of genetics in prediction of disease course and response to therapy. World J Gastroenterol 2010;21:2609–15.

29. Booth RA, Ansari MT, Loit E, et al. Assessment of thiopurine S-methyltransferase activity in patients prescribed thiopurines: a systematic review. Ann Intern Med 2011;12:814–23, W–295–8

30. Weersma RK, Stokkers PC, van Bodegraven AA, et al. Molecular prediction of disease risk and severity in a large Dutch Crohn's disease cohort. Gut 2009;3:388–95.

31. Henckaerts L, Van Steen K, Verstreken I, et al. Genetic risk profiling and prediction of disease course in Crohn's disease patients. Clin Gastroenterol Hepatol 2009;9:972–80.e2.

32. Vermeire S, van Assche G, Rutgeerts P. Review article: altering the natural history of Crohn's disease—evidence for and against current therapies. Aliment Pharmacol Ther 2007;1:3–12.

33. Arijs I, Li K, Toedter G, et al. Mucosal gene signatures to predict response to infliximab in patients with ulcerative colitis. Gut 2009;12:1612–9.

34. Lee JC, Lyons PA, McKinney EF, et al. Gene expression profiling of CD8+ T cells predicts prognosis in patients with Crohn disease and ulcerative colitis. J Clin Invest 2011;10:4170–9.

35. Lewis JD. The utility of biomarkers in the diagnosis and therapy of inflammatory bowel disease. Gastroenterology 2011;6:1817–26, e2.

36. Tamboli CP, Doman DB, Patel A. Current and future role of biomarkers in Crohn's disease risk assessment and treatment. Clin Exp Gastroenterol 2011;4:127–40.
37. Lichtenstein GR, Targan SR, Dubinsky MC, et al. Combination of genetic and quantitative serological immune markers are associated with complicated Crohn's disease behavior. Inflamm Bowel Dis 2011;12:2488–96.
38. van Limbergen J, Philpott D, Griffiths AM. Genetic profiling in inflammatory bowel disease: from association to bedside. Gastroenterology 2011; 5:1566–71, e1.

Index

Note: Page numbers of article titles are in **bold face** type.

A

Abdominal radiography, versus capsule endoscopy, 318
Abscess
  in perianal fistula, 380
  of pouch, 356–357
Absorptive dyes, for chromoendoscopy, 293
ACCAs (chitobioside antibodies), 468–469
ACCENT trial, 432
Acriflavine, in confocal laser endoscopy, 298–299
ACT (Acute Ulcerative Colitis Treatment) studies, 278, 413
Acute self-limited colitis, versus inflammatory bowel disease, 275–276
Acute Ulcerative Colitis Treatment studies, 278
Adalimumab
  for perianal fistula, 380
  in combination therapy, 411–428
  optimizing therapy with, 399–405
Adenomas, chromoendoscopy for, 291–292
Adhesions, 358
Advancement flap, endorectal, for perianal fistula, 387
Afferent limb syndrome, 356–357
Age factors, in disability, 434
Aggressive IBD
  definition of, 444
  predictors of, **443–462**
    clinical, 447–451, 455–458
    colectomy, 444–446
    mortality, 446, 455
    natural history of disease, 444, 453–454
    surgery, 454–455
ALCAs (laminarbioside antibodies), 468–469
Allopurinol, for Crohn disease, 398–399
AMCAs (mannobioside antibodies), 468–469
Americans with Disabilities Act, 432
Anal sphincter, injury of, 358
Anastomotic leaks, of pouch, 356–357
ANCAs (antineutrophilic cytoplasmic antibodies), 465–466, 471–473, 519
Anemia, in pouch disorders, 363, 367
Anesthesia, examination under
  for perianal fistula, 384–385
  for pouch disorders, 369–370
Anismus, 361–362

Gastroenterol Clin N Am 41 (2012) 523–537
doi:10.1016/S0889-8553(12)00052-0
0889-8553/12/$ – see front matter © 2012 Elsevier Inc. All rights reserved.

gastro.theclinics.com

Moving?

Make sure your subscription moves with you!

To notify us of your new address, find your **Clinics Account Number** (located on your mailing label above your name), and contact customer service at:

Email: journalscustomerservice-usa@elsevier.com

800-654-2452 (subscribers in the U.S. & Canada)
314-447-8871 (subscribers outside of the U.S. & Canada)

Fax number: 314-447-8029

Elsevier Health Sciences Division
Subscription Customer Service
3251 Riverport Lane
Maryland Heights, MO 63043

*To ensure uninterrupted delivery of your subscription, please notify us at least 4 weeks in advance of move.

Printed and bound by CPI Group (UK) Ltd, Croydon, CR0 4YY

03/10/2024

01040449-0007